Psychiatry and Religion

Psychiatry and Religion: Context, Consensus and Controversies works to eradicate the distinction between spiritual and psychological welfare and promote greater understanding of the relationship between the two.

This book brings together chapters from fifteen mental health practitioners and pastoral workers to explore what their different philosophies have to offer the individuals in their care. As well as all the major world religions, the text also provides detailed information about newer religions and the significance of their belief systems for mental health management. The book examines the positive and negative effects that strict moral codes and religious rituals can produce and shows how awareness of these effects is crucial to the treatment of these patients.

This classic edition of *Psychiatry and Religion*, with a new introduction from Dinesh Bhugra, will continue to provide an important resource to practicing and training psychiatrists.

Dinesh Bhugra is Emeritus Professor of Mental Health and Cultural Diversity at the IoPPN, King's College, London. He is Past-President of the Royal College of Psychiatrists (2008–2011) and the World Psychiatric Association (2014–2017). He is President of the British Medical Association (2018–2019).

Routledge Mental Health Classic Edition

The *Routledge Mental Health Classic Edition* series celebrates Routledge's commitment to excellence within the field of mental health. These books are recognized as timeless classics covering a range of important issues, and continue to be recommended as key reading for professionals and students in the area. With a new introduction that explores what has changed since the books were first published, and why these books are as relevant now as ever, the series presents key ideas to a new generation.

The Therapeutic Use of Self
Counselling practice, research and supervision (Classic Edition)
Val Wosket

Depression
The Evolution of Powerlessness (Classic Edition)
Paul Gilbert

Human Nature and Suffering (Classic Edition)
Paul Gilbert

Individuation and Narcissism (Classic Edition)
Mario Jacoby

Shame and the Origins of Self-Esteem (Classic Edition)
Mario Jacoby

Psychiatry and Religion (Classic Edition)
Context, Consensus and Controversies
Edited by Dinesh Bhugra

For more information about this series, please visit: www.routledge.com.

Psychiatry and Religion

Context, Consensus and Controversies

Classic Edition

Edited by Dinesh Bhugra

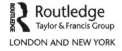

Routledge
Taylor & Francis Group

LONDON AND NEW YORK

Classic edition published 2019
by Routledge
2 Park Square, Milton Park, Abingdon, Oxon OX14 4RN

and by Routledge
711 Third Avenue, New York, NY 10017

Routledge is an imprint of the Taylor & Francis Group, an informa business

First edition published by Routledge 1996

British Library Cataloguing-in-Publication Data
A catalogue record for this book is available from the British Library

Library of Congress Cataloging-in-Publication Data
A catalog record for this title has been requested

ISBN: 978-1-138-59116-5 (hbk)
ISBN: 978-1-138-59121-9 (pbk)
ISBN: 978-0-429-49057-6 (ebk)

Typeset in Times New Roman
by Apex CoVantage, LLC

For My Mother

Contents

PART III
Psychopathology, psychiatry and religion

Contributors

Eileen Barker is Professor of Sociology with Special Reference to the Study of Religion at the London School of Economics. She has over 120 publications to her name. In 1988, with the support of the Home Office and mainstream Churches, she founded INFORM, a charity which helps enquirers by providing up-to-date and objective information about new religions.

Dinesh Bhugra, M.Sc., MBBS, MRCPsych., M.Phil., is Senior Lecturer in Psychiatry at the Institute of Psychiatry. His research interests include cross-cultural psychiatrists and sexual dysfunction. He has authored two books and co-edited two volumes on management for psychiatrists and principles of social psychiatry. He is one of the authors of the Royal College of Psychiatrists' 'Caring in the Community' policy.

Khalipha M. Bility, MPH, Ph.D., is Senior Lecturer in Public Health at the University of the Western Cape in South Africa. He was formerly a Postdoctoral Fellow at the Center for Health Policy and Research, Yale University School of Medicine, and upon completion of that held a position with the United Nations Development Program in Botswana, Africa. Dr Bility is currently participating in establishing the first Graduate School of Public Health in South Africa.

Howard Cooper is a rabbi, a psychotherapist in private practice, and a lecturer in biblical, psychological and spiritual themes. He is the editor of *Soul Searching: Studies in Judaism and Psychotherapy* (SCM Press, 1988) and is co-author of *A Sense of Belonging: Dilemmas of British Jewish Identity* (Weidenfeld & Nicolson/Channel 4, 1991).

John L. Cox, BM, B.Ch., DM, FRCPsych., FRCP (Ed.), is Professor of Psychiatry at the School of Postgraduate Medicine, Keele University and Consultant Psychiatrist, North Staffordshire. He is a former senior lecturer at Edinburgh University and lecturer at Makerere University, Kampala. He has a longstanding interest in transcultural and perinatal psychiatry and is an active member of the Methodist Church.

Padmal de Silva is Senior Lecturer in Psychology at the Institute of Psychiatry, University of London, and Consultant Clinical Psychologist for the Maudsley and Bethlem National Health Service Trust. He has a special interest in Buddhist psychology and is the author of several papers on the subject.

Aziz Esmail, who holds a doctorate from the University of Edinburgh, was for many years a lecturer in Philosophy, Comparative Religion and Islamic Studies at the University of Nairobi. He was twice a visiting Fellow at the Committee on Social Thought at the University of Chicago, and then at Harvard. He now lives in London.

Peter Fenwick, MB, B.Ch., DPM, FRCPsych., is Consultant Neuro-psychiatrist at the Maudsley Hospital, the John Radcliffe Hospital, and the Broadmoor Special Hospital for Violent Offenders. He holds a research post as Senior Lecturer at the Institute of Psychiatry in London and is Honorary Consultant at St. Thomas's Hospital, London.

John Foskett was Anglican hospital chaplain to the Bethlem Royal and Maudsley Hospitals and NHS Trust from 1976 to 1994. He is a Canon Emeritus of Southwark Cathedral and a pastoral counsellor and consultant. He is the author of a number of articles on pastoral care and counselling, ethics and mental health, including *Meaning in Madness: The Pastor and the Mentally Ill* (SPCK, 1984).

K.W.M. (Bill) Fulford is Professor of Philosophy and Mental Health, Department of Philosophy, University of Warwick, and Director of the Oxford Practice Skills Programme at the Medical School, University of Oxford. He is also a research fellow, Green College, Oxford. He has published widely on the philosophy and ethics of medicine and psychiatry and on medical education, in particular *Moral Theory and Medical Practice* (CUP, 1990). He is the editor of a new journal for philosophy and mental health, *PPP – Philosophy, Psychiatry and Psychology*.

Ezra E. H. Griffith, MD, is Director of the Connecticut Mental Health Center and Professor of Psychiatry and of African and African-American Studies at Yale University. He has broad consultation experience in the area of mental health service systems and has written extensively in the areas of cultural and forensic psychiatry. Dr Griffith has consulted to several universities, as well as to Project HOPE and to the Pan American Health Organization. He currently directs a university-based mental health centre with about 50 full-time faculty and well over 400 staff and students.

Maurice Lipsedge, M.Phil., FRCP, FRCPsych., was born in 1936 and is the Consultant Psychiatrist at Guy's Hospital. He is also Senior Lecturer in the Department of Psychiatry and Psychological Medicine, United Medical and Dental Schools of Guy's and St. Thomas' Hospitals. He is co-author with Roland Littlewood of *Aliens and Alienists; Psychiatry and Ethnic Minorities*, 2nd edition (Routledge, 1989).

Roland Littlewood, B.Sc., MB, BS, D.Phil., MRCPsych., is Professor of Anthropology as Applied to Medicine at University College, London University. He is Director of the UCL Medical Anthropology Centre and author of *Aliens and Alienists* (with Maurice Lipsedge, 1982/1989), *Intercultural Therapy* (with Jafar Kareem, 1992) and *Pathology and Identity* (1993, winner of the Wellcome Medal for Anthropology).

Tony Nayani, B.Sc., MBBS, MRCPsych., is Senior Registrar at the Maudsley Hospital. His research interests include insight and psychosis as well as social factors in the genesis of mental illness.

Mark Sutherland is the Chaplain to the Maudsley NHS Trust and has been in the post for the last four years. He has a background training in theology and psychoanalytic counselling. His general concern is with the care of persons with mental health problems, and this leads him to struggle with the relationship between religious experience and psychotic levels of mental functioning. He is the author of several papers on the role of religion.

Preface for the Classic Edition:
Psychiatry and Religion

The word *religion* is said to originate from Latin *religionem*, meaning respect for what is sacred, reverence for gods, conscientiousness and a sense of right or wrong, moral obligation, religious observance and mode of worship, and in late Latin it means monastic life or a state of life bound by monastic vows. It has been argued that the word may have been a derivative of *relegre*, meaning re-reading, or *religare*, meaning to bind fast or a bond between the gods and human beings. Dating back to the 1300s, the English meaning related to a sense of allegiance and recognition of a higher unseen power or powers. Religion is an integral part of many cultures and cultural identities. Spirituality on the other hand is said to date from 1300 from old French pertaining to or concerning the spirit or from Latin meaning or pertaining to breath, breathing or air. Attitudes related to religion are often a result of child rearing and cultural factors which formulate the world view. Religion has three particular qualities: awesomeness, mysteriousness beyond human beings which then leads on to clear social implications and causation and provides a relationship with a superhuman being or object, which then develops attitudes which are important in an individual's functioning.

Why should psychiatrists be interested in religion or spirituality? There are many reasons. Firstly our patients are interested in religion and participate in various religious activities and taboos, but more importantly, religion contributes significantly to many people's identities and concepts of the self.

Religious rituals, attending churches, mosques, temples and gurudwaras, not only provide a common safe space to meet and belong, but also these institutions provide structures to many people's lives. These institutions provide group space and forum for mutual understanding and caring. It can be argued that certainly in the UK where numbers of people attending churches have been falling, the impact on social networking and interactions has been felt in a number of areas. Across the globe there are different world views related to mono-theistic or polytheistic religions. These combined with notions of ego-centricity and socio-centricity, or individualism and collectivism, respectively, affect formation of individual identities which people tend to carry with them wherever they go. Religion is important for both believers and non-believers. Thus religion goes beyond simple collection of beliefs, rituals and taboos and provides a sense of identity, meaning to life and a sense of purpose and belonging along with a sense of community. Community and communication add to a sense of purpose and belonging as well as attempting to understand the world and cosmos around us. The polarisation of the world as a result of globalising economic and political factors has meant that, in many parts of the world, a sense of religious belonging has become extreme because that may provide a stability and belonging which may be unobtainable otherwise.

Human spirit helps the individuals to face adversity and deal with it. It may be spirituality that provides a far-reaching insight into the meaning of living and life. Spirituality can be seen at personal, social and political levels. Anti-psychiatrists have argued that psychiatrists have taken over from church leaders, but that is a very simplistic observation. Psychiatrists have a role to play in identifying causation and management using biopsychosocial models, and in many countries and settings the model is supplemented by an anthropological–spiritual model. Human beings are surrounded by family and community, and the ties that bind families and communities are important sources of support and purpose.

Psychiatry and Religion, first published in 1997, followed the first ever meeting on the subject to be held in the Institute of Psychiatry at that time. The interest was such that several meetings followed. The Royal College of Psychiatrists established a special interest group on spirituality and mental health which has been very active and thriving. The World Psychiatric Association too created a section on the subject, thus highlighting the importance of religion, spirituality and mental health. Both organisations launched Position Statements on spirituality and mental health. It is worth emphasising that it is not essential that the clinicians follow their or any religion as long as they are sensitive to patients' religious values and views and are willing to work with patients, their carers and families. There appears to be no need for religious matching between the clinician and the patient. Both the clinicians and the clinical services they provide need to be sensitive and empathic and aware of religious similarities and differences. It is important not to carry discriminatory attitudes if the patients and their carers and families are to be engaged in building therapeutic alliances. There is serious danger in the times of economic downturn; chaplaincy services in hospitals will be hit hard. Clinicians need to make alliances with community organisations, churches and other religious organisations with sensitivity and respect towards people of all faiths and none.

A recent example from India (Shields *et al.* 2016) has demonstrated that working with religious healers in a Muslim *dargah* (holy place) where people with mental illness go to pray can improve therapeutic adherence. The government invested in the project and over a two-year period worked with religious healers who then allowed establishment of a clinic on the premises, thereby reducing stigma and increasing accessibility.

This book recognises the importance of religious and spiritual beliefs and asserts that part of good clinical practice is to explore the patient's views, as well as those of their carers and families, by recognising their spiritual and religious beliefs.

I am grateful to Joanne Forshaw and Charlotte Taylor at Taylor & Francis for their ongoing support. Once again thanks to all the contributors who made this venture possible.

Professor Dinesh Bhugra
CBE
MA, MSc, PhD, MBBS, FRCP, FRCPE, FRCPsych, FRCPsych (Hon), FHKCPsych (Hon), FAC-Psych (Hon), FAMS (Singapore), FKCL (Hon), MPhil, Emeritus Professor of Mental Health and Cultural Diversity, Kings College, London, SE5 8AF

Reference

Shields, L., Chauhan, A., Bakre, R., Hamlai, M., Lynch, D. and Bunders, J. (2016) 'How can mental health and faith-based practitioners work together? A case study of collaborative mental health in Gujarat, India', *Transcultural Psychiatry 53*(3):368–391.

Part I

Introduction and history

Chapter 1

Religion and mental health

Dinesh Bhugra

Man's faith in religion is as old as humankind itself. The need for a greater force that could be seen as immortal developed as man struggled to survive physiologically and then psychologically and started to make sense of traumatic and not so traumatic experiences. As a result, all illness in the beginning was seen as a responsibility of priests and shamans. They would not only provide descriptions and enable the individual to make sense of this experience but also help the individual and his family to manage the illness in different ways. Priests and physicians were often the same individuals in different civilisations across the world. Physicians did not appear to have any confusion about their dual functioning.

In different medical systems, whether Graeco-Roman or Hindu, psychiatric illnesses were often seen to be due to different types of possession. Management involved dietary restrictions, the use of herbs and prayers (see Bhugra, 1992, for a discussion of Hindu systems). In classical Greece and Rome, with the development of more secular states, a split appeared to have occurred between the profession of priest and physician (Ball, 1985). However, the overlap did continue for a time and physicians continued to work in temples within a single religious framework. Furthermore, a change developed with limited use of religious factors, and outstanding, secular physicians emerged.

The fall of the Roman Empire and the growth of the Catholic Church led to the dual role of priest–physician, with the church becoming a repository for all knowledge. The Galenic principles held a monopoly on medical ideas for a considerable length of time, which meant that the development of medicine as a separate individual system was sluggish. Ball (1985) argues that the chaotic political situation and problems of the Church also contributed to this sense of a lack of innovation or exploration.

The secularisation of medicine has been linked with the parallel development of other professions. Ideas of contagion and possession continued to plague aetiological discourses of psychiatric illness. Ball (1985) blames the resurgence of possession of phobic attitudes towards women along with sexual anxieties and morbid hostility. The persecution of witches was a kind of mass psychosis where charity and compassion vanished and social class, intelligence and education counted for nothing. Until the fifteenth century, medicine and the priesthood could work together but several reasons, chiefly secularisation, led to the two professions going their separate ways. The development of pathology and the discovery of bacterium led to the 'scientification' of medicine and left psychiatry in the realm of philosophy. The growth of psychiatric asylums and the isolation of the mentally ill from society were a sign of the quarantine where a possibly 'contagious' individual was shunted away and a new class of 'carers/warders' emerged. This has led some authors, notably Szasz, to argue that psychiatrists emerged as the new priests, dealing with confessions and giving absolutions. Taking the imagery further, one could argue that the development of pills added to the communion scenario where the patient is asked to put the pills on their tongue and a small tumbler with perhaps about 20 mls of water is used as 'communion wine'.

Increasingly, mental health practitioners are assuming the three functions traditionally recognised as being in the domain of religion. First, an explanation of the unknown. Second, ritual and social function, and, third, the definition of values (Nelson and Fuller Torrey, 1973). When priests interpreted earthquakes, epidemics and droughts, they were focusing on the explanations of the unknown, and this explanation was responsible for reassuring the masses that things were under control. With the advent of scientific inventions and theories, these mysteries of nature have largely been explained. Whereas formerly, the mentally ill were seen by the priests as possessed by spirits, demons and devils, their odd behaviour was subsequently explained away by psychiatry as 'illness of the mind'.

The competition between the priest and the psychiatrist for the mind and the soul of the individual continued. Psychiatrists were the father figures who gave sage advice and occasionally controlled the patient without appearing to do so. The strength of psychiatry is not as unlimited as that of religions, or rituals. As Crenshaw (1963) comments, there are enough similarities between medicine and religion partly because both serve moral and humanitarian purposes. Science without religion can be destructive, and religion without science can become superstition according to Feibleman (1963). He then goes on to argue that, since the problems of today do not draw a sharp demarcation between what is medical and social or religious, the treatment should cover cooperation of all these disciplines. Although the training, expertise and views of physicians and priests may be different, their sensitivity to various factors affecting the individual in psychic or spiritual pain brings them together on the same level. Neither of the two is, nor should be, morally or scientifically superior. Cooperation between doctor and clergyman is essential in ministering to the total needs of the person (Sholin, 1962). There is, of course, an ongoing debate to ascertain whether mental health is a state leading towards the goal of religious growth, or whether religion is only one part of a mentally healthy person whose goal may be biological or social adaptation (see Sutherland, 1964). The *raison d'être* of the psychiatrist is to alleviate suffering of the mentally ill and support, treat and manage such an individual along with managing members of the family and the community that such an individual affects. The Church and the priest, on the other hand, also have to provide a therapeutic environment, intercede for the sick, administer the sacrament, help man prepare for death, and in general inculcate the somewhat personal faith that upholds one in difficult times (Feilding, 1964). Thus, it would appear that, as the psychiatrist prepares the individual with an array of coping strategies, the priest can do exactly the same. The process of psychic immunisation can thus be approached in two ways, which do not have to be in competition with each other for the individual's soul.

The interaction between religion and psychiatry can be at several levels. Psychiatric patients may have religious beliefs that may need to be taken into consideration when planning any management. They may also seek help from religion and religious healers, using different models of distress. The interaction of the therapist's religious views and the patient's religious views may cause conflict. The patient's religious values may affect acceptance of psychotherapy and other treatments. Furthermore, symptoms of one kind may be understood completely differently by someone else. Possession states are a classic example of this. In a recently completed study, Campion and Bhugra (1994) found that 75 per cent of their psychiatric patients had consulted religious healers about possession and similar findings have been reported from other parts of India. On the other hand, while looking at possession syndromes, Teja *et al.* (1970) and Varma *et al.* (1970) reported that these conditions were seen in women, and were largely hysterical in origin. Spirit possession remains a 'culturally sanctioned, heavily institutionalized and symbolically invested means of expression in action for various egodystonic impulses and thoughts' (Kiev, 1961). Life events have been linked to the onset of these states. Their management has to include clear understanding of the cultural background and the explanations of the experience.

Morris (1987) argues that, with the growth of materialistic interpretations of social reality, the general interest in comparative religions emerged. The phenomenological approach of religion made its appearance. Phenomenology is (its) instrument of hearing, recollection, restoration, and of meaning, as are the underlying meanings of religion. Jung (1938) went so far as to suggest that religion is not only a sociological or historical phenomenon but that it also has a profound psychological significance. He defines religion as a numinous experience that seizes and controls the human subject (Morris, 1987). The Jungian approach too is phenomenological. Although Jung (1938) argues that the phenomena are true thoughts – these can be understood by relating these to 'collective unconscious' – a psychic reality shared by all humans.

Religion, its psychological aspects, and its practice all affect mental health. Beliefs about mental illness and its treatment may be closely tied to beliefs about sin and suffering and views that mental illnesses may result from some kind of separation from the divine, or even possession, by evil (Loewenthal, 1995). Psychiatry may be mistrusted and religious healers may use modified versions of cognitive–behavioural approaches.

Loewenthal (1995) suggests that good mental health may go with religiously encouraged social support, religious ideas, feelings, experiences and orientation.

The continuing collaboration and consensus between religion and psychiatry are essential for the well-being of patients, but it is also important to be aware of the conflict between two disciplines.

REFERENCES

Ball, J. R. (1985) 'Psychiatry/medicine/religion – union, association – symbiosis?', paper presented at Psychiatry and Religion Conference, Melbourne, Australia, 27–28 June 1985.

Bhugra, D. (1992) 'Psychiatry in ancient Indian texts: a review', *History of Psychiatry* 3: 167–86.

Campion, J. and Bhugra, D. (1994) 'Religions healing in south India', paper presented at World Association of Social Psychiatry Meeting (June), Hamburg.

Crenshaw, C. P. (1963) 'Medicine and religion', *Journal of the Mississippi State Medical Association* 4: 383–5.

Feibleman, J. B. (1963) 'Men of God and Science', *Journal of the Mississippi State Medical Association* 15: 29–39.

Feilding, C. R. (1964) 'Some misunderstandings in spiritual healing', *Pastoral Psychology* 15(143): 29–39.

Jung, C. (1938) *Psychology and Religion*, New Haven: Yale University Press.

Kiev, A. (1961) 'Spirit possession in Haiti', *American Journal of Psychiatry* 118: 133.

Loewenthal, K. (1995) *Mental Health and Religion*, London: Chapman & Hall.

Morris, B. (1987) *Anthropological Studies of Religion*, Cambridge: Cambridge University Press.

Nelson, S. H. and Torrey, E. F. (1973) 'The religious functions of psychiatry', *American Journal of Orthopsychiatry* 43: 362–7.

Sholin, P. D. (1962) 'Medical–religious liaison', *Arizona Medicine* 19: 31A–34A.

Sutherland, R. L. (1964) 'Therapeutic goals and ideals of health', *Journal of Religion and Health* 3: 119–35.

Teja, J. S., Khanna, B. C. and Subrahmanyam, T. S. (1970) '"Possession states" in Indian patients', *Indian Journal of Psychiatry* 12: 71–87.

Varma, L. P., Srivasrva, D. K. and Sahay, R. N. (1970) 'Possession syndrome', *Indian Journal of Psychiatry* 12: 58–70.

Chapter 2

Religion and psychiatry
Extending the limits of tolerance

K. W. M. Fulford

INTRODUCTION

Religion and psychiatry occupy the same country, a landscape of meaning, significance, guilt, belief, values, visions, suffering and healing. This indeed is the
world of the psyche, itself interchangeably soul or mind (Bettelheim, 1982). Yet
the relationship between the two disciplines, which in the past has ranged from
mutual suspicion to open hostility (Lipsedge, this volume), is even in today's more
liberal times hardly more than one of tolerant indifference. Pastoral counselling
has brought the two sides closer (Sutherland, this volume), but the 'religiosity
gap', in Lukoff *et al.*'s (1992) apt phrase, remains: psychiatric history taking, as
John Cox (this volume) notes, although covering many of the most intimate details
of a patient's life, normally does not include enquiries about religious beliefs, not-
withstanding the fact that these are likely to be important for up to three-quarters
of patients. Conversely, while priests may nowadays be willing to engage the help
of psychiatrists, there is little in the way of formal guidance on where spiritual or
psychological interventions are appropriate, with even those closest to psychiatry
acknowledging significant tensions (Foskett, this volume).

So far as psychiatry is concerned, there are a number of prejudices standing
in the way of a closer relationship with religion. Many of these are dealt with in
this book. It is said that religions attract the mentally unstable – but the mental
health of the followers even of new religious sects is if anything above rather
than below average (Barker, this volume). It is said that religions may have their
origins in madness (Littlewood, this volume) – but madness can also be a source
of creativity in art and science (Storr, 1972). It is said that religious experience is
phenomenologically similar to psychopathology (visions are like hallucinations,
for example) – but this is to confuse form and content: normal and pathological
varieties of religious experience stand to be differentiated by essentially the same
criteria as normal and pathological varieties of non-religious experience (Jackson
and Fulford, forthcoming). It is said that paranormal experiences are a product
of definable patterns of brain functioning – but as Fenwick (this volume) points
out, paranormal experiences are no less invalidated by their grounding in neurophysiology than are normal experiences. It is said that religions are harmful, that

they induce guilt, for example (Nayani and Bhugra, this volume) – but religion, no more than psychiatry, is not harmful as such. It is also said, conversely, that religious belief is ineffective – but there is empirical evidence that it is not, improved 'coping', for instance, being correlated with religious faith in a variety of adverse situations (Griffith and Bility, this volume; Koenig *et al.*, 1992). The effectiveness of religion in this respect is no proof of its metaphysical claims (a delusion could be just as effective). Also, it is unclear from published work whether it is specifically religious faith which is required (there have been no double blind faith trials). But this work none the less does dispose of the question of efficacy as such.

There are, though, deeper reasons for the separation between psychiatry and religion. These have to do with the identification of psychiatry with what is sometimes called the 'medical' model (Macklin, 1973). According to this model, medicine is, essentially, a science. Psychiatry, therefore, in identifying with the medical model, has come to think of itself as a branch of science, and hence, by common implication, as separate from religion both epistemologically and ethically. Thus as a science, psychiatry is assumed to be based on observation and experiment, and, in principle, open to objective testing. Religion, on the other hand, is taken to be 'revealed', its knowledge claims being rooted in authority and upheld through faith. Again, as Littlewood notes in this volume, the identification of psychiatry with science implies a naturalistic ethic. Psychiatry employs an essentially deterministic model of human thought and behaviour within which actions are morally neutral. Whereas religion, in most Western traditions at least, assumes freedom of action as the basis of moral responsibility. Though, by contrast, the guiding ethic of psychiatry, along with the rest of medicine, is the principle of autonomous individual patient choice, whereas that of religion is subordination of individual choice to the will of God.

The separation between science and religion is perhaps a peculiarly Western phenomenon (Cox, this volume). In the first two sections of this chapter we will find that viewed in either of its aspects, epistemological or ethical, it is considerably less clear cut than it is commonly assumed to be. Contrary, though, to recent attempts at reconciliation, it will be argued here that the separation between science and religion is genuine and, ultimately, irreducible. This is because it reflects an essential ambiguity in our natures as human beings, namely that we occupy simultaneously a world of facts (in which science is mainly operative) and a world of values (in which religion is mainly operative). Recognising the reality of the divide between fact and value does not lead to a widening of the gap between religion and psychiatry, however. On the contrary, it shows that psychiatry, just to the extent that it is concerned with human beings, rather than merely with mental machines, is intrinsically connected with religion as well as with science. Religion and psychiatry should therefore move from tolerant indifference to tolerant engagement as the basis of good practice in both disciplines.

EPISTEMOLOGICAL ASPECTS OF THE DIVIDE

Along with the rest of medicine, psychiatry has developed in the twentieth century largely as a scientific discipline (Zilboorg and Henry, 1941). The work of Karl Jaspers, Emil Kraepelin and others helped to establish a firm basis for descriptive psychopathology and classification, these being further elaborated and formalised in recent decades through such innovations as structured examinations of the mental state (Wing *et al.*, 1974) and operational criteria for the diagnosis of a wide range of mental disorders (American Psychiatric Association, 1980; World Health Organisation, 1992). Building on this careful descriptive work a number of important advances have been made in treatment, through psychopharmacology, through the development of counselling and psychotherapeutic skills, and by applying the principles of behavioural and cognitive science to symptom modification. Moreover, following the classical pattern of the development of a new science (Hempel, 1961), causal brain-based theories of mental disorder – although still somewhat tentative and preliminary – are beginning to emerge from the new technologies of dynamic brain imaging and molecular genetics.

All this appears very different from religion, then. Indeed, the development of psychiatry as a science, with all its attendant successes, is widely perceived as having been made possible in part only by the shedding of religious mysticism and dogma. As Lipsedge notes (this volume), the case has often been overstated. Moreover, religious and psychological explanations of mental distress are not necessarily counterposed: in the Jewish and Hindu traditions, in particular, they are complementary (see, respectively, Cooper and Bhugra, this volume). But modern causal theories of mental illness, as disturbances of mental functioning, are none the less generally regarded as displacing the possession theories on which religious explanations of the phenomena of mental illness have often been based. Science, it could be said, has, literally, cast out the demon, replacing the moral categories of madness with the value-neutral categories of scientific disease theory. Freud went so far as to explain religion away as a form of pathology: it represented a neurotic avoidance of the demands of a mature relationship through the substitution of an ideal father figure for the imperfect biological father (Freud, 1927).

This account of the development of psychiatry is one with which perhaps a majority of psychiatrists would identify. They would recognise, perhaps, the historical contribution of religion to the development of humane treatment of the insane, in the work of Tuke and others at the end of the eighteenth century. They would acknowledge, increasingly, the significance of the ethical and experiential aspects of clinical work in psychiatry. But at the heart of their subject they would identify an emergent psychiatric science, undogmatic, transparent, testable; replacing acts of faith with empirical investigations, ineffable mystery with understanding, revelation with the cautious development of objective theory through prediction, test and falsification.

Closer inspection of this picture shows, however, that it is at best over-simplified. This is partly because, as we will see later, there is more to psychiatry than just science. More fundamentally though, the point is that even as a science, psychiatry is not like this at all. This is essentially because, on all three points – freedom from presupposition, transparency and objectivity – science itself is not like this either.

Thus in the first place, there is a clear sense in which science, no less than religion, depends on certain presuppositions, certain 'acts of faith'. It must be assumed, for the scientific endeavour to get going at all, that induction 'works' – for there can be no scientific (i.e., inductive) test of this (Russell, 1912). It must be assumed, similarly, that there is no limit to the explanatory power of science, no question which science cannot answer. For this can be shown only by default, in the sense that the question itself cannot (in principle, cannot) be susceptible to scientific test. Moreover, the core virtue of science, the supposed objectivity of its observations, depends on a tacit fiction. For an observation requires an observer; an observer, as the philosopher Thomas Nagel (1986) has put it, has a 'point of view'; and the fiction of science is to suppose that its account of the world is somehow from no point of view at all, that in Nagel's phrase, it is a 'view from nowhere'.

Fiction or not, though, it may be said, science does work, it makes the world more transparent, less mysterious, for science explains things that before were inexplicable. But the effect of this, at least in the paradigm science of physics, has been to reveal a deeper level of mystery beneath the mysteries of the every-day world. What is involved here is not the plain difficulty of modern physics, the impenetrable mathematics of some of its formulations, and the difficulty of translating these mathematical concepts into visualisable images (12-dimensional spaces!); still less is it the popular extrapolations of these concepts into metaphors of 'holism', 'connectedness', 'indeterminacy', and so forth. The mystery revealed by physics is rather in the world view to which we are led by physics itself, on its own territory, and by way of its own mathematics.

This is nowhere more dramatically illustrated than in quantum mechanics. As a mathematical tool kit, for predicting the behaviour of matter and energy on the smallest scales, this is widely regarded as the most successful physical theory ever devised. Yet the world view to which it points is one in which reality is (within limits) determined by the observations which we choose to make. Again, we need to be careful to see just how mysterious this is. It is not merely that observations at the atomic level disturb the world to an extent of which we can never be exactly sure. There is indeed uncertainty in this sense built into quantum mechanics. But more than this, a quantum mechanical measurement (in part) actually determines what is there. Observer and observed are thus woven together in quantum mechanics in a way which is wholly contrary to the spirit, not to say the letter, of a classical understanding of science. The classical, indeed the common sense, way of understanding a measurement is that it extracts infor-mation from a pre-existing and in principle independent system. But a quantum mechanical measurement (in part) determines the state of the system. And this is no longer a matter merely of speculation. The two ways of understanding measurement – 'extracting information' and 'determining the state of' – may under certain circumstances produce measurably different results (d'Espagnat, 1976). This was used by Einstein as the basis of a thought experiment designed to show that quantum mechanics is incomplete. But when the experiment was done, it showed, on the contrary, that quantum mechanics was right and Einstein was wrong (Aspect, 1986)!

The world as revealed by science is thus no less mysterious than the world as revealed by religion. This, moreover, has been most clearly recognised by those who have contributed most to the development of modern physical theory (Bell, 1986; Einstein, 1960; Feynman, 1965). We can add, then, that the world as revealed by science is mysterious, not to the extent that we lack deliberative understanding, but, on the contrary, in direct proportion to the extent of our deliberative capacity.

The natural response of the scientific hard-liner to all this is to fall back on the third supposed characteristic of science, its objectivity. The world view derived from science may be mysterious, so this line of argument might go, it may indeed require certain presuppositions, but it differs from that of religion in being based on objective data, on the facts, rather than on divine revelation. Yet even this is not as straightforward as it seems. For as Quine first put it, scientific theories are always underdetermined by the data (Quine, 1948). Any set of data can be explained by more than one theory. And when we look at what more is required to establish a given theory, we find ourselves involved, at best, in aesthetics, with concepts like simplicity, elegance and economy, and at worst in the personal and political value structures within which science as a human endeavour necessarily proceeds.

The post-empiricists have made much of this (see e.g., Kuhn, 1962; Lakatos, 1970). It is not merely, they claim, that the practice of science requires a certain ethic (though of course it does – not 'rigging the data', for instance). It is rather that the very theories we adopt, and hence the world view to which science leads, are a product of the values of the scientific community. All world views, then, scientific and non-scientific, are, according to post-empiricism, on a par, valid within the community in which they arise, but none more nor less true to 'reality'. This may seem far-fetched. But even in physics, at the leading edge of hard science, we find hints of the value-embeddedness of knowledge to which post-empiricism has pointed. In writing of the measurement problem in quantum mechanics, for instance, the physicist and philosopher Bernard d'Espagnat concludes that Bohr's interpretation of quantum mechanics (which is the standard interpretation) 'ultimately defines instruments with reference to *our desires*' (d'Espagnat, 1976, p. 95, emphasis in the original).

All this is not to suggest that science is, somehow, unsound. Clearly, by the (biblical) measure of its fruits, it is not. Nor is it to suggest that science is no different from religion. We will see later that, on the contrary, there is an essential gap between them. The point is rather that if we are to come to an understanding of the relationship between psychiatry and religion, we must first see that science is not the assumptionless, demystifying and wholly objective method for discovering the 'truth' that it is often assumed to be.

ETHICAL ASPECTS OF THE DIVIDE

A post-empiricist view of science may seem especially apposite in relation to psychiatry. In physical medicine, our theories, like those in biology, at least appear to be (though they are not, Fulford, 1989, ch.3, also see Fulford 1991) value-free and objective. But in psychiatry, it would seem, theory choice has indeed been governed to a large extent by the prevailing orthodoxies – the history especially of psychoanalysis reads like a history of religion, with competing camps periodically at war. There is something of a truce at present, albeit an 'armed truce' (Storr, 1989). Even in mainstream psychiatry, the biological and social, analytic and cognitive schools have often been in open competition. Moreover, the very concept of mental disorder, as against that of physical disease, is overtly valueladen. This is evident in differential diagnosis – alcoholism is close to drunkeness, hysteria to malingering, psychopathy to delinquency. Certain disorders (e.g., conduct disorder in the *Diagnostic and Statistical Manual of Mental Disorders* (DSM-III), American Psychiatric Association, 1980, and the paraphilias in *ICD-10*, World Health Organisation, 1992) are actually defined in our 'scientific' classifications, by reference to social–evaluative norms.

Where psychiatrists have emphasised the scientific aspects of psychiatry, the value-ladenness of the subject has been taken by anti-psychiatrists, such as Szasz (1960), to suggest that it is, really, a 'moral' discipline, and closer therefore to law and ethics than to science. Szasz might, perhaps, have taken the value-ladenness of psychiatry to point to a post-empiricist interpretation of psychiatric science. But given the classical view of science, as *prima facie* concerned with a value-free world of facts, he is surely right that psychiatry is, in this classical sense, less scientific than physical medicine. There is an extension of his argument, however, one perhaps even less palatable to scientifically-minded psychiatrists. For the more overtly value-laden nature of the subject brings it closer not only to law and ethics, but also to religion.

This is a point at which we have to go carefully. Values, even moral values, are not the exclusive property of religion. Humanism and communism, for instance, are both partly moral creeds even though neither depends on belief in God; both, indeed, reject this belief, in part on moral grounds. And, indeed, much that is most wicked in the world has been done in the name of religion. Yet as against science, religion is, for good or ill, overtly concerned with values. Again, religion is not exclusively concerned with values: it offers an ontology; it makes claims to knowledge. In the past it has been the primary authority on the way the world is. But even in the modern world, in which science is generally accepted as the authority on the facts, religion is still perceived as at least one important authority on ethics, on the world of values generally, on the way the world ought to be. In these terms then, and to this extent, psychiatry, as an overtly value-laden discipline, is closer to religion than are most other branches of medicine.

The response of the scientific hard-liners in psychiatry to observations of *this* kind is to reject the connection with values. We will see in the next section that even if this were possible, its effect would be to impoverish psychiatry, rather than (as these hard-liners suppose) to protect its scientific virtue. This is not to say that the anti-psychiatrists are right. Psychiatry is not, like aesthetics, a matter solely, nor even primarily, of values. But there is a vital point behind the anti-psychiatric move. For what is implied by the connection with values is no less than that psychiatry is concerned essentially with people.

Baldly stated, this may seem like a truism. It leads, however, to some important conclusions about the very nature of psychiatry as a medical discipline. To reach these conclusions we need, first, to look more closely at what it is to be a person. Thus, as we noted at the start of this chapter, the (classical) scientific model of a person is of an object governed by natural law, different only in degree of complexity from simple mechanical objects, and indeed from non-mechanical objects like stones and stars, in principle predictable (within the limits set by the sensitivity of a complex system to its starting conditions), and subject to the same laws as anything else in nature. How different, then, from at least the dominant 'Western' religious view of persons as essentially free agents, as beings who are ultimately responsible for their actions.

We will see later that even in religion things are not quite as simple as this. But to the extent at least that religion is concerned with values, it implies a model of this free-agent kind. For the very possibility of making ethical claims depends on the assumption that what we do is not predetermined. The basis of the distinction between 'ought to do' and 'do', is that we are free to do other than we do: 'ought (in the well-worn aphorism) implies can' (see, e.g., Warnock, 1967). Unless I could have done something different I can be neither praised nor blamed for what I do as something that, respectively, I ought or ought not to have done.

There are many philosophical difficulties with freedom of the will (see, e.g., Lucas, 1993), difficulties with which theology, too, has been concerned. We will return to these in the next section. At a practical level, too, freedom is a mixed blessing. Treating people as machines is the root cause of much of the dissatisfaction with modern 'scientific' medicine (Fulford, 1988): and to the extent that psychiatry has taken over this view, it has taken over the dehumanising aspects of technological medicine. But, on the other hand, with responsibility goes liability, with praise goes blame, with reward goes punishment, and with all these goes guilt. The attachment of guilt to a religious world view has indeed often been advanced as one of the 'grounds' for the rejection of religion by psychiatry (Nayani and Bhugra, this volume).

The scientific hard-liner in psychiatry might be tempted to draw from the difficulties about freedom of the will support for an exclusively scientific model of the subject. Far from connecting psychiatry with the world of values, the hard-liner might say, these difficulties provide us with good pragmatic grounds for adopting a mechanistic view of persons. This argument could back-fire, however. For if freedom is a property which is essential to our status as moral agents, as beings concerned with values, it could also be a property which is essential to our status as epistemological agents, as beings concerned with knowledge. Science, as we noted earlier, has to assume a deterministic model, not in the sense of taking everything to be fully predictable, but in the sense that events, including those initiated by people, are lawful. Yet as John Lucas has argued (1993), in so far as science can be taken to yield knowledge, it, too, like ethics, must assume freedom of action.

This, of course, is not at all the kind of thing that the scientific hard-liner in psychiatry would say. Psychiatrists have identified rather with positivism, perceiving this to be offering an apparently straightforward picture of science. Yet scientists themselves, at the hardest cutting edge of the subject, in physics, have rejected the positivist account of what science is about. As John Polkinghorne (1984), a theoretical physicist and ordained priest, has put it, science is not about discovering ever more comprehensive correlations between the patterns of results from measuring instruments; it is about discovering the truth about the world, or at any rate getting closer to the truth. But if this is correct, Lucas' point is that the epistemology of science cannot itself be deterministically governed. For if it were, there would be no (real) difference between a true and a false scientific theory. Truth and falsehood would be no more than different kinds of deterministically driven beliefs.

The possibility of knowledge, then, as distinct merely from belief, goes beyond the scope of deterministically governed conclusions. It is not enough that I come to a conclusion, the truth of which I firmly believe (any hypnotist can achieve that); it is not enough that I come to a conclusion which happens to be true (philosophers have given us a number of intriguing cases of accidental true belief; Nozick, 1981); it is not enough that a belief which happens to be true is useful (biologically or otherwise). Knowledge, as Plato first put it, is justified true belief. And when we look at what the justification of true belief amounts to, we find ourselves struggling with the requirement for a freedom which is at least closely similar to that which is essential to moral agency. There is a nice irony here, then, in that the possibility of knowledge, including scientific knowledge, depends on rejecting the deterministic assumptions necessary to the scientific endeavour.

FROM DIVIDE TO DIALECT

The ideas discussed in the last two sections could be seen as bringing science and religion closer together. Starting from the perceived epistemological divide, we found science to be no less ineffable, theory-laden and dependent on unprovable presupposition than religion. And starting from the perceived ethical divide we have now found religion, in its connection with ethics, to imply a model of agency, expressing freedom of choice, upon which the very existence of science as a discipline concerned with knowledge depends.

A number of authors have indeed taken arguments of this kind to point to a reconciliation between science and religion. Polkinghorne (1983) has made an eloquent case for the knowledge claims of religion to be hardly less well founded than those of science. And a number of theologians have argued that hermeneutics – giving meaning to events – is necessary alike to religious revelation and scientific advance (Mitchell, 1991). Again, the Cambridge theologian, Janet Soskice, has pointed out that metaphors are as important in scientific thinking as in religious (Soskice, 1991).

This merging or conflation of science and religion can be seen as part of a movement towards reductionism in modern philosophical thinking. This has influenced a number of areas of philosophy. We have touched already on post-empiricism which, in the philosophy of science, amounts to an attempt to reduce facts to values. The corresponding move in ethics has been the descriptivists' attempts to reduce values to facts (see e.g., Warnock, 1971). In the philosophy of mind, as McGinn (1982) notes, so anxious have philosophers been to avoid what they see as the errors of Cartesian dualism, they have retreated to one or other reductive extreme, reducing either mind to brain (as in physicalism) or brain to mind (as in idealism). The former, reflecting the success of empirical science, has been the more popular recently. Mind, so the functionalists have claimed, is no more than the running of a software programme on cytoplasmic hardware (Fodor, 1981); freedom is an illusion, reasons (the reasons by which our rationality is constituted) are no more than a species of cause, actions are a species of event (Davidson, 1963).

Reductionism might seem to offer an attractive philosophical strategy for psychiatry, spanning as it does the mind/brain divide. However, there are a number of philosophers who have resisted the reductive trend. In the philosophy of science the Cambridge philosopher, Mary Hesse, has taken an anti-reductionist stand against post-empiricism (1980). Theory, she says, may be underdetermined by data; but this is not to say that our theories have nothing at all to do with what is there, that they are driven solely by the power structures within which science is set. It is high time, she says, for a post-post-empiricist realist backlash!

Stephen Clark, writing of Dennett's *Consciousness Explained*, points out that his (Dennett's) attempt to construct a fully naturalised account of consciousness, would make him (Dennett) as fictional as the detective Holmes: 'each person (would become) a disparate set of programs, Joycean machines, enjoying a virtual existence in the parallel architecture machines constructed by DNA in its pursuit of being' (Clark, 1993). Thomas Nagel, similarly, has argued that attempts to capture mind scientifically, by, in effect, inventing a new element of the physical, must fail. For such attempts necessarily leave out a key feature of the mental. As we noted earlier, Nagel has emphasised the subjective point of view as the cardinal feature of mind. Our awareness of things, as he says, is always from a particular perspective. Science, on the other hand, advances through progressive attempts to detach understanding from the point of view of the individual. Objectivity in science, therefore, is approached in proportion as our view shifts from the particular to the general (Nagel, 1986).

Anti-reductionist arguments of this kind are well illustrated by recent advances in cognitive science. Developments in this field have provided for the first time mathematical models of at least some of our cognitive capacities. Prior to this, our models of mind (mechanical, telegraphic, behavioural) either ignored consciousness or were so far from offering a convincing picture of its physical basis, that we could still harbour a comforting dualism, a suspicion that mind existed in a realm somehow separate from that of the body, perhaps even connected with the 'soul stuff' of religion. But now machines built on well-understood (if not always wholly predictable) mathematical principles, can do some of the things that minds can do. They can reproduce some of the operations of mind, and, more remarkably perhaps but of particular interest to psychiatry, they can reproduce some of the characteristic ways in which minds can fail (Park and Young, 1994). Yet this is not to abolish the problem of consciousness, it is rather to sharpen it. For it makes inescapable the central mystery of the mental, how patterns of blind molecular movements in my brain and yours, are, at the same time, the conscious experiences of me writing and you reading these words.

If reductionism is important in psychiatry, as the scientific hard-liners recognise, so too is anti-reductionism. 'Biological' psychiatry is impoverished if it seeks to detach itself, other than for the heuristic purposes of particular experiments, from the subjective experiences of particular patients. Social psychiatry, similarly, if pursued solely as an 'objective' science, attending to behaviour as though it could be analysed wholly without regard to meaning and significance, is empty (Wing, 1978). This was well recognised not least by Karl Jaspers, one of the founders of modern scientific psychiatry (1913); and it has been emphasised in the context of cross-cultural psychiatry (Esmail, this volume). It is reflected in recent philosophical work pointing to the need for a richer conception of rationality, a pre-Cartesian conception in which affection figures equally with cognition (Clark, 1992; Radden, 1994; Wallace, 1993). While as to post-modern science, the factional rivalries noted earlier in the development of modern psychiatry (between the analytical and biological, social and behavioural, and so forth) provide a clear warning of what happens when theory choice really is driven primarily by the force of personality of its proponents, of what happens when theory really is allowed to become detached from data.

But the need for both in psychiatry, for both poles of the traditional dualisms, is shown perhaps most decisively by the fact/value, description/evaluation divide. For this divide is directly reflected in the form of the debate in recent years about the very concept of mental illness. As we noted earlier, the origin of this debate is the more value-laden nature of mental illness compared with the physical. And the debate itself can be shown to have taken the form of an either/or reduction, either of fact to value or of value to fact (Fulford, 1989, ch. 1). Thus Szasz's argument amounts to the claim that the value element in mental illness is irreducible. This is the basis of his conclusion that mental illnesses are really to be understood as moral categories. The pro-psychiatrists, on the other hand, have run the reductionist argument in reverse. They have sought to eliminate the value element from mental illness in order to tidy up mental illness, to make it into a concept which is properly 'scientific', as, they suppose, the concept of physical illness to be.

In terms of philosophical reductions, these two strategies – the anti-psychiatry and pro-psychiatry strategies – can be understood, respectively, as counterparts of the reduction of fact to value in the philosophy of science and of value to fact in descriptivist moral theory (Fulford, 1989, ch.12). There is, however, a third, a non-reductive, possibility, the 'non-descriptivist' position first made explicit by the eighteenth-century empiricist philosopher, David Hume (1962), and developed recently in particular by R. M. Hare (see, e.g., Hare, 1952; 1963). Hume argued that there is an irreducible logical gap between fact and value, that we could not get an 'ought' from an 'is'. This is not to deny that in ordinary language these two elements, fact and value, description and evaluation, are closely connected. It is rather to claim that the relationship between them should be understood, not by reduction of one to the other, but as distinct strands woven together in a single fabric.

Applying this to medicine, then, we have the *prima facie* plausible idea, first set out in detail by Sedgewick (1973) and explored recently by a number of authors (Agich, 1983; Engelhardt, 1975; Fulford, 1989; Nordenfelt, 1987), that concepts like illness and disease are essentially mixed factual and evaluative concepts. The language of medicine is thus to be understood as a fact+value language, made up (*inter alia*) of description and evaluation, in different proportions and different patterns in different contexts, but both equally necessary to the overall pattern.

There are points to be made for and against this account (Fulford, 1989, ch. 2). In my own work I have shown that among other points in favour of a fact+value view of the medical concepts is the observation that even the most enthusiastic supporters of an exclusively scientific picture of medicine continue to use the medical concepts with clear evaluative connotations (ibid., ch. 3). But at all events, the fact+value picture turns out to be highly productive from a practical point of view. It puts mental illness and physical illness on an equal footing (ibid., ch. 12); it helps us to understand the vulnerability of psychiatry to abuse (Fulford et al., 1993); it gives us a more sophisticated understanding of psychiatric diagnosis and classification (Fulford, 1994a); it provides important new insights into a number of key psychopathological concepts, including that of delusion (Fulford, 1993a; 1994b); and perhaps most important of all, it suggests a model of clinical practice (and hence, too, of medical education) which is more closely attuned to the needs of patients (Hope and Fulford, 1993).

A fact+value model, it should be said, is no sinecure. Even at the level of practice it makes life considerably more complicated in some ways: it requires a more sophisticated view of the role of the psychiatrist as an expert witness, for instance (Fulford, 1993b). But it is, at least, both theoretically cogent and practically useful. And if it is right, it suggests that psychiatry, so long as it is concerned with persons, must be capable of tolerating a non-reductive philosophy. For the very notion of a person, as no less an empiricist than John Locke first pointed out (Locke, 1960), and as a number of philosophers have argued recently (Frankfurt, 1971), has both factual and evaluative aspects. Just how these aspects are related is an open question. P. F. Strawson in his book, *Individuals* (Strawson, 1977), has argued that so far as consciousness and corporeal characteristics are concerned, the concept of a person is logically primitive. Persons, he says, are a type of (logical) entity of which, uniquely, predicates attributing both consciousness and corporeal characteristics are equally appropriate. There is evidence from the psychopathology of delusions that persons may, similarly, be logically primitive for descriptions and evaluations (Fulford, 1989, ch.10). This suggests, then, that we should understand the relationship between fact and value, not as it were horizontally (i.e., by transverse reduction of one to the other), but vertically, that is, as twin and equally essential attributes of persons.

Persons, then, are of a fact+value nature, not merely contingently, in the sense that persons just happen to be concerned with questions of value as well as with questions of fact. This would be sufficient to require psychiatry, so long as it is concerned with persons, to engage in the world of values as well as in the world of facts. But persons, if Strawson is right, are actually defined by the property of dual attribution of both values and facts. To deny either is thus to deny the very (logical) nature of our status as human beings. Psychiatry, therefore, so long as it claims to be concerned with persons, can deny either side of human nature, its evaluative or factual side, only at the price of self-contradiction. Psychiatry cannot (logically cannot) both claim to be concerned with persons and reject a fact+value model of the conceptual framework within which it operates. Moreover, to the extent that fact and value are logically irreducible, psychiatry, rather than seeking (with the anti-psychiatrists) to reduce fact to value, or (with the pro-psychiatrists) to reduce value to fact, must engage in a dialectic, an open, progressive exploration of science and ethics, as reflecting two incompatible, yet equally essential, aspects of what it is to be a person.

CONCLUSIONS: PSYCHIATRY, SCIENCE AND RELIGION

The arguments of this chapter suggest that the psychiatric tendency to ignore religion and to identify with science reflects a one-sided understanding of its own nature. It stems from a picture of psychiatry as a science, and hence as divided off from the world of values occupied by religion. The opposition between science and ethics, as we have seen, is considerably less clear cut than it is often supposed to be. This has led some authors to seek a conflation of science and religion, in line with modern philosophical reductions of the traditional dualisms – mind/brain, reason/cause, subject/object, fact/value. Such reductions, if they could be carried through successfully, would bear directly on the relationship between psychiatry, science and religion. Here, though, in line with anti-reductionist thinking, it has been suggested that description and evaluation, at least, reflect a genuine immiscibility of two equally essential aspects of what it is to be a person – engagement in a natural world of causal law, and, at the same time, engagement in a moral world of free action. Thus it has been concluded that since psychiatry is concerned essentially with persons, it, too, must engage equally in these two worlds, not by conflation, nor by reductive elimination of one or the other, but by way of an active dialectic.

It is important to see that there is nothing here which is, somehow, anti-scientific. There is a tendency to assume that an argument for there being a value element in the conceptual structure of psychiatry is an argument against the possibility of psychiatric science (Boorse, 1975). In this chapter I may inadvertently have reinforced this tendency by emphasising the weaknesses in the conventional medical model. This emphasis was necessary precisely because the medical model assumes that psychiatry is an exclusively, or at any rate centrally, scientific discipline. But the emphasis might just as well have been the other way. In this chapter, in responding to the prejudices of psychiatry, we first undermined the common picture of science as providing a value-free account of the world, and then showed that science itself assumed a model of free agency more widely associated with ethics. But had we been responding to the prejudices of religion, we could have shown, first, that values require facts about the world (since value judgements always involve the adoption of descriptive criteria, Hare, 1963), and then, second, that the very possibility of moral agency is dependent on an assumption of the natural lawfulness of events (for without this we could have no idea of the outcome of our actions). The two worlds in which we live, then, the natural world of lawful events and the moral world of free agency, although mutually exclusive are none the less mutually dependent. We really do need both.

This is not a tidy conclusion, of course. The conventional 'scientific' psychiatric reduction of persons to machines is much tidier. As indeed is the anti-psychiatric reduction of madness to morals. And there is, certainly, nothing here for the tidy-minded, no simple path, no stable solution, no final beaching. But then there is nothing tidy about human beings. Philosophers have often puzzled over the possibility of irrationality. Yet confusion, complexity, even self-contradiction, are our characteristic, not exceptional, states. There is a need for steady scholarship, of course, for critical reflection, for rigorous appraisal, for the careful accumulation of data. But these virtues have too readily been hijacked by the mundane, the domesticated and the prim. Philosophy, especially in recent years, has sometimes followed this path, seeking respectability in common sense. We should avoid a merely destructive dialectic, 'the smug deconstruction of other people's certainties' (Clark, 1992). We should avoid a merely local investigation of concepts, seeking instead, as Esmail (this volume) puts it, 'the cultural basis of meaning'. But properly understood, the very purpose of philosophy, the very aim of its disciplines, is to challenge common sense, to show the insecurity of our assumptions, to stretch our imaginations.

It is this stretching of our imaginations which is perhaps one of the most important contributions of philosophy to psychiatry. In allying itself with

physical medicine, psychiatry has been through a period of aloofness from philosophy. There was some excuse for this at a time when philosophers themselves
tended to hold aloof from 'practical' disciplines. Even J. L. Austin, whose work is
relevant to psychiatry at several levels (Fulford, 1990), saw the role of philosophy
as developing a subject to the point where it could be taken over by science (Warnock, 1989). But now we begin to see that psychiatry still has need of philosophy.
At the most basic of practical levels, the lesson of recent history is that some
of the worst abuses of psychiatry occur when, in place of imaginative renewal,
the discipline is allowed to lapse into ideology and dogma. This has been true,
not least, where the dogma is the dogma of materialistic science (Fulford *et al.*,
1993). Philosophy can contribute to good practice in this area by helping us to
retain an imaginative, flexible, adaptive approach to clinical work, sensitive to
the values, wishes and experiences of the users of psychiatric services, and open
to the diverse paradigms of the multidisciplinary team (Fulford and Hope, 1993).

At the level of theory, the importance of imaginative stretching is perhaps even
greater. The plain difficulty of the subject, and the muddles generated when we
seek to mould psychiatry too closely to the relatively simple models appropriate
to physical medicine, have sometimes been taken, even by psychiatrists, as a sign
of deficiency. Psychiatry is thought to be in some way lagging behind scientifically. But as we have seen here, a proper understanding of science shows that, at
the very limits of the hardest of hard sciences, in theoretical physics, there are
deeply embedded problems with the relationship between observer and observed.
And problems of this kind are at the surface in psychiatric science. This is an area
where physics may come to the aid of psychiatry, then. But there is no reason,
other than the self-imposed restrictions of a nineteenth-century view of science,
why things should not go the other way, why psychiatry should not come to the
aid of physics. In the future development of science, therefore, psychiatry, given
a bold enough imaginative grasp, instead of trailing behind could be in the very
front line of the action.

None of this is necessarily to make a claim for religion: there is no proof here
that God exists, or, indeed, does not exist. Still less is it to claim for this or that
particular religion a unique understanding of His nature and purpose. Scientific
advance, as we have seen, increases rather than decreases our awareness of the
mysteriousness of things. This certainly removes one of the barriers to belief, the
mysteriousness of the idea of God. Indeed, if anything, it encourages belief. For
a sense of the mysteriousness of things has traditionally been one of the main-
springs of the religious as well as of the scientific impulse. But there is no actual
requirement for religion in the identification of psychiatry with the world of facts,
however mysterious science shows this world to be.

There is no actual requirement, either, for religion in the identification of psychiatry with the world of values. The need for psychiatry to be identified with
both worlds, with the world of values as well as with the world of facts, arises as
we have seen, from the claim that persons (with whom psychiatry is essentially
concerned) occupy both worlds. But religion has no exclusive claim on the world

of values. It has a claim, a claim which is not ruled out *a priori*, or indeed by the findings of science, and a claim which is highly significant for many patients. This is why psychiatry should move closer to religion in its day-to-day practice. But this is a contingent requirement, one arising from the plain fact that religion happens to be an important part of the world of values. The stronger, logical requirement is that psychiatry, so long as it is concerned with persons, must be engaged in the world of values.

So there is no proof here, and no disproof either, of religion as such. Though it is worth adding, finally, that in the necessity of freedom as a condition of our engagement as agents in either world – as moral agents or as epistemological agents – there is a parallel between religion and psychiatry. For in both, freedom, as the defining characteristic of agency, is something which arises not *de novo* but through relationship. In religion this is often expressed mystically: to be subject to the will of God is not to lose one's freedom of choice, it is rather the very basis of true freedom. And in psychiatry this same idea is repeated, in psychological rather than metaphysical terms, in the recognition of the dependence of adult autonomy on secure relationships in childhood (e.g., Bowlby, 1969, 1973, 1980). We should not confuse these two freedoms, the psychological freedom (of developmental psychology) and the metaphysical freedom (necessary to the status of persons as agents). A reduction of the latter to the former has been common in recent philosophy, as yet another aspect of modern reductionist thinking. But there is a parallel here, a parallel, moreover, in which there is perhaps a clue to the otherwise paradoxical idea of a personal God.

REFERENCES

Agich, G. J. (1983) 'Disease and value: a rejection of the value-neutrality thesis', *Theoretical Medicine* 4: 27–41.

American Psychiatric Association (1980) *Diagnostic and Statistical Manual of Mental Disorders*, 3rd edition, Washington: American Psychiatric Association.

Aspect, A. (1986) Ch. 2 in P. C. W. Davies and J. R. Brown (eds) *The Ghost in the Atom*, Cambridge: Cambridge University Press.

Bell, J. (1986) Ch. 3 in P. C. W. Davies and J. R. Brown (eds) *The Ghost in the Atom*, Cambridge: Cambridge University Press.

Bettelheim, B. (1982) *Freud and Man's Soul*, London: Penguin.

Boorse, C. (1975) 'On the distinction between disease and illness', *Philosophy and Public Affairs* 5: 49–68.

Bowlby, J. (1969) *Attachment and Loss: Volume I, Attachment*, London: The Hogarth Press and the Institute of Psychoanalysis.

—— (1973) *Attachment and Loss: Volume II, Separation, Anxiety and Anger*, London: The Hogarth Press.

—— (1980) *Attachment and Loss: Volume III, Loss, Sadness and Depression*, New York: Basic Books.

Clark, S.R.L. (1992) 'Descartes' debt to Augustine', in M. McGhee (ed.) *Philosophy, Religion and the Spiritual Life*, Cambridge: Cambridge University Press.

—— (1993) 'Minds, memes and rhetoric', *Inquiry* 36: 3–16.

Davidson, D. (1963) 'Actions, reasons and causes', *Journal of Philosophy* 60: 685–700.

d'Espagnat, B. (1976) *Conceptual Foundations of Quantum Mechanics*, 2nd edition, Reading, MA: W.A. Benjamin.

Einstein, A. (1960) *Relativity: The Special and the General Theory*, trans. R. W. Lawson, London: Methuen.

Engelhardt, H. T.Jr. (1975) 'The concepts of health and disease', in H. T. Engelhardt Jr. and S. F. Spicker (eds) *Evaluation and Explanation in the Biological Sciences*, Dordrecht, Holland: D. Reidel.

Feynman, R. (1965) *The Character of Physical Law*, London: BBC.

Fodor, J. (1981) *Representations*, Cambridge, MA: MIT Press.

Frankfurt, H. G. (1971) 'Freedom of the will and the concept of a person', *Journal of Philosophy* LXVIII(1): 15–20.

Freud, S. (1927) 'The future of an illusion', in J. Strachey and A. Freud (eds) *The Complete Psychological Works of Sigmund Freud*, London: The Hogarth Press.

Fulford, K. W. M. (1988) 'Is medicine a branch of ethics?', in G. Gillett and A. Peacocke (eds) *Personality and Insanity*, Oxford: Blackwell.

—— (1989) *Moral Theory and Medical Practice*, Cambridge: Cambridge University Press.

—— (1990) 'Philosophy and medicine: the Oxford connection', *British Journal of Psychiatry* 157: 111–15.

—— (1991) The concept of disease', in S. Bloch and P. Chodoff (eds) *Psychiatric Ethics*, 2nd edition, Oxford: Oxford University Press.

—— (1993a) 'Mental illness and the mind-brain problem: delusion, belief and Searle's theory of intentionality', *Theoretical Medicine* 14: 181–94.

—— (1993b) 'Value, action, mental illness and the law', in K. Gardner, J. Horden and S. Shute (eds) *Criminal Law: Action, Value and Structure*, Oxford: Oxford University Press.

—— (1994a) 'Closet logics: hidden conceptual elements in the DSM and ICD classifications of mental disorders', in J. Z. Sadler, M. Schwartz and O. Wiggins (eds) *Philosophical Perspectives on Psychiatric Diagnostic Classification*, Baltimore and London: Johns Hopkins University Press.

—— (1994b) 'Insight, delusion and the intentionality of action: framework for a philosophical psychopathology', in G. Graham and G. L. Stephens (eds) *Philosophical Psychopathology*, Cambridge, MA: MIT Press.

Fulford, K. W. M. and Hope, R. A. (1993) 'Psychiatric ethics: a bioethical ugly duckling?', in G. Raanon (ed.) *Principles of Health Care Ethics*, Chichester: John Wiley.

Fulford, K. W. M., Smirnoff, A. Y. U. and Snow, E. (1993) 'Concepts of disease and the abuse of psychiatry in the USSR', *British Journal of Psychiatry* 162: 801–10.

Hare, R. M. (1952) *The Language of Morals*, Oxford: Oxford University Press.

—— (1963) Descriptivism, *Proceedings of the British Academy* 49: 115–34, reprinted in R. M. Hare (1972) *Essays on the Moral Concepts*, London: Macmillan.

Hempel, C. G. (1961) 'Introduction to problems of taxonomy', in J. Zubin (ed.) *Field Studies in the Mental Disorders*, New York: Grune & Stratton.

Hesse, M. (1980) *Revolutions and Reconstructions in the Philosophy of Science*, Brighton: The Harvester Press.

Hope, R. A. and Fulford, K. W. M. (1993) 'Medical education: patients, principles and practice skills', in G. Raanon (ed.) *Principles of Health Care Ethics*, Chichester: John Wiley.

Hume, D. (1962) 'Of personal identity', Book I, Part IV, Section IV, in D. G. C. Macnabb (ed.) *A Treatise of Human Nature*, Glasgow: Collins.

Jackson, M. and Fulford K. W. M. (forthcoming) 'Religious experience and psychopathology', in *PPP – Philosophy, Psychiatry and Psychology*.

Jaspers, K. (1913) 'Causal and meaningful connexions between life history and psychosis', in S. R. Hirsch and M. Shepherd (eds) (1974) *Themes and Variations in European Psychiatry*, Bristol: Wright.

Koenig, H. G., Cohen, H. J., Blazer, D. G., Pieper, C., Meador, K. G., Shelp, F., Goli, V. and Di Pasquale, B. (1992) 'Religious coping and depression among elderly, hospitalised medically ill men', *American Journal of Psychiatry* 149: 1693–700.

Kuhn, T. S. (1962) *The Structure of Scientific Revolutions* second edition, *International Encyclopedia of Unified Science*, vol. 2, no. 2, Chicago: University of Chicago Press.

Lakatos, I. (1970) 'Falsification and the methodology of scientific research programmes', in I. Lakatos *The Methodology of Scientific Research Programmes*, J. Worrall and G. Currie (eds), Cambridge: Cambridge University Press.

Locke, J. (1960) 'Of identity and diversity', *Essays*, Book II, in A. D. Woozley (ed.) *John Locke: An Essay Concerning Human Understanding*, London: Collins.

Lucas, J. R. (1993) *Responsibility*, Oxford: Clarendon Press.

Lukoff, D., Francis, L. and Turner, R. (1992) 'Towards a culturally sensitive DSM-IV. Psychoreligious and psychospiritual problems', *Journal of Nervous and Mental Disease* 180: 673–82.

McGinn, C. (1982) *The Character of Mind*, Oxford: Oxford University Press.

Macklin, R. (1973) 'The medical model in psychoanalysis and psychotherapy', *Comprehensive Psychiatry* 14: 49–69.

Mitchell, B. (1991) 'Philosophy and theology', in A. Loades and L. D. Rue (eds) *Contemporary Classics in Philosophy of Religion*, Illinois: Open Court Publishing Company.

Nagel, T. (1986) *The View from Nowhere*, Oxford: Oxford University Press.

Nordenfelt, L. (1987) *On the Nature of Health: An Action – Theoretic Approach*, Dordrecht, Holland: D. Reidel.

Nozick, R. (1981) *Philosophical Explanations*, Oxford: Oxford University Press.

Park, B. and Young, J. (1994) 'Neural nets and psychopathology', in *PPP – Philosophy, Psychiatry and Psychology* 1: 51–8.

Polkinghorne, J. (1983) *The Way the World is: The Christian Perspective of a Scientist*, London: SPCK.

—— (1984) *The Quantum World*, London and New York: Longman.

Quine, W. (1948) 'On what there is', *Review of Metaphysics*, 2, reprinted in W. Quine, *From a Logical Point of View*, Cambridge, MA: Harvard University Press (1953).

Radden, J. (1994) 'Philosophical aspects of psychiatric nosology: a review', in *PPP – Philosophy, Psychiatry and Psychology* 1: 193–200.

Russell, B. (1912) *The Problems of Philosophy*, London: Williams & Norgate.

Sedgwick, P. (1973) 'Illness – mental and otherwise', *The Hastings Center Studies* I, 3: 19–40, Hastings-on-Hudson, New York: Institute of Society, Ethics and the Life Sciences.

Soskice, J. M. (1991) 'Model and metaphor in science and religion', in A. Loades and L. D. Rue (eds) *Contemporary Classics in Philosophy of Religion*, Illinois: Open Court Publishing Company.

Storr, A. (1972) *The Dynamics of Creation*, London: Secker & Warburg.

—— (1989) *Freud*, Oxford: Oxford University Press.

Strawson, P. F. (1977) *Individuals: An Essay in Descriptive Metaphysics*, Oxford: Oxford University Press.

Szasz, T. S. (1960) 'The myth of mental illness', *American Psychologist* 15: 113–18.

Wallace, K. (1993) 'Reconstructing judgment: emotion and moral judgment', *Hypatia* 8: 61–83.

Warnock, G. J. (1967) *Contemporary Moral Philosophy*, London and Basingstoke: Macmillan.

—— (1971) *The Object of Morality*, London: Methuen.

—— (1989) *J L Austin*, London: Routledge.

Wing, J. K. (1978) *Reasoning about Madness*, Oxford: Oxford University Press.

Wing, J. K., Cooper, J. E. and Sartorius, N. (1974) *Measurement and Classification of Psychiatric Symptoms*, Cambridge: Cambridge University Press.

World Health Organisation (1992) *The ICD-10 Classification of Mental and Behavioural Disorders: Clinical Descriptions and Diagnostic Guidelines*, Geneva: World Health Organisation.

Zilboorg, G. and Henry, G. W. (1941) *A History of Medical Psychology*, London: Allen & Unwin.

Chapter 3

Religion and madness in history

Maurice Lipsedge

> Religion is another fertile cause of insanity. Mr Haslam,[1] though he declares it sinful to consider religion as a cause of insanity, adds, however, that he would be ungrateful did he not avow his obligation to Methodism for its supply of numerous cases . . . it cannot fail, however, that a minute description of the consequences of sin, of the horrors of hell, and the dreadful sufferings of the damned, in the most glowing colours, should make a deep impression on weak minds and that those who are not naturally predisposed to insanity should lose the free actions of their will.
>
> (J. G. Spurzheim, 1817:142–3)

INTRODUCTION

This chapter compares religious and medical interpretations of unusual subjective experience.[2] My examples are mainly European, Christian and Jewish, and I have not been able to draw on the rich Islamic literature on the Holy Madman (see, e.g., Dols, 1992). Visions, trances, possession and Messianic beliefs have been construed in various historical periods in either secular or religious terms. At times the particular choice of interpretation appears to have been influenced by factional, class or professional interests as well as by individual piety. In some cases personal ambitions and rivalries appear to have been the dominant motive.

I begin with contemporary reactions to possession in a Third World rural community where modernist, orthodox and spiritistic ideas co-exist and compete. I move on to consider medical as opposed to theological interpretations of possession in the early modern period in France, England and North America. Both possession and 'holy anorexia' are currently analysed in terms of women's struggle for autonomy in an oppressively patriarchal religious society.

Retrospective medical reductionist psychobiographies (Hildegard of Bingen as a migraineuse, etc.) are rejected in favour of the more historically illuminating interpretations of extreme behaviour offered by the mystic's own contemporaries. The use of dreams and visions, on the one hand, and the label of insanity, on the other, to promote a secular cause or to discredit political and religious opponents are contrasted with the exploitation of mental illness in mitigation by persecuted religious heretics. Examples are drawn from sixteenth-century Madrid, counter-reformation Italy and South Africa in the 1920s.

As psychological medicine became professionalised in the eighteenth and nineteenth centuries, ecstatic experiences were blamed for outbreaks of collective insanity, while mystical experience itself was increasingly pathologised. In parallel with these developments, suicide became secularised, and the chapter ends with a case of late eighteenth-century deliberate self-harm. Apprentice physicians construed this patient's self-mutilation, which was based on an injunction found in the New Testament, in terms of mental illness rather than malign supernatural influence.

'AUTO-SUGGESTION' AND THE APOSTLES OF INFINITE LOVE

Over a period of one week just before Easter 1977, the Guadeloupe daily newspaper, *France-Antilles*, carried a series of sensational reports from their Religious Affairs correspondent. The headline of the first article read: 'Scandal among the Apostles of Infinite Love', and the journalist declared his intention to find out whether the Apostles' work was divinely inspired or just pure humbug (*une baudruche vulgaire*).[3]

At the centre of the scandal was a 15-year-old girl who had assumed the name Sister Anne Andrée de Jésus Marie. Over the previous year Sister Anne had reported a series of visions of the Virgin Mary and of a giant crucifix. According to her mother, since early childhood Anne had been prone to swoon and faint, especially at school. Their doctor had advised the parents to slap her with a wet towel to revive her and this invariably worked. After coming round from one of these fainting spells she claimed to be able to see and hear the Holy Virgin. At first the family were sceptical and refused to believe her but after they had all heard a sudden, terrifying noise, like an earthquake, which was the sound of 'the Holy Mother shaking her veil', the incredulous family became convinced of her presence. After that, Sister Anne's mother was also able to see visions of the giant crucifix at the same time as her daughter and she also felt the Holy Virgin's presence, but unlike Anne she could not actually see or hear her. Sister Anne had also seen *une dame vêtue en blanc*, near a church who had commanded her to be baptised. As her mother was concerned about Anne's frequent temper tantrums which she attributed to *esprits* tormenting her, she asked a local Roman Catholic priest to baptise Anne. The priest established that Anne was having *relations surnaturelles* and that she had diabolical knowledge of secret information, so he agreed to baptise her.

Shortly afterwards Anne joined the Apostles of Infinite Love, a Canadian evangelical Catholic sect which had recently established a mission on the island. Anne started to have frequent *états et extases* in which she would suddenly fall to the ground. She would then have a vision, get up and walk around in a twilight state (*état de veille*) during which she would enunciate messages from the Holy Virgin. Anne's mother did not approve of her membership of the Apostles. On one occasion Anne became paralysed while visiting the Apostles' *foyer-cénacle* (upper room of the Last Supper). The Apostles' leader, Père Serge de l'Enfant Jesu, declared that the Holy Virgin had caused the paralysis and convinced her mother that Anne had a sacred mission to fulfil among the Apostles, and he advised her to pray for Anne for six hours non-stop. Anne then made a miraculous recovery from her paralysis. At this point her mother consulted a *gadédzafée* (an occult healer),[4] a Madame Coco at Baie-Mahaut. Madame Coco warned Anne's mother that it was Father Serge rather than the Holy Virgin who had paralysed her daughter. He had achieved this by using his special 'magnetic powers'. Anne's mother reported this to her own parish priest who in turn informed the police and the newspaper. As a result, Anne's mother was denounced by the Apostles as 'mad and inspired by the Devil'.

The Religious Affairs correspondent claimed that the Apostles were secretly in league with the *gadédzafée* and her coven of 'white witches' who had the power to communicate with spirits but who did not actually practise *sorcellerie* (black magic). In a later article headed 'The Church of Lies and Terror', the reporter described the Apostles both as 'heretics' because of their claim to be Catholic, and as 'impostors' because of their alleged links to the *école de magie* run by Mme Coco.

At an open-air mass prayer meeting lasting several days and nights at Pointe Noire in January 1977, the assembled Apostles, who had had to crawl to the meeting place on the summit of a hill on their hands and knees, were promised miracles and healing: 'The blind will see again'. The Apostles' leaders declared that they were being persecuted 'just like Christ', and the penitents were encouraged to abandon their houses and to live among the Apostles. Eventually Sister Anne's mother asked the police to rescue her daughter from the Apostles, claiming that she was being held in the community against her will. The diocesan authorities also requested the police to investigate the sect, who were accused of kidnapping their followers. Anne was removed and taken to a psychiatrist. He concluded that she had been 'brain-washed' and eventually Anne herself admitted that her visions had been based on 'auto-suggestion'.

PHYSICIANS AND POSSESSION

The elements of this scandal – ecstatic visions, possession, and accusations of heresy and witchcraft – are recurrent themes in the history of religion, as are the tension between official beliefs and popular culture, and the appeal to secular authority to defend the established church. Of particular interest is the involvement of physicians who since the early modern period have been requested from time to time to provide a medical invalidation of heterodox belief and practice.

The story of Sister Anne Andrée de Jésus Marie in Guadeloupe in 1977 resembles that of the typical possessed adolescent in early modern Europe and New England (Demos, 1982; MacDonald, 1991; D. P. Walker, 1981). She would generally be a teenager who has become intensely preoccupied with her own spiritual condition and who is aware of God's displeasure. She might begin to have spontaneous fainting spells or disturbances of sight and of hearing. Protracted fits might follow, accompanied by imaginary confrontations with Satan or his agents. The possessed girl could go into bizarre contortions and have periods of apparent paralysis alternating with frenetic activity. She might be unable to eat and she would have 'vocalisations' when she would speak with Satan's voice. The physician's task was to distinguish between 'natural maladies' and witchcraft-induced disease (Demos, 1982:167). Doctors would be asked to examine a patient or victim and to provide a differential diagnosis. At times both natural and supernatural interpretations were regarded as valid concurrently.[5] Keith Thomas (1973:640) gives examples from the sixteenth and seventeenth centuries of cases in which a diagnosis of witchcraft was made by physicians, generally in the absence of any identifiable natural cause for an illness. Conversely, of the 148 patients who complained of demonic persecution when they consulted Richard Napier, the astrological physician, he concluded that only eighteen were actually possessed (MacDonald, 1981). His near contemporary, the Norwich physician, Dr Browne, actually contested a diagnosis of witchcraft and was accused in 1578 of 'spreading a misliking of the laws by saying there are no witches' (Thomas, 1973:693).[6]

If the symptoms were interpreted as evidence of possession, a special powerful status would be conferred on the girl and this would be reinforced when some of her utterances were attributed to the Devil (D. P. Walker, 1981:16). In due course both fits and vocalisations would tend to occur in front of a specially assembled audience.

John Putnam Demos (1982) has described the possession of a young woman called Elizabeth Knapp in a small Massachusetts town in the late seventeenth century. She was a girl of 16 and her bewitchment is recorded in a treatise written by her spiritual adviser, the Reverend Samuel Willard, entitled: 'A Brief Account of the Strange and Unusual Providence of God Befallen to Elizabeth Knapp of Groton'. Her possession started in October 1691 with severe seizures. This was attributed to affliction by local witches. Her seizures persisted and in November she was examined by a physician who offered a medical diagnosis: 'A main part of her distemper . . . [was] natural, arising from the foulness of the stomach and corruptness of her blood, occasioning fumes in her brain and strange fantasies' (Demos, 1982:106). The physician prescribed physic and she went into temporary remission. However, about ten days later the fits recurred and she claimed to have been on horseback journeys with the Devil who accompanied her in the form of a black dog with eyes in his back. When reassessed by the physician a couple of weeks later, he 'contended that her distemper was diabolical, refused further to administer, [and] advised . . . extraordinary fasting; whereupon some of God's ministers were sent for' (ibid.: 106). Elizabeth continued to identify neighbours as witches responsible for her possession and the Rev. Willard went on to demonstrate to his own satisfaction that Elizabeth's fits had a demonic aetiology.[7]

Possession might be exploited in the interests of a particular religious faction. D. P. Walker (1981:17) offers a politico-ecclesiastical explanation for the fact that for orthodox Christians the possessing spirit is generally evil.[8] Possession with a divine spirit (as with Sister Anne) would carry supreme authority and its revelations might then threaten the stability of the Church, as occurred with the Montanist heretics.[9]

A fascinating example of the relationship of psychological medicine to magico-religious beliefs and political conflict is to be found in Michael Mac-Donald's explication of the medical controversy surrounding the bewitchment of Mary Glover as the struggle for power between the anti-exorcism established Church and its Catholic and Puritan adversaries, who abrogated to themselves the power to cast down devils and who used their thaumaturgical prowess to attract converts (MacDonald, 1991). For Anglicans all miraculous occurrences, including the casting out of devils by command, were no longer possible and exorcism was regarded as a perfect example of Catholic magic and priestcraft (Midelfort, 1977). Puritans, however, maintained that fasting and prayer to God to expel the devil were still legitimate. Mary Glover was a young Puritan woman who had developed convulsions after alleged bewitchment by a bad tempered, irascible old woman, Elizabeth Jackson, who was convicted in 1602 of witchcraft.[10] Mary Glover's possessing spirit was 'dispossessed' by a group of Puritan preachers who held a ritual session of prayer and fasting in Mary Glover's presence. After a final paroxysm of convulsions the devil left her body as she declared that the Lord had delivered her.

Edward Jorden, a senior and highly respected physician, was commissioned as a medical witness by the Bishop of London to advance scientific arguments for challenging the authenticity of the witchcraft-induced possession, which was being exploited for propaganda purposes by members of the religious opposition. The medical and theological arguments for and against possession were adopted explicitly 'to validate the claims to religious authority of both sides' (MacDonald, 1991: xliv).

According to Jorden, hysteria, epilepsy and possession might all be present with convulsions which could be triggered by the presence of a specific person, leading to apparent loss of consciousness and dysphagia. Jorden warns against the use of prayer and fasting in the treatment of hysteria, although he recognises that they might be appropriate in cases of true possession. In France during the same period the medical response to the fake possession of Marthe Brossier indicates a similar shift towards natural explanations for witchcraft and possession (Mandrou, 1968:163–73). While Jorden had testified that Mary Glover was suffering from a natural disease, i.e. hysteria and that she was not the victim of witchcraft, Marthe was dismissed by some leading physicians as a fraud. Until that time, i.e. a century before the possession of Elizabeth Knapp, the role of physicians had generally been restricted to demonstrating insensitive areas of skin made by the devil in a suspected witch, or showing supernumerary teats for nourishing the familiar demon. Doctors in the sixteenth century were not routinely asked for an opinion regarding the authenticity of a possession (Mandrou, 1968). Marthe was a 25-year-old woman from Romorantin where, a few years previously, some possessed women had denounced a number of witches, whose execution had allegedly relieved them of their possessing devils.

Subsequently a further twenty women had claimed to be possessed. In 1598 Marthe declared that she was also possessed by a demon and she made witchcraft accusations against one of her neighbours, who was embroiled with her in a family feud. This unfortunate woman, Anne Chevrot, was thrown into prison. Anne Chevrot appealed to the Paris authorities to be released, attributing Marthe's malevolent denunciation to 'a frenzied passion' caused by the prospect of remaining a spinster (Marthe was the third unmarried daughter of an impecunious merchant). However, both the local priest and the doctor declared that Marthe was possessed rather than sick. She was escorted to Paris by her father and their journey from the Loire Valley was punctuated by repeated diabolic convulsions. Marthe underwent public exorcisms which attracted large crowds.[11] Once established in Paris her vehement denunciations of the Huguenots, vocalised by her possessing demon, soon gave her the status of a prophet and a visionary. The Archbishop of Paris summoned both theologians and doctors to examine her. Although two doctors claimed to demonstrate the pathognomonic witch's anaesthetic patch on her hand, she failed the other diagnostic test of prodigious linguistic skills and the court physician, Dr Marescot, concluded that she was not truly possessed.[12] He demonstrated this by defying the exorcists 'at peril of his life' and restrained Marthe during one of her convulsions and managed to halt her wild thrashing fits. Marthe, whose anti-Huguenot diatribes threatened the fragile armistice brought about by the Edict of Nantes, was eventually arrested as a fraud.[13] However, the Capuchins then summoned another group of doctors who declared that she was indeed possessed. Eventually, the sceptics prevailed and she was banished from Paris. Her anti-Calvinist ecclesiastical and medical supporters fought a rearguard action, publishing a pamphlet which rehearsed the evidence in favour of possession – notably the fact that her condition fluctuated between perfectly normal behaviour and frantic convulsions which were accompanied by ugly and unseemly grimaces. The pro-Marthe doctors concluded that she was not suffering from a natural illness such as epilepsy or hysteria nor was she faking because she could tolerate pricking with long needles during her convulsions and the puncture sites did not bleed. According to these medical supporters, only possession by the devil could account for the convulsions. However, in this and in other contemporary French cases described by Mandrou (1968), only simulation could reasonably account for the protracted outpouring of sectarian diatribes such as anti-Huguenot propaganda during the seizures (D. P. Walker, 1981:15). In 1599 John Darrell, a Puritan, was actually convicted for teaching two demoniacs how to fake the symptoms of possession. The book published in defence of Darrell in the same year argued that denial of the phenomena of possession and witchcraft might in turn lead to accusations of atheism: 'If neither possession nor witchcraft, contrary to hath bene so longe generally and confidently affirmed, why should we thinke that there are Divells? (If no Divells, no God)' (ibid.: 71–2).

'HOLY ANOREXIA'

If possession was a 'culture-bound syndrome' (Littlewood and Lipsedge, 1987) found in young European and North American women in the sixteenth and seventeenth centuries and even later, conferring power and prestige on certain members of an under-priviledged social group, holy anorexia had served a similar function in the preceding centuries. Rudolph Bell (1985) has proposed that the holy anorexia of saints such as Catherine of Siena, Veronica Giuliani and Mary Magdalen de'Pazzi was at least in part a response to the patriarchal social structure of medieval Catholicism. Unlike contemporary anorexia, this was no self-conscious unremitting pursuit of thinness. The unwillingness to eat in holy anorexia was driven by the desire to be saintly: 'Nothing so pleases God as a thin body; the more it is emaciated by sharp mortifications, the less will it be subject to corruption in the grave and it will thus be resurrected all the more gloriously' (de Montargon, 1752:6). Protracted fasting was a sign of interior strength bestowed as a special divine favour (Bell, 1985:116).

In contemporary rural North West Portugal there is still a cult of reverence for women who eat very little except the Eucharistic host and who appear to lack normal bodily functions. They are regarded as women of great sexual purity and they resemble the Virgin who was conceived without the stain of original sin and who ascended to Heaven without physical corruption (de Pinha-Cabral, 1986).

The holy anorexic's struggle against her bodily urges also gave her freedom from the patriarchy that tried to

> impose itself between the holy anorexic and her God . . . the holy anorexic rebels against passive vicarious dependent Christianity . . . once she convinces herself that her spiritual bridegroom communicates directly with her and she thereby achieves true autonomy, the commands of earthly men become trivial.
>
> (Bell, 1985:116)[14]

With the Reformation the male clerical hierarchy became increasingly hostile to and critical of autonomous female religiosity which could be 'dangerous to herself and to all the faithful' (ibid.: 152) and so 'female piety came to be seen variously as insane, demoniacal and heretical' (ibid.: 178). Dominica del Paradiso at the end of the fifteenth century who fasted, prayed and flagellated herself was accused of having the evil eye: 'She was cited by the curial nuncio before the vicarial tribunal on charges of witchcraft and suspected heresy . . . she was placed under the direction of the Vicar to *correct her and restore her mental health*' (ibid.: 170, emphasis added).

Her contemporary, Columba da Rieti, was charged with not eating and therefore of being in league with the devil. Her self-induced vomiting allegedly 'relieved her of her evil spirits'. An inquisitor labelled her as 'areptitia', i.e. 'out of her mind' and/or 'in error' (ibid.: 157).

As sanctions against holy anorexia intensified, an alternative strategy was employed by women to achieve 'public and influential vocal sanctity' (ibid.: 57). This goal could be reached via a 'good possession' disguised as, or sometimes combined with, a 'diabolical one', as in the case of Louise Capeau in Sainte Baume in the early seventeenth century (D. P. Walker, 1981:77).

MYSTICAL EXPERIENCE, PSYCHOPATHOLOGY AND MEDICAL REDUCTIONISM

In his address to the Leo Baeck College in 1968 entitled 'Psychiatry and the Jewish tradition', Aubrey Lewis made reference to the trances, visions and voices experienced by Isaiah, Jeremiah and other prophets of the Old Testament, but he concluded with modest caution that 'it would be presumptuous to equate the prophetic afflatus with the psychopathic disorders of consciousness to which it bears a resemblance' (Lewis, 1978). Lewis then gave a brief psychobiography of Joseph Caro, the sixteenth-century cabalistic compiler of the Shulchan Aruch. Caro was the recipient of regular messages from a spirit guide, a *maggid*, who spoke through the Jewish visionary as his medium. Again, Lewis was reluctant to ascribe psychopathology to a mystic whose behaviour fell within the normal range for his historical period, for the cultural setting and for Caro's 'personal qualities'. Like the medieval historian, Gurevich (1988), Lewis withholds judgement on whether prophets and pseudoprophets, false christs, miracle workers, self-proclaimed saints and messiahs, mystics and messengers were 'conscious hoaxers and impostors, self-deluded visionaries or psychologically unstable, abnormal people' (Gurevich, 1988:69). Lewis adopts a cultural-relativist position in the tradition of Ackerknecht (1943) and Devereux (1956). William James (1985:333) had warned against 'medical materialism' which would reduce St Paul's vision to an abnormal cortical discharge, and would designate St Theresa an hysteric and St Francis an hereditary degenerate. James condemned the dismissal of George Fox's pining for spiritual veracity as merely a symptom of a disordered colon.

Physiological reductionism of this type still surfaces from time to time as in the attribution of witchcraft fantasies to ergotism and the ecstatic visions of Hildegard of Bingen to migrainous fortification spectra (Flanagan, 1989).

The psychobiographies of historical figures who have experienced religious visions, trances and other transcendental happenings also rely on more or less reductionistic interpretations of this type. Recent examples include the prophecies of Arise Evans whom Hill and Shepherd (1976) tentatively labelled as a case of Kleist's 'Revelatory Psychosis'; while the elevations and descents of Evans' contemporary, the seventeenth century false messiah, Sabbatai Sevi, as well as those of the eighteenth century Hasidic *zaddiq* Nahman of Bratzlav, the English mystic Marjory Kempe, and the Belgian nun Beatrice of Nazareth, were all manic-depressive according to some historians (Scholem, 1973:126–8; Green, 1979:174; Freeman *et al.*, 1990 and Kroll and de Ganck, 1986).

VISIONS, INSANITY AND SIN IN THE MIDDLE AGES

A range of subjective phenomena that may be considered pathological by contemporary psychiatry might have been attributed in the Middle Ages to a religious experience, whether ordinary or extraordinary, and only rarely would they be regarded as evidence of insanity. Medieval visions were not regarded as a homogeneous type of experience, as shown by Kroll and Bachrach's exhaustive examination (1982) of the lives of eight saints, eight historical chronicles and an autobiography, plus correspondence and the records of St Bartholomew's church in Smithfield. These sources cover both England and France in the period 600 to 1300. All the descriptions of visions, voices and dreams which were recorded by contemporaries as a *visio* were scrutinised. Nearly half of these 134 visionary experiences occurred in a dream or twilight state (dream-visions seem to have the same status of credibility or sanctity as other types of visions). Of the remainder, about 50 per cent occurred in the course of an organic confusional state associated with fever, starvation, terminal illness, etc. Thirty-three of the visionary experiences which occurred in a setting of clear consciousness have no obvious medical explanation, half of them as an apparent response to extreme circumstances (combat, shipwreck, etc.) while half occurred in normal everyday circumstances, such as the vision of the Mother of Mercy seen and heard while at prayer by the Monk Herbert. These visions were typically regarded as communications from God or his emissaries, or, in a minority of cases, as messages from the Devil. However, some of the visions, especially those seen by people of low status, were greeted with disbelief and scepticism by the local nobility or high clergy (Kroll and Bachrach, 1982).[15] In this series one of the four cases of probable psychosis is that described by Guibert of Nogen – a penitent who mutilates himself in response to commands from the Devil in the guise of St James the Apostle (ibid., 1982).

Thus, only a tiny proportion of the visions occurred during an episode of mental illness. Conversely, few descriptions of major psychiatric disorder in these records actually refer to visionary experiences, suggesting that the standard symptomatology of psychosis did not include hallucinations at that time. The salient features of those recorded as mentally ill included incoherence, irrational speech, melancholia and delirium.

In the Middle Ages a possessed person behaved 'like a raging madman' (Neaman, 1975:32). The demoniac, the possessed man or woman, was recognisable by both their appearance and their highly stereotyped behaviour. Just as in the biblical accounts, the demoniac's face would be distorted in a hideous grimace, foaming at the mouth, eyes rolling or staring. There would be convulsions, speech in another person's voice and inability to pray or to take the Eucharist. The demoniac would show abhorrence of the name or image of Christ. This ordeal would be followed by amnesia (ibid.: 31–2).

Exorcists expelled the devil by praying, by eliciting his name, invoking the name of God and by applying the crucifix to the forehead and breast of the victim and by the laying on of hands. Medical theologians, lawyers and physicians distinguished clearly between insanity and possession, which might precede or follow each other in any particular case but which were not identical (ibid.: 40). Both possession and madness caused the destruction of order, the devil wreaking havoc on the cosmic scale, insanity causing chaos within the individual; loss of 'reason' meant erosion of the soul.

Insanity was defined as corruption of 'reason', i.e. of order, stability and the instinct for virtue which is part of the soul, residing in the brain (ibid.: 41). God punished unrepentant sinners with madness and other diseases, which were also a test of faith, a purgation and a warning to repent (ibid.: 48–9). Saul's madness (1 Kgs: 15–16) was attributed to sin and God warned (Deut. 28:15–28) that he would strike with madness those who failed to obey his Commandments. However, post-biblical Jewish literature conceptualised sin as mental illness: 'No man sins unless the spirit of madness [Ruach Shtus] overtakes him' (T. Sotan 3A in Spero, 1978:275).

In her study of the literary uses of madness in Middle English literature, Doob wrote:

It was commonly recognised in the Middle Ages that disease was a fitting punishment for the wicked because it inflicted misery in life as a token of the pains of Hell, it symbolised the deformity of a sinful soul, it provided a forceful example to deter others and it conveniently dispatched sinners to the greater punishments of death and Hell.

(1974:3)

As the most extreme form of irrationality, insanity carried the threat of damnation because it implied a sinful rejection of divine order and a turning away from God. Deprived of reason, Man became a wild beast like Nebuchadnezzar in Daniel 4. With the Fall, Man had become susceptible to both sin and madness. According to Hildegard of Bingen (ibid.: 8), the Fall changed every man's constitution by leading to the creation of the melancholy humour, the major cause of both madness and disease. There was thus both a physiological and psychological deterioration which led to sin and hence to disease and madness (ibid.: 10). The Devil could not only invade the body and upset the balance of humours, he could also invade and destroy the mind. Furthermore, he could tempt a man to excessive indulgence which might in turn lead to illness.

Insanity, like leprosy and plague, aroused terror and revulsion. The Church 'felt obliged to determine whether folly was a sin, disease or a state of blessedness and, finally, to decide whether a visionary was a true mystic or a charlatan deluded by the devil' (Neaman, 1975:56).

In a systematic review and quantitative analysis of a sample of secular and religious biographies, 'Lives of the Saints' and chronicles from pre-crusade sources, Kroll and Bachrach (1984) extracted every reference to mental illness. Of the fifty-seven episodes of mental illness, the medieval clerical authors described roughly equal number of bouts of madness alone, possession alone and madness combined with possession. Only about a sixth of these episodes were attributed directly to sin as the proximal cause of the illness. Sin was most commonly implicated as the cause in those cases of madness or epilepsy which were combined with possession, while possession alone was attributed to sin in only a single case. The commonest combination was madness/possession/sin. Madness without possession was rarely attributed to sin (ibid.: 1984).

In summary, sin could cause insanity or insanity could lead to sin. Both led to deviation from God's pattern. Neaman (1975:54) points out that pride ramifies to wrath and wrath to *tristitia* or melancholic despair. Despair implied lack of faith in God's mercy.

Zilboorg's influential *History of Medical Psychology* (1941) which was based on printed rather than manuscript sources, dominated psychiatric teaching for forty years giving generations of students the impression that in the medieval and early modern period virtually all the mentally ill were regarded as being either witches, or their victims or in league with the devil or his agents. Neugebauer's examination of the Court of Wards archives and Chancery records which date from the fourteenth to the seventeenth century and which cover a wide range of social classes, provide little evidence of a supernatural or demonological explanation for mental disturbances and the diagnosis of insanity seems to have been based entirely on naturalistic criteria (Neugebauer, 1979).[16] Aetiological explanations included physical illness, cerebral trauma and major adverse life events and the documents examined by Neugebauer contain only a single case (1383) where a demonological explanation of mental illness appears. Unexpected or inexplicable illness was attributed to a 'visitation of God', a pious and conventional idiom which is not to be confused with a demonological explanation. (The corresponding idiom in our own secular practice of psychiatry would be the term 'idiopathic'.)

The naturalistic explanations for mental illness contained in these medieval and early modern English legal documents are not necessarily inconsistent with the literary and ecclesiastical sources examined by Doob (1974) and Neaman (1975) respectively. This might just be an historical example of the simultaneous belief in numerous apparently incompatible explanatory models of disease, in this case the theological, the popular, the literary and the legal (see Luhrmann, 1989).

THE SOCIAL AND POLITICAL RESPONSE TO ECSTATIC EXPERIENCES

Over the past twenty-five years or so historians influenced by George Rosen (1968) have turned away from the retrospective diagnosis of individual psychopathology towards an emphasis on the social and political response to individual and collective ecstatic experience, as adumbrated originally in William James' lecture on 'The Value of Saintliness' (James, 1985). Referring to George Fox's auditory hallucinations, James wrote:

A genuine first-hand religious experience like this is bound to be a heterodoxy to its witnesses, the prophet appearing to be a mere lonely madman. If his doctrine proves contagious enough to spread to any others, it becomes a definite and labelled heresy.

(ibid.: 337)[17]

Enthusiasts during much of the seventeenth century were treated by their opponents either as conniving hypocrites or as collaborators with the Devil. DePorte (1974) refers to a book published in 1646 with a chapter entitled 'The Anabaptists are a lying and blasphemous sect, falsely pretending to divine Visions and Revelations'.

At times, psychiatric labels have been used to discredit the religious innovator and the political radical, while on other occasions the prophet has evaded his secular or ecclesiastical persecutors by invoking madness. Alternatively, his visions might be used to further a political cause. In his account of radical ideas and movements during the English Revolution, Christopher Hill (1991 a) gives examples of all three processes, with the confinement in Bedlam of Lady Eleanor Davis who predicted the violent overthrow of Charles I, the expression of seditious ideas under cover of feigned insanity by the Ranter Abiezer Coppe, and the political exploitation of Arise Evans' prophecies (Hill, 1991b: 227–86).

Eighty years ago the Liberian charismatic prophet and visionary, William Wade Harris, went to the Ivory Coast to pursue a mission which he believed was divinely inspired, namely to convert the African population to Christianity. In a few months he converted over 100,000 people, a tenth of the population of the country (S. Walker, 1983). While travelling on his proselytising mission, Harris was arrested by colonial officials. It is believed that a group of traditional leaders were afraid that Harris would undermine their influence and they informed the colonial administrator that Harris was a false prophet who was deceiving the people in order to take their money. In the event, the French concluded that he was a 'harmless maniac' and released him (ibid.: 1983).

Rivalry between innovative religious leaders might lead to accusations and counter-accusations of witchcraft or of insanity. The Muslim fundamentalist theologian and jurist Ibn Taymiyya, who died in 1328, attacked the principle that Muhammad and the saints were intercessors with God and he castigated pilgrimages and the veneration of saints as idolatrous. He was condemned and imprisoned for his reformist views and was publicly discredited as mentally unbalanced (Little, 1975).

A vision or a dream could be utilised to test the authenticity of a rival's claims to exceptional spiritual status. In her account of the conversion to Judaism of a rural Catholic community in Apulia by the patriarchal figure Donato Manduzio in the 1930s, Cassin describes the visit of a young man to the community. He declared that he was 'an envoy of the Lord, come to announce the approach of the Kingdom of Heaven' – and he added: 'I am the White Horse [of the Apocalypse].'

Manduzio suspected the visitor of being a false Apostle, and prayed to God to let him know in a vision the truth about him.

> That night he dreamt that he saw a tree and on it was a young girl with a pruning fork. She showed him a dead branch, and told him to cut off that branch which was rotten . . . Manduzio concluded that the young man must be sent away.
>
> (Cassin, 1957)

As Thomas Hobbes (1914) put it: 'If men were at liberty to take for God's Commandements their own dreams and fancies . . . scarce two men would agree upon what is God's Commandement.'[18]

PROPHETIC DREAMS, RELIGIOUS MADNESS AND POLITICAL SUBVERSION

The soldier – prophet, Miguel de Piedrola Beaumonte, identified himself with Elijah and Malachi and issued sibylline statements on the streets of counter-reformation Madrid. His prophecies were based on a series of dreams which he attributed to God (Kagan, 1990). The prophecies were all highly critical of the monarch and Piedrola was eventually denounced by a Franciscan friar as 'an agent of Lucifer . . . possessed by a demon that was responsible for everything he said and did' (Kagan, 1991:113). Piedrola was arrested by the Holy Office in 1587 but pleaded insanity in mitigation and was sentenced to a term of imprisonment and exile rather than execution.

A plea of insanity was also used in attempted mitigation at the trial of Minochio the miller, born in 1532 in the Friuli region of Italy. In 1583 he was denounced by the Holy Office, accused of uttering 'heretical and most impious words' about Christ (Ginzberg, 1992). According to Minochio's cosmogony, the universe had been created out of a giant putrefying cheese, with angels evolving from worms within this cheese while God himself was an angel created out of chaos. During the preliminary hearing, because of the strange tales reported by witnesses, the Vicar-General asked if Minochio was of sound mind. Minochio himself asserted that he was sane, but after the beginning of the trial one of his children spread the word that Minochio was 'mad' or 'possessed'. However, the Vicar rejected this interpretation. The miller's family had hoped that Minochio's opinions and his eccentric cosmogony would be tolerated as insane fantasies. In the event, the counter-reformation interpreted these idiosyncratic notions as heresy rather than as madness (ibid.: 6). Seventy years later an English prophet, James Nayler, was treated less leniently than either Piedrola or Minochio. Nayler recorded his own divine commission in 1653 in an Appleby court:

> I was at the plough, meditating on the things of God and suddenly I heard a voice saying unto me: 'Get thee out from thy kindred and from thy father's house' and I had a promise given in with it whereupon I did exceedingly

rejoice that I had heard the Voice of that God which I had professed from a child but had never known him.

(Reay 1985:51)

As Roy Porter has written, 'there was nothing odd . . . for a seventeenth-century Christian to expect direct personal revelation; what would have been abnormal, indeed spiritually terrifying, was if God never communicated His Will' (Porter, 1986:511).

Thirteen years later in 1666, the year when the millennium was expected, 'Nayler entered Bristol on a donkey, his hair and beard styled in the manner attributed to Christ. His companions, mostly women, walked beside him singing "Holy, holy, holy, Lord God of Israel." He was arrested and severely punished' (Reay, 1985:53).

The seditious prophetic dreams of Piedrola's contemporary, Lucrecia de Leon, were subjected to all three processes of political exploitation, psychiatric exculpation and dismissal as the products of a disordered mind. She was a young Spanish woman whose 400 prophetic dreams were examined in the course of a five-year trial by the Inquisition in the last decade of the sixteenth century. These dreams had been transcribed and circulated widely in manuscript form by two clergymen and were used to bolster the cause of an anti-Philip political faction. While Lucrecia's supporters represented her as a divinely inspired prophet, she was charged by the Holy Office with both heresy and sedition. Kagan (1990) shows how the dreams voiced criticism of the government of the monarch, including an attack on ecclesiastical corruption, oppressive taxes and social injustice.[19]

Some of the dreams have a millennial theme predicting the imminent destruction of the kingdom, and the issue at Lucrecia's trial was whether her dreams were indeed divinely inspired prophecies or communications from the Devil.

Kagan suggests that a number of the dreams fell within the genre of 'fictive dreams in which an individual uses the dream form to communicate ideas that, conveyed by other means, might prove dangerous' (Kagan, 1990:58).[20] As Keith Thomas has indicated, since women were denied public means of expression, their most effective way of obtaining an audience was to represent their views as the product of divine revelation. This might account for the prominence of women among religious prophets in England in the first half of the seventeenth century (Thomas, 1973:163). Two of Lucrecia's inquisitors concluded that the dreams were not of divine origin 'because true prophets never contradict themselves' (Kagan, 1990:120), while a third (ibid.: 121) attributed them to a 'vertiginous spirit' and recommended exorcism. One of the inquisitors concluded that much of her testimony to the secret tribunal had been designed to convince the judges that she was a madwoman who could not be held responsible for the content of her dreams (ibid.: 144). She had told a fellow prisoner that she was contriving to be compared with Balaam's Ass, and thus be regarded as insane.

One of Lucrecia's dream-transcribers, Alonso de Mendoza, similarly invoked a psychiatric defence when he appeared before the Inquisition, claiming that he was eccentric and mentally unstable. (Lucrecia's father described him as a madman.) In the event, the Supreme Council of the Inquisition concluded that Mendoza was suffering from 'a lack of judgement' and he was transferred from prison to a monastery (ibid.: 99). In summary, prophetic dreams were used as an ideological weapon by opposition groups and radical reformers, but the dreamer ran the obvious danger of severe punishment. She might be discredited as insane or bewitched or both. Thus, in 1654 Anne Trapnel, a Fifth Monarchist prophet and visionary, who poured forth prophecies in verse when in a state of trance and who was imprisoned as a radical opponent of Cromwell for her fierce anti-government polemics, complained in the introduction to her 'Report and Plea' that: 'England's rulers and clergy do judge the Lord's handmaid to be mad and under the administration of evil angels and a witch' (Trapnel, 1654:2).

The Zulu prophetess, Josephina, suffered a similar fate. Her African separatist speeches attracted large audiences at meetings of the South African Native Congress. In 1923 a police inspector reported that Josephina had alleged

> that the word of the Lord had come to her in the form of a vision at night, in that she saw a hand writing on the wall with an indelible pencil to the effect that she, Josephina, should go out to the people of South Africa and tell them that it would be dark for twelve days, that the locusts would come in the winter and that these locusts would have the faces of men. She stated that the time had arrived for Europeans, Indians and Chinese to quit this country and go back to their respective lands.

Another police inspector concluded that 'there can be no doubt that Josephina is not mentally normal as she keeps on repeating the same phrases over and over', and eventually she was confined in a lunatic asylum (Sapire, 1993).[21]

THE REACTION AGAINST ENTHUSIASM

In the sixteenth and seventeenth centuries phenomena such as ecstatic visions, witchcraft confessions and mental illness were attributed either to the supernatural or to an excess of black bile at high temperature, or to both. By 1750, however, those who claimed direct divine inspiration were increasingly stigmatised as melancholic or even insane: 'In so doing, the intellectuals and ecclesiastical elite redefined not only the phenomenon of "enthusiasm" but also the boundaries of "normal" behaviour' (Heyd, 1981:279). As beliefs in Satan, Hell, magic, witchcraft and divination declined (Weber's 'disenchantment of the world'), religious enthusiasm began to be regarded with incredulity. As early as 1646, when William Franklin, a rope-maker, proclaimed himself to be Jesus Christ, a sceptical physician recommended bleeding (Hill, 1993:418), while ten years later Henry More in 'Enthusiasmus Triumphatus' defined enthusiasm as 'a false persuasion' and as 'nothing else but a misconceit of being inspired' (More, 1656:6). More attributed the misconceit or delusion to melancholy, in which the sufferer was prone to misinterpret his passions as divinely inspired. He claimed that true religious experience is never opposed to the faculty of Reason. From then on, according to DePorte,

> it became more and more common to see fanatics as men fitter for Bedlam than for Bridewell, and to speak of enthusiasm as a state in which the force of fancy caused one to lose touch with the real world.
>
> (DePorte, 1974:39)

Samuel Johnson in his *Dictionary of the English Language*, published in 1755, sceptically defined enthusiasm as 'a vain belief of private revelation' and described an enthusiast as 'one who has a vain confidence of his intercourse with God'. Johnson cites Locke: 'Enthusiasm is founded neither on reason nor divine revelation, but rises from the conceits of a warmed or over-weening brain.'

The English dictionary edited by Thomas Dyche and William Pardon, published in 1774, defined an enthusiast thus: 'Commonly means a person poisoned with the notion of being divinely inspired, when he is not, and upon that account commits a great number of irregularities in words and actions' (Tucker, 1972).

In 1802 George Nott preached a series of eight sermons on the subject of enthusiasm. He declared 'despair and madness in every age have been the common attendance upon the preachings of enthusiasts.' Methodism itself was linked to madness and John Wesley's Enthusiasm was described as a hereditary disease of the Mind (ibid.).

Those who claimed direct supernatural inspiration, such as the Cevennes prophets in England at the beginning of the eighteenth century, were increasingly perceived as a menace to social and political stability (Schwartz, 1978) and they were rejected by the established Church. Charismatic individuals who spoke of personal revelation were opposed by Anglican polemicists who sought to explain enthusiasm in naturalistic terms as the manifestation of melancholy and the result of 'vapours going up into the brain and affecting the imagination' (Heyd, 1981:266).[22]

The early Quakers believed in the potential power of the divine inner light and this could lead to bizarre behaviour including going naked as a sign, as testimony to the spiritual nakedness of the world (Reay, 1985), but towards the end of the seventeenth century there was a gradual waning of enthusiasm; fasting was forbidden and 'dreams and pretended visions' had to be approved by Quaker meetings (ibid.: 112).

For about fifty years after the scandal of the French prophets and their 'mysterious effluvium' (Schwartz, 1978) overt displays of religious enthusiasm were frowned upon and there was little mystery or emotion in Anglican churches (Obelkevich, 1993).[23]

In MacDonald's view 'The governing classes' intense antipathy to radical religion and miracle-mongering sectarians and priests, cast doubt on supernatural explanations for events and enhanced the appeal of philosophy and science' (MacDonald, 1986:94). However, enthusiasm revived with the rise of Envangelical public conversions and the extemporary prayers and cries of distress, praise and rejoicing (the 'outpouring of the spirit') at emotional Methodist services and open-air meetings. The medical response to the nineteenth-century revivals was no less partisan than that of the physicians mobilised 260 years earlier by the opposing factions in the cases of the possessed teenagers, Mary Glover and Marthe Brossier. The anti-revival medical journal, *The Lancet*, anticipating the critical view expressed by the Established Church of Ireland took an anti-enthusiasm stance when it described the convulsions and stupors of the participants in the 1859 Ulster Revival as due to hysteria and epileptiform convulsions. Conversely, the Presbyterian medical opponents of the hysteria theory concluded that 'the great majority of the stricken cases were genuinely religious' (Donat, 1988:144).

THE REVIVAL OF MILLENARIANISM AND THE REACTION TO PROPHETS AND MESSIAHS

From the end of the eighteenth century there was a revival of millenarianism, orchestrated by a number of self-proclaimed messiahs who claimed to be divine and endowed with the gift of prophecy and the power to save mankind. Joanna Southcott, daughter of a Devonshire farmer, claimed to be 'the woman clothed with the sun and the moon under her feet, and upon her head a crown of twelve stars' as in Revelation 12. She promised to give birth to Shiloh, the divine child. She died childless in 1814 (Harrison, 1979). John Rowe, who claimed to be the lawful successor of Joanna Southcott, also declared that he had been divinely commanded to start his career as a prophet and missionary among the Jews (Taylor, 1983). Richard Brothers, a former lieutenant in the Royal Navy, became convinced that he was 'the nephew of the Almighty'. He believed that he had been charged with a divine mission to rescue the Jews of the Diaspora and that he was destined to be revealed as the Prince of the Hebrews and ruler of the world. In 1795 he was confined to a lunatic asylum (Harrison, 1979). John Nichols Tom, alias Sir William Courtenay, Knight of Malta, was a radical social reformer who claimed to be the Saviour. (He physically resembled the traditional image of Christ.) He preached that the land must be taken from the rich and redistributed among the poor. Like Rowe and Brothers, he had a mission to reclaim the Jews and he was soon incarcerated in the county lunatic asylum where he remained from 1833 to 1837. One year after his release, together with his band of disciples, he led an insurrection which ended in his death at the Battle of Bossenden Wood (Rogers, 1961). Harrison (1979) has shown that while the religious preoccupations of respectable Protestant society might include the Books of Daniel and Revelation, to actually behave as if the end of the world was imminent was to invite condemnation and ostracism. Whether penal or medical sanctions were applied to blasphemers seems to have been somewhat arbitrary.

Thus John Ward, the founder of a sect, who described himself as the 'Son of God' and who rejected Heaven, Hell and the biblical Jesus, was sentenced to eighteen months in prison for blasphemy in 1832. The judge evidently regarded him as a threat to political stability: 'To endeavour to induce man to believe that there were no rewards and punishments hereafter, and that he was not an account-able being, would produce the most serious effect upon society, and ultimately overturn our excellent institutions' (Oliver, 1978:167). Two generations later the law on blasphemy was redefined. Lord Chief Justice Coleridge, in a judgement delivered in 1883 ruled: 'If the decencies of controversy are observed, even the fundamentals of religion may be attacked without a person being guilty of blas-phemous libel' (Webster, 1990:23–4).

Ward's contemporary, John Perceval, the evangelical son of an assassinated Prime Minister, spent fourteen years in private asylums because he was convinced that he had a personal divine mission to proclaim the Second Coming and he had visual and auditory hallucinations with a religious content (Harrison, 1979). Some of the voices ordered him to kill himself to hasten his own resurrection. Perceval's 'Narrative of the Treatment Experienced by a Gentleman During a State of Mental Derangement', published in two volumes in 1838 and 1840, is a bitter attack on the way the supposedly enlightened Brislington Asylum regime, based on moral therapy, both infantilised and dehumanised the patients with its patronising 'Quaker quackery' (Porter, 1987:185).

SUICIDE AND THE CHURCH

From the Middle Ages the clergy had taught that suicide happened as a result of the temptations of the Devil. Keith Thomas (1973) gives an account of a law student named Briggs whose possession occurred in 1574 and was recorded by the Puritan martyrologist, John Foxe. Briggs convinced himself that he had com-mitted the 'sin against the Holy Ghost' and that he was a 'reprobate whose prayers were in vain'. He made several suicide attempts and then became aware of an ugly dog which was following him. He realised that the dog was in fact the Devil waiting for his soul. A physician made a diagnosis of melancholy and prescribed blood letting and a purge. 'But Briggs fell into a trance and from his lips came forth his part of a dialogue between himself and the Devil which was eagerly recorded by the godly onlookers.' He was subsequently 'dispossessed' by Foxe himself (Thomas, 1973:574).

Suicides were buried at some distance from the community and their bodies were pierced with a stake to offer protection against their malevolent souls. In his detailed study of the decisions reached by coroner's juries, MacDonald (1986) shows how attitudes to suicide changed in the century and a half following the English Revolution with increasing official lenience and public sympathy. Coro-ner's juries decriminalised suicides by bringing in more frequent *non compos mentis* verdicts (ibid.: 60). In contrast, sixteenth-and early seventeenth-century juries tended to reject the opportunity presented by ambiguous deaths such as drownings to avoid declaring a person a suicide, and according to MacDonald less than 7 per cent of the suicides reported to the King's Bench were declared to have been insane in the early 1660s (ibid.: 6).

Nevertheless, the Reverend Ralph Josselin, a seventeenth century Essex clergyman, treated suicide leniently. McFarlane's analysis of his diaries (McFarlane, 1970) shows that Josselin

> never seems to have contemplated taking such a step himself, but showed neither anger or horror when someone else committed this, theoretically, most heinous offence. On three occasions he merely noted that someone had drowned or hanged himself and added no comment. In the other cases his instinctive response was pity. He spoke of the 'sad end of one Rust, who drowned himselfe' and of 'sad sins, judgements, one made away himselfe for feare of want'.
>
> (ibid.: 169)

The proportion of suicides categorised as insane between 1660 and 1680 more than doubled in the next two decades and by the early eighteenth century lunacy verdicts exceeded 40 per cent (MacDonald 1986:60).

As MacDonald points out (ibid.: 75–6), the *non compos mentis* verdicts implied a secularisation of suicide with a rejection of both religious and folkloric interpretations of self-destruction in favour of medical explanations that excused it rather than condemned it. By the late eighteenth century, physicians assumed that the causes of suicide were entirely physical or psychological.

The attribution of self-harm to mental illness rather than to the Devil, and the medically undesirable influence of Methodist enthusiasm are alluded to in a case presented to the Guy's Physical Society in October 1790.

> Mr Wilson read the case of a man about thirty years of age of a spare habit but general good health active and ingenious who for sometime past had been very dissipated and extravagant by which he became reduced in his circumstances and depress'd in mind; in this situation he fell in with an old companion who had now become a Methodist[24] and with whom he was observ'd to have long and frequent conversation – his conduct and behaviour was become chang'd, he was morose, violent, thoughtful and sometimes appear'd remarkably agitated – these circumstances increas'd to such a degree that he told the people with whom he lodg'd that the enormity of his crimes was such that he despair'd of pardon or any mitigation of his punishments – on the morning after this his reason became evidently deranged, he utter'd the most horrid imprecations and those incoherently. He refused nourishment and requir'd four strong men to secure him from mischief – on the third day in the afternoon he very calmly desired his keeper to loosen his right hand as the cords hurt him. This being done he applied the forefinger to his eye and thrusting it to the bottom of the orbit tore it out with amazing violence after which he exclaim'd 'it is done'[25] and then desired a surgeon might be sent for . . . the eye lids were brought over the orbit and superficial dressings applied – the antiphlogistic plan was adopted[26] and the patient recover'd without one symptom that could be attributed to the accident – he at length in a great degree recover'd from his

Mania but never could be made sensible of the injury he had done himself always asserting when told of it that he still possessed both Eyes.

(Physical Society, Guy's Hospital, 30th October 1790)[27]

NOTES

1 This is a reference to John Haslam who had published *Observations on Insanity* in 1798.

2 I am grateful to Samantha Bland-Rudderham for secretarial and research assistance. Andrew Baster and Karen Lipsedge provided invaluable bibliographic support. James Watson, Simon Dein and Andrew Hodgkiss have offered helpful comments and Hilary Sapire provided the information about the prophetess, Josephina.

3 This summary is based on the translation of the articles in *France-Antilles* which I made in Pointe-à-Pitre at the time (1977). The newspaper archives were destroyed in the cyclone of 1989. I recently (1993) obtained additional information about the scandal from Commissaire Joseph Prauca of the Police Judiciaire in Pointe-à-Pitre.

4 In Guadeloupe, an island with a population of 350,000, there are several hundred *gadédzafées (Lesne, 1990)*.

5 The differential diagnosis of violent convulsions followed by stupor lay between epilepsy, hysteria, and possession. However, the presence of hysteria or epilepsy would not necessarily exclude possession by the Devil since he might be the cause of those symptoms in the first place or he might even use a naturally occurring disorder to conceal his presence or to torment the victim (D. P. Walker, 1981).

6 The debate about the nosological status of trance and possession continues to this day – see Leavitt (1993) and Bilu and Beit-Hallahmi (1989).

7 Willard was also prepared to consider malingering, as well as insanity, as the differential diagnosis in cases of apparent loss of reason. He wrote that when his parishioners suffered from a 'smiting in their intellectuals' they might be fantasising or even 'dissembling' (Demos, 1982:168).

8 Contrast the present-day possessed Muslim women described in Somalia by Lewis (1989) where the spirit is often benign.

9 Montanus was a second-century native of Phrygia who claimed to be the voice of the Holy Spirit and proclaimed the coming of the millennium. His followers routinely had ecstatic seizures and spoke in strange languages (glossolalia). His emphasis on individual religious inspiration and ecstatic expression was condemned as heresy by the Orthodox Latin and Greek Churches who rejected Montanus' claim to supplement the New Testament, which was perceived as a threat to the uniformity of the hierarchical organised Church (Greenslade, 1972).

10 Johann Weyer, ducal physician at the court of Julich-Clevens, published *De praestigius demonum* (1563) in which he asserted that melancholia was prevalent among old women who were accused of witchcraft. But he also claimed that the devil actually had greater powers than were generally acknowledged and that he delighted in deceiving and deluding feeble and gullible old women into thinking that they had magical powers. Such women needed Christian instruction rather than persecution (Midelfort, 1972).

In1611 the Spanish scholar, Pedro de Valencia, while not denying the reality of witchcraft, recommended that exceptional care must be taken to prove offences: 'The accused must be examined first to see if they are in their right mind or possessed or melancholic.' He asserted that their conduct 'is more that of madmen than of heretics and should be cured with whips and sticks rather than with San Benitos' (Kamen, 1985:213).

11 Demos (1982:28) emphasises the entertainment value of public performances such as these.

12 D. P. Walker (1981:12) enumerates the pathognomonic features of possession as amazing linguistic ability, knowledge of secret information and a horrified recoiling from sacred texts or objects such as holy water.

13 Le Roy Ladurie (1987) cites three physicians in late seventeenth-century Toulouse who wrote detailed accounts of fraud in girls who claimed to be possessed.

14 In situations of deprivation or frustration where recourse to personal jural power is not available, the principal is able to adjust his or her situation by recourse to 'mystical pressure' (A. Lewis, 1978:1–89).

15 Pedro Navarro, a seventeenth-century Spanish commentator said: 'Women easily believe in any spirit, and sometimes tell, as revelations that occurred in the daytime, the foolish things they dreamed at night; and so it is necessary to hear them with a prudent, mature and cautious mind' (Christian, 1981:197).

16 These naturalistic criteria for the attribution of insanity resemble the 'folk' criteria for the diagnosis of mental illness in rural Laos noted by Westermeyer (1979) and by Edgerton (1966) in four East African societies. They include verbal abuse, talking nonsense, unprovoked assault or destructive acts, social isolation, self-neglect, socially disruptive or inappropriate behaviour and inability to do productive work.

17 In his research published over the past decade, Roland Littlewood has shown how individual psychopathology can give rise to social and cultural innovation (Littlewood, 1984; 1993).

18 In the late twelfth century a Jewish messianic pretender in the Yemen who had attracted numerous followers was arrested by the Muslim authorities. Believing that he would survive decapitation, he requested that his head be cut off (Sharot, 1982).

19 Political visions which foretold the fate of a ruler in the Other World had been specifically addressed in the Middle Ages to the bearers of state authority, warning them that their fate depended on their attitude to the clergy. These prophetic visions were a common means of coercing secular rulers in the Carolingian period (Gurevich, 1988).

20 The rural Kaliai of West New Britain have dreams which reveal themselves being cannibalised by colonial administrators (Lattas, 1993). 'In dreams, whites can be cut up into small pieces without the risk of gaol. Dreams transcend the structures of present power which whites have built up to police and protect their privileges and their bodies. In dreams there are no courts. An alternative space of justice is opened up where the black man can seek his own revenge for the sickness and death which consume the lives of his children and villagers' (ibid.: 66).

21 Central Archives Depot, Pretoria, Archives of the South African Police, file 41 6/953/23/3: Inspector C.I. Officer, Witwatersrand Division to the Deputy Commissioner, South African Police, Witwatersrand, 15th August 1923 and Inspector, Divisional Officer, Witwatersrand Division to the Deputy Commissioner, South African Police, Witwatersrand Division, 21st August 1923. (I am grateful to Hilary Sapire, of Birkbeck College, for this information about Josephina.)

22 Harrison (1979:212–61) refers to a physician named Browne who published a comparison of the 'beliefs and conduct of noted religious enthusiasts with those of patients in the Montrose Lunatic Asylum' (*Phrenological Journal and Miscellany*, 9:1834–1836 and 10:1836–1837). Browne attributed religious delusions to hypertrophy of the 'organ of veneration'.

Dowbiggin (1990) has suggested that French anti-clerical physicians in the period 1840 to 1870 emphasised the physiological basis of dreams and visions because they wished to discredit practices like mesmerism and hypnosis which they believed, 'celebrated superstitious, immoral and politically subversive forms of experience' (p. 287).

23 'Preferring "rational" forms of religion, shunning zealotry and superstition, and fearing the subversive potential of claims to possess divine inspiration, the upper classes
increasingly repudiated popular supernaturalism, and with it the language of religious
psychology and the practice of spiritual healing' (Scull, 1993:178).
24 'The doctrines of the Methodists have a greater tendency than those of any other sect
to produce the most deplorable effects on the human understanding' (Pargeter, 1792).
25 Matthew 5:29: 'And if thy right eye offend thee, pluck it out and cast it from thee: for
it is profitable for thee that one of thy members should perish, and not that thy whole
body should be cast into Hell.'
    St John 10:20–1: 'And many of them said, He hath a devil and is mad; why hear ye
him? Others said, These are not the words of him that hath the devil. Can a devil open
the eyes of the blind?'
    One of the twenty-six patients admitted to Omagh Asylum during the 1859 Ulster
revivalist campaign, which emphasised sin and damnation, tried to pluck out her eyes
because they were 'offending members' (Robins, 1986:120).
26 'The avoiding these [irritations] as much as possible, or, the moderating their force,
constitute what is rightly called the Anti-phlogistic Regimen, proper to be employed in
almost every continued fever . . . absolutely necessary for moderating the violence of
reaction' (Cullen, 1816:73).
27 For a modern case history and a review of the literature on self-inflicted blindness, see
Tapper *et al.* (1979).

REFERENCES

Ackerknecht, E. H. (1943) 'Psychopathology, primitive medicine and primitive culture',
Bulletin of the History of Medicine 14: 30–69.
Bell, R. M. (1985) *Holy Anorexia*, Chicago: University of Chicago Press.
Bilu, Y. and Beit-Hallahmi, B. (1989) 'Dybbuk-possession as a hysterical symptom: psy-
chodynamic and socio-cultural factors', *Israeli Journal of Psychiatry and Related Sci-
ences* 26: 138–49.
Cassin, E. (1957) 'San Nicandro: histoire d'une Conversion', quoted in E. J. Hobsbawm
(1959) *Primitive Rebels: A Study in Archaic Forms of Social Movement in the 19th and
20th Centuries*, Manchester: Manchester University Press.
Christian, W. A. (1981) *Apparitions in Late Medieval and Renaissance Spain*, Princeton,
NJ: Princeton University Press, quoted from P. Navarro (1622) *Favores de el Rey de el
Cielo*, Madrid, p. 7.
Cullen, W. (1816) *First Lines of the Practice of Physic*, 1, Edinburgh: Bell, Bradfute &
Adam Black.
de Montargon, H. (1752) *Dictionnaire Apostolique 3*, article I, quoted in J. Delumeau
(1991), trans. E. Nicholson, *Sin and Fear: The Emergence of a Western Guilt Culture,
13th to 18th Centuries*, New York: St Martin's Press.
Demos, J. P. (1982) *Entertaining Satan: Witchcraft and the Culture of Early New England*,
Oxford: Oxford University Press.
de Pinha-Cabral, J. (1986) *Sons of Adam, Daughters of Eve: The Peasant World View of the
Alto Minho*, Oxford: Clarendon Press.
DePorte, M. V. (1974) *Nightmares and Hobbyhorses: Swift, Sterne and Augustan Tales of
Madness*, San Marino: The Huntington Library.
Devereux, G. (1956) 'Normal and abnormal: the key problem in psychiatric anthropology',
in J. Casagrande and T. Gladwin (eds) *Some Uses of Anthropology: Theoretical and
Applied*, Washington, DC: Anthropological Society of Washington.
Dols, M. W. (1992) *Majnun: The Madman in Medieval Islamic Society*, Oxford: Clarendon
Press.

Donat, J. G. (1988) 'Medicine and religion: on the physical and mental disorders that accompanied the Ulster Revival of 1859', in *The Anatomy of Madness: Essays in the History of Psychiatry*, London: Routledge.

Doob, P. (1974) *Nebuchadnezzar's Children: Conventions of Madness in Middle English Literature*, Newhaven and London: Yale University Press.

Dowbiggin, I. (1990) 'Alfred Maury and the politics of the unconscious in 19th century France', *History of Psychiatry* 1: 255–87.

Edgerton, R. B. (1966) 'Conceptions of psychosis in four East African societies', *American Anthropologist* 68: 408–25.

Flanagan, S. (1989) *Hildegard of Bingen, 1098–1175: A Visionary Life*, London: Routledge.

Freeman, P., Bogarad, C. R. and Sholomskas, D. E. (1990) 'Margery Kempe, a new theory: the inadequacy of hysteria and post-partum psychosis as diagnostic categories', *History of Psychiatry* 1: 169–90.

Ginzberg, C. (1992) *The Cheese and the Worms: The Cosmos of a 16th Century Miller*, trans. J. A. Tedeschi, Harmondsworth: Penguin.

Green, A. (1979) *Tormented Master: A Life of Rabbi Nahman of Bratslav*, Alabama, GA: University of Alabama Press.

Greenslade, S. L. (1972) 'Heresy and schism in the later Roman Empire', in D. Baker (ed.) *Schism, Heresy and Religious Protest*, Cambridge: Cambridge University Press.

Gurevich, A. (1988) *Medieval Popular Culture: Problems of Belief and Perception*, trans. J. M. Bak and P. A. Hollingsworth, Cambridge: Cambridge University Press.

Harrison, J. F. C. (1979) *The Second Coming: Popular Millenarianism 1780–1850*, London and Henley: Routledge & Kegan Paul.

Heyd, M. (1981) 'The reaction to enthusiasm in the 17th century: towards an integrative approach', *Journal of Modern History* 53: 258–80.

Hill, C. (1991a) *Change and Continuity in 17th Century England*, Newhaven and London: Yale University Press.

—— (1991b) *The World Turned Upside Down: Radical Ideas during the English Revolution*, Harmondsworth: Penguin.

—— (1993) *The English Bible and the 17th Century Revolution*, Harmondsworth: Penguin.

Hill, C. and Shepherd, M. (1976) 'The case of Arise Evans: a historico-psychiatric study', *Psychological Medicine* 6: 351–8.

Hobbes, T. (1914) *Leviathan*, London: Dent & Dutton.

James, W. (1985) *The Varieties of Religious Experience in Human Nature*, Harmondsworth: Penguin (first published in 1902).

Johnson, S. (1755) *A Dictionary of the English Language*, London: Knapton, Longman, Hitch & Hawes, Miller & Dodsley.

Kagan, R. (1990) *Lucrecia's Dreams: Politics and Prophecy in 16th Century Spain*, Berkeley, Los Angeles and Oxford: University of California Press.

—— (1991) *Politics, Prophecy and the Inquisition from Cultural Encounters: The Impact of the Inquisition in Spain and the New World*, M. A. Perry and A. J. Cruz (eds) Berkeley, Los Angeles and Oxford: University of California Press.

Kamen, H. (1985) *Inquisition and Society in Spain in the 16th and 17th Centuries*, London: Weidenfeld & Nicolson.

Kroll, J. and Bachrach, B. (1982) 'Visions and psychopathology in the Middle Ages', *Journal of Nervous and Mental Disease* 190: 41–9.

—— (1984) 'Sin and mental illness in the Middle Ages', *Psychological Medicine* 14: 507–14.

Kroll, J. and de Ganck, R. (1986) 'The adolescence of a thirteenth century visionary nun', *Psychological Medicine* 16: 745–56.

Lattas, A. (1993) 'Sorcery and colonialism: illness, dreams and death as political languages in West New Britain', *Man* (N.S) 28: 51–77.

Leavitt, J. (1993) 'Are trance and possession disorders?', *Transcultural Psychiatric Research Review* 30: 51–7.

Le Roy Ladurie, E. (1987) *Jasmin's Witch*, trans. B. Pearce, New York: Braziller George Inc.

Lesne, C. (1990) *Cinq Essais d'Ethnopsychiatrie Antillaise*, Paris: Editions l'Harmattan.

Lewis, A. (1978) 'Psychiatry and the Jewish tradition', *Psychological Medicine* 8: 9–19.

Lewis, I. M. (1989) *Ecstatic Religion: A Study of Shamanism and Possession*, 2nd edition, London: Routledge.

Little, D. P. (1975) 'Did Ibn Taymiyya have a screw loose?', in M. W. Dols *Majnun: The Madman in Medieval Islamic Society*, Oxford: Clarendon Press.

Littlewood, R. (1984) 'The imitation of madness: the influence of psychopathology upon culture', *Social Science and Medicine* 19: 705–15.

—— (1993) *Pathology and Identity: The Work of Mother Earth in Trinidad*, Cambridge: Cambridge University Press.

Littlewood, R. and Lipsedge, M. (1987) 'The butterfly and the serpent: culture, psychopathology and biomedicine', *Culture, Medicine and Psychiatry* 11: 289–335.

Luhrmann, T. M. (1989) *Persuasions of the Witch's Craft: Ritual Magic and Witchcraft in Present-day England*, Oxford: Blackwell.

MacDonald, M. (1981) *Mystical Bedlam: Madness, Anxiety and Healing in Seventeenth Century England*, Cambridge: Cambridge University Press.

—— (1986) 'The secularisation of suicide in England, 1660–1800', *Past and Present* 111: 50–100.

—— (1991) *Witchcraft and Hysteria in Elizabethan London: Edward Jorden and the Mary Glover Case*, London: Routledge.

McFarlane, A. (1970) *The Family Life of Ralph Josselin: An Essay in Historical Anthropology*, Cambridge: Cambridge University Press.

Mandrou, R. (1968) *Magistrats et Sorciers en France au XVIIe Siècle: Une Analyse de Psychologie Historique*, Paris: Plon.

Midelfort, H. C. E. (1972) *Witch Hunting in South Western Germany, 1562–1684: The Social and Intellectual Foundations*, Stanford: Stanford University Press.

—— (1977) 'The renaissance of witchcraft research', *Journal of the History of Behavioural Sciences* 13: 294–7.

More, H. (1656) 'Enthusiasmus Triumphatus or a discourse of the natural causes, kinds and cure of enthusiasme', in R. Hunter and I. MacAlpine, *Three Hundred Years of Psychiatry 1535–1860*, London: Oxford University Press (1963).

Neaman, J. S. (1975) *Suggestion of the Devil: The Origins of Madness*, New York: Anchor Press/Doubleday.

Neugebauer, R. (1979) 'Medieval and modern theories of mental illness', *Archives of General Psychiatry* 36: 477–83.

Obelkevich, J. (1993) *The Cambridge Social History of Britain, 1750–1950*, Cambridge: Cambridge University Press.

Oliver, W. H. (1978) *Prophets and Millennialists: The Use of Biblical Prophecy in England from the 1790s to the 1840s*, Auckland: Auckland University Press.

Pargeter, W. (1792) *Observations on Maniacal Disorders*, 31, Reading.

Physical Society, Guy's Hospital (1790) '5th meeting of the 9th session', *Public Minutes*, 30th October 1790.

Porter, R. (1986) 'Diary of a madman, 17th century style: Goodwin Walton, MP and communer with the fairy world', *Psychological Medicine* 16: 503–13.

—— (1987) *A Social History of Madness: Stories of the Insane*, London: Weidenfeld & Nicolson.

Reay, B. (1985) *The Quakers and the English Revolution*, London: Temple Smith.

Robins, J. (1986) *Fools and Madmen: A History of the Insane in Ireland*, Dublin: Institute of Public Administration.

Rogers, P. J. (1961) *Battle in Bossenden Wood: The Strange Story of Sir William Courtenay*, Oxford: Oxford University Press.

Rosen, G. (1968) *Madness in Society: Chapters in the Historical Sociology of Mental Illness*, London: Routledge & Kegan Paul.

Sapire, H. (1993) Personal communication.

Scholem, G. (1973) *Sabbatai Sevi: The Mystical Messiah, 1626–1676*, London: Routledge & Kegan Paul.

Schwartz, H. (1978) *Knaves, Fools, Madmen and That Subtle Effluvium: A Study of the Opposition to the French Prophets in England, 1706–1710*, monograph no. 62, Yale: University of Florida, Social Sciences, Board of Regents of the State of Florida.

Scull, A. (1993) *The Most Solitary of Afflictions: Madness and Society in Britain 1700–1900*, New Haven and London: Yale University Press.

Sharot, S. (1982) *Messianism, Mysticism and Magic*, Chapel Hill, North Carolina: University of North Carolina Press.

Spero, M. H. (1978) 'Sin as neurosis – neurosis as sin: further implications of a Halachic meta-psychology', *Journal of Religion and Health* 17: 274–87.

Spurzheim, J. G. (1817) *Observations on the Deranged Manifestations of the Mind, or Insanity*, London: Baldwin, Cradock & Joy.

Tapper, C. M., Bland, R. C. and Danyluk, L. (1979) 'Self-inflicted eye injuries and self-inflicted blindness', *Journal of Nervous and Mental Disease* 167: 311–14.

Taylor, B. (1983) *Eve and the New Jerusalem: Socialism and Feminism in the 19th Century*, London: Virago Press.

Thomas, K. (1973) *Religion and the Decline of Magic: Studies in Popular Beliefs in 16th and 17th Century England*, Harmondsworth: Penguin.

Trapnel, A. (1654) 'Anna Trapnel's report and plea, or, a narrative of her journey from London into Cornwall, for Thomas Brewster', in E. Graham, H. Hinds, E. Hobby and H. Wilcox (eds) *Her Own Life: Autobiographical Writings by 17th Century English Women*, London: Routledge (1989).

Tucker, S. I. (1972) *Enthusiasm in Semantic Change*, Cambridge: Cambridge University Press.

Walker, D. P. (1981) *Unclean Spirits. Possession and Exorcism in France and England in the Late 16th and Early 17th Centuries*, Philadelphia: University of Pennsylvania Press.

Walker, S. S. (1983) *The Religious Revolution in the Ivory Coast: The Prophet Harris and the Harris Church*, Chapel Hill: University of North Carolina Press.

Webster, R. (1990) *A Brief History of Blasphemy; Liberalism, Censorship and the 'Satanic Verses'*, London: The Orwell Press.

Westermeyer, J. (1979) 'Folk criteria for the diagnosis of mental illness in rural Laos: on being insane in sane places', *American Journal of Psychiatry* 136: 755–61.

Zilboorg, G. and Henry, G. W. (1941) *A History of Medical Psychology*, London: Allen & Unwin.

Part II

Religions: East and West

Chapter 4

Christianity and psychiatry

John Foskett

Of Jesus, 'Many of them said, "He has a demon, he is mad, why listen to him?"' (John 10:20). The relationship between psychiatry and Christianity begins inauspiciously, with the words of the founder discredited because of his madness. In the centuries since that relationship has fluctuated often. People with mental health problems and peculiarities have been persecuted and praised, cared for and cast out by Christians and their churches. Psychiatry has protected the weak from some of the excesses of Christian ministry, but sometimes has undermined the faithful's precarious beliefs while living off their dis-ease. On occasion, Christianity and psychiatry have ignored one another. Religion rarely appears in the pages of psychiatry's text books, and psychiatry goes unmentioned in theological journals. At other times there has been fruitful cooperation between people in both fields. Two of the earliest and most prestigious asylums, the Bethlem Royal Hospital and the Retreat at York, have Christian origins. However, neither priests nor physicians have been conspicuous listeners to the words of the sufferers themselves. In this chapter the relationship between psychiatry and Christianity is described, and an analysis offered of the effect this relationhip has upon people diagnosed as mentally ill and those who treat and care for them.

In contemporary Western society there are similarities between Christianity and psychiatry: both are preoccupied with subjective phenomena and with internal and illusive realities. Each depends upon the testimony of individuals, as difficult to refute as they are to believe. And despite the rationalism of our culture, both have a considerable effect upon it. Christianity has largely forsaken the search for objective confirmation of its beliefs. Recognising the irrationality of drawing twentieth-century conclusions from first-century writings, theologians (Houlden, 1991; Sanders, 1987) have turned their attention to the historical and critical exploration of the culture and context from which their religion emerged, and good use has been made of anthropology, archaeology and history. At the same time only a minority of Christians take notice of this critical development, popularised in the United Kingdom by John Robinson (1963), David Jenkins (1976) and Don Cuppitt (1986). The majority of the faithful remain loyal to their own dogmas irrespective of the doubts cast by theologians. Scripture and tradition are selectively harnessed to the vehicle which best bears their beliefs, be they the preservation of the Book of Common Prayer, the infallibity of the Pope, or the literal interpretation of the Bible. For better and for worse Christianity has survived. Christians claim this is because God wills it to survive, others point to the churches' facility in seducing human beings by offering them what they want. At present this is exemplified in the thirst for certainty, security and a return to Victorian values. Although the numbers of active Christians slowly dwindle, groups offering a simple faith flourish (Brierley, 1991).

Historians, social and political analysts have an explanation of this. Starting with the Emperor Constantine, dominant authorities have hijacked religions for their own ends. Prelates and reformers have conspired with monarchs and presidents, capitalists and communists to shape and reinforce societies in their own image, justified more by works than by faith, and by those who exploit rather than love their neighbours. Churches are as vulnerable to the spirit of the age, and as addicted to competition as anyone, and soon our airways will be awash with holy rivalry. It is difficult to value things, including health and salvation, in anything but monetary terms. No wonder people turn to the certainties of a simple faith to ease the burdens of their faithlessness (Pattison, 1989).

Over the same period psychiatry has moved, according to its adherents, from a discipline of faith and a little science, to a more objectively grounded enterprise, both medically and psychologically. Of course, the advances in biochemistry, genetics and psychology could deceive one into believing that faith plays only a small part in the work of the mental health professions. Some, particularly those in academic psychiatry, would like it to be that way. Others like Michel Foucault (1967) and Thomas Szasz (1974) dispute these claims altogether. For the majority, much still depends upon the hunches and hopes, the fears and the faith of the clinician, who 'has not a lot of gold dust to show for over a century of sifting and sieving the mud of human experience' (Clare, 1976:213). Psychiatry too has its 'denominations' organic and dynamic, behavioural and social to help protect it from its ignorance. There are 'heretics' and 'inquisitors', the pure and the eclectic, and in such an uncertain science there is room for many different points of view, and evidence of a kind to support them all. According to one school of thought, splitting and projecting are natural ways to manage anxiety, and both psychiatry and Christianity have their share of anxiety. If religion really is psychiatry's last taboo (Kung, 1986), then perhaps it is anxiety which spawns the reticence they show towards one another.

THE HISTORICAL RELATIONSHIP

History throws some light on the relationship, its problems and its potential. Henry VIII's sexuality, fruitful and dysfunctional as it was, has something to answer for. Some would say that the present sexual crisis in the Church of England owes much to Henry's narcissism. By dissolving the monasteries, he inadvertently removed society's asylums from the care of the churches. In the rest of Europe the Church has continued to be one of the major resources for those diagnosed as suffering from madness. In this country, no such tradition survives, and it is only individual Christians, like Tuke and Lord Shaftesbury, who were conspicuous in their contribution to care and treatment. More recently, Frank Lake (1966), an evangelical and a psychiatrist, established the Clinical Theology Association, Elly Jansen, a theological student from King's College in London, founded the Richmond Fellowship, an association of therapeutic communities, and Jane Lindon, whose letters in the religious press unleashed a torrent of offence at the churches' neglect, formed the Association for the Pastoral Care of the Mentally Ill.

The Church, once the dispenser of healing, gave way to medicine – physicians needed a bishop's licence to practise until the beginning of the eighteenth century but by 1800 it was doctors who authorised clergy to minister in their asylums. The General Court of the Bethlem Hospital sought guidance of a committee of physicians regarding the appointment of a chaplain. Their report (1816) noted that, 'actual injury has not been satisfactorily proved to have arisen from religious instruction at Bethlem, and secondly that positive good has, on the contrary, been proved to have resulted in many instances'.

Most notable among the reasons for religion and psychiatry's uneasy relationship is the different meaning each has placed upon the phenomena of madness. The former identified the causes of madness as both natural and supernatural; good and bad madness (Boisen, 1936; James, 1902; Pattison, 1989). The good was to be cherished and revered, the bad treated and exorcised. The latter, with little knowledge of or interest in the supernatural, has concentrated upon the pathology of madness. Medicine diagnoses mental illnesses, which like other illnesses are open to treatment and cure. 'The corporeal or the material is the fundamental fact; the mental or spiritual the effect', wrote Henry Maudsley in 1918. Unproven as this hypothesis remains, religion's ambivalence has jarred with medicine's conviction. The relative ineffectiveness of both has not dampened the ardour of either's contempt for the other's efforts, but it has left the sufferers confused as to where help and consolation are most likely to be found. Paul Halmos in his seminal work *The Faith of the Counsellors* (1965) traces the evolution of secular counsellors, including mental health professionals, to the demise of the clergy. Halmos recognises in the former group an implicit faith in their work, but one which they are reluctant to own, for they prefer to stress the technical and scientific basis for what they do. Are they perhaps a new kind of priesthood administering their own mysteries and conversing in their own 'religious' language? I have spoken with hospital chaplains of various denominations during the twenty-five years of psychiatric admissions and I have found their perspectives increasingly valuable. Nevertheless, their contribution always seems marginal to the main purpose of psychiatric hospitals (Campbell, 1993:11).

The current relationship between Christianity and psychiatry exists in a number of forms. There is conflict, cooperation and collusion, and, at its most creative, intercourse; each will be explored in turn. Cox (this volume) talks about explanatory models and the collaborations between physicians and priests.

CONFLICT

Conflict, active and passive, is a common feature of the relationship. The clash of cultures between religion and science, different understandings of the nature of madness and the theories of care and treatment derived from them, and the relative status and power of the professions all contribute to the hostilities which simmer beneath the surface, and explode from time to time. Of course, conflict is familiar to each discipline in its own right. Case conferences, especially the grand academic ward rounds, could be mistaken for debates in the councils of the early Church. As in Corinth, there are parties and charismatic figures to lead them. Some come to the arena brandishing statistics and video recordings of significant interventions, while others are empty-handed when the president calls for a formulation. At its best this conflict is about worth and value, as represented by sacred or secular symbols. What weight can be given to them, how far do they unravel the mystery confronting priest or physician, or clothe the nakedness of their ignorance? Just as Christians strive for purity in doctrine so psychiatrists look for the validity of research in diagnosis and preferred treatment. Here there will always be room for conflict, indeed, a need for it. What else can protect us against the subjectivism which Christianity abhors as idolatry, and psychiatry disowns in anecdotalism?

The taking apart of each other's illusions and false claims is as essential as it is painful (see also Sutherland, this volume). What is not so helpful about conflict is the distraction it becomes when used to cloak a common sense of inadequacy in the face of madness. It remains so much a mystery from all points of view. Like those who built the Tower of Babel, an idol if ever there was one, different tongues speak the languages of biochemistry, psychology, neuropathology, let alone theology.

The abuses of both Christianity and psychiatric practice provide inflammable fuel for the more explosive conflicts. The popular imagination holds all psychiatrists to be atheists bent upon saving people from the guilt-induced miseries of religion. Thus when mental health workers do appear to be disinterested in their patients' religious ideas (Campbell, 1993) or discouraging of the practice of faith, Christians are quick to condemn. Some studies support this fear. On average, psychiatrists hold far fewer religious beliefs than their parents did or their patients do (Neeleman and King, 1993), and little if any attempt is made to explore the relevance of faith to illness or health (Hambidge, 1990; Neeleman and King, 1993).

Meanwhile the horrors of religion, the Jones and Waco massacres being the most extreme, excite the fear and anger of mental health services. Jeanette Winterson (1985) in her first novel, *Oranges Are Not the Only Fruit*, explores the primitive and destructive power of fundamentalism, while Solignac paints a grim picture of Catholicism in these words from a priest sent to him with severe psychosomatic problems:

Very soon I had nightmares; I saw myself burning in the fires of hell . . . I can remember a text from the catechism. It was entitled 'I deserve hell for my sins'. I read it and re-read it so often that I still know it almost off by heart: 'Terrible are the tortures of the damned in hell . . . . They suffer in a fire a thousand times hotter than fires on earth . . . . Hell is a terrible place, and that is where mortal sin brings us. Perhaps at this very moment I may have mortal sins in my heart. So if I were to die now, I would be cast down into hell.'

(Solignac, 1976:4)

Latterly, creative tension has been conspicuous by its absence. Psychiatry and Christianity appear to be going their separate ways. While the churches ignore the plight of those suffering from mental health problems (Pattison, 1988), psychiatry sometimes quietly disposes of religion. There is no reference to religion in the index of *The Essentials of Postgraduate Psychiatry* (Hill *et al.*, 1979) or in the Mental Illness Handbook, *The Health of the Nation* (1993), and in the *Oxford Textbook of Psychiatry* (Gelder *et al.*, 1989) religiousness is confined to the chapter on delusions. Hambidge (1990) in his recent study of the training of both clergy and psychiatrists shows how little they know about one another's speciality, despite having to be involved with many of the same people in their future work. He estimates that religious belief and practice will be important to one in eight people seen by a consultant psychiatrist, and that a similar number of any congregation will have a major psychiatric illness. Neeleman and King (1993:5) too voice their concern. 'However it appears that psychiatrists are undecided about the the role of religious and spiritual belief in the development of, or the recovery from, mental illness and are reluctant to directly liaise with clergy or other religious leaders.' Pattison (1989) explains this development by following the demise in contacts between doctors and priests since a high point in the 1960s. Then the Institute of Religion and Medicine fostered an atmosphere of tolerance and cooperation. Recent social, economic and political crises have changed all that. Professions are fighting for their livelihoods, and in a cost-conscious environment the value of anything or anyone is a threat to someone else's survival.

Working in any professional ghetto fosters omnipotence, and the sin of narcissism (Capps, 1993). This affects both clergy and doctors, when they keep their parishioners and their patients in a paternalistic embrace. Concentrating their expertise on the relevant aspect of a person's problem is really all that overworked professionals can do. The danger is in the divisions this may create and the destructive conflict it can occasion. One very common element of mental suffering is its internal psychic disharmony, and professional rivalry will aggravate this aspect of madness. At their best, multidisciplinary teams will utilise their conflicts as signs of their clients' internal battles or of the open political and social warfare which rages around us all. If religious leaders are excluded or exclude themselves from multidisciplinary working, the danger of destructive splitting is more likely.

A creative response to conflict between psychiatry and religion owes most to a tradition which stems from the work of William James. James, himself a sufferer from clinical depression and psychosomatic hypochondria, began to explore the relationship of mind and soul. In his classic study *The Varieties of Religious Experience*, he writes:

> The same sense of ineffable importance in the smallest events, the same texts and words coming with new meanings, the same controlling by extraneous powers . . . . It is evident that from the point of view of their psychological mechanism, the classical mysticism and these lower mysticisms spring from the same mental level . . . of which so little is really known. That region contains every kind of matter: seraph and snake abide there side by side.
>
> (James, 1902:426)

James touches upon the notion of divine madness of which St Paul writes in his first letter to the Corinthians. More recently researchers at the Alister Hardy Centre in Oxford have looked further into the idea of 'good' and 'bad' madness, in an attempt to understand the relationship between psychopathology and religious experience. Michael Jackson, in a project entitled 'Divine Madness', studied the relationship between the spiritual and psychotic experiences in the 5,000 accounts reported to the centre. He found similar phenomena among those with and without psychiatric histories. In order to discover why apparently similar experiences had such different results, he interviewed people nearest the centre of a continuum from psychotic to spiritual. At one end were those who had never received psychiatric treatment, but whose accounts contained some psychotic features. At the other end were those who had been diagnosed as having a major psychiatric illness, but nevertheless felt that their experience had been spiritual and religious as well as pathological. Although there were exceptions in each group the following picture emerged:

> The benign experiences of the first (healthy) group collectively met criteria for 17 psychotic symptoms. Although in the short term, the psychotics' ability to function had been seriously impaired by their experiences, over a longer period, they led to dramatically spiritual 'fruits' in their lives: all members of this group were deeply involved in altruistic, creative, ecological or spiritual activities. There was an important association between the quality of early family life, and that of adult spiritual experiences; in general, the psychotics had experienced severe emotional trauma as children, while the healthy group came from more stable backgrounds.
>
> (Jackson, 1992:4)

The author's use of labels like 'psychotics' for people is as unacceptable as it is common amongst professionals. However, labelling is not the only 'sin' of which the research accuses them. Jackson's interviews revealed the significance for good and ill of the professionals' reactions to these experiences; if they were listened to and accepted, individuals found ways to integrate even the most disturbing ideas and emotions. If they were ignored or pathologised by others then the trauma was aggravated.

The study suggests that the social context in which a relatively schizotypal individual has potentially spiritual experiences may influence the form, content and consequences of their experiences; and that a purely psychiatric approach which explains them in terms of dysfunction may actually be instrumental in producing pathological syndromes (Jackson, 1992:4).

No doubt there is more to psychosis than either spiritual or medical explanations suggest, but the idea that it may be a way of resolving critical mental trauma makes a lot of sense to those who listen to patients' stories, and brings a degree of dignity and respect to what is so often symptomatised and then ignored. For the diagnosed group this was their major disappointment with both psychiatry and religion.

The relationship of spiritual/psychotic experience and creativity, which Jackson recognises, is confirmed in Felix Post's (1989:3) retrospective study of genius. He noted that mental illness was more common among outstanding artists, authors and dramatists than either in the general population, or among leading scientists. A study by Moody (1990) of a small group of people of Afro-Caribbean origin, who had a psychiatric diagnosis, illustrates the distorting effect of psychiatry's, and indeed black activists', ignorance of religion. Hearing the voice of God can mean one thing coming from the mouth of a chief constable and quite another from a black person on an inner city housing estate. According to Jackson, the traditional churches are as bound by the taboo on religious experience as psychiatry is. Clergy approached by those wishing to discuss what they have felt or seen are often redirected to a psychiatrist, and vice versa. Gaining a better understanding of the varieties of religious experience is clearly a priority for priest and psychiatrist. The work of James Fowler (1987) on faith development, of Jacobs (1988), McGlashan (1989) and Fleischman (1990) on the understanding of religious experience, and of Weiss (1991) and Allison (1992) on methods of presentation to other professions, all illustrate ways in which this can be done and applied in practice utilising the clinical, therapeutic and pastoral skills already available.

COOPERATION AND COLLUSION

Cooperation, though the most obvious basis for a profitable relationship between psychiatry and religion, has been in practice the most elusive. The exceptions to this afford us important examples of the conditions which can create and sustain effective cooperation, and the rewards which that will bring. The most potent example is in the life and work of Anton Boisen. He set out to explore the mysterious territory which James (1902) had identified between classical mysticism and psychosis. Boisen, a lifelong sufferer from a form of schizophrenia, was for thirty years chaplain to psychiatric hospitals in Massachusetts and Illinois. It was while he was trying to establish his vocation that he had the breakdown which he records as the turning point in his life:

First of all came the thought that I must give up the hope that meant every-thing to me. Following this came the surging in upon me with overpowering force a terrifying idea about a coming world catastrophe . . . . I myself was more important than I have ever dreamed of being: I was also a zero quantity. Strange and mysterious forces of evil . . . were also revealed. I was terrified beyond measure and in my terror I talked, and I soon found myself in a psycho-pathic hospital. There followed three weeks of violent delirium which remain indelibly on my memory.

(Boisen, 1936:3)

Initially Boisen found that neither clergy nor physicians were much use to him:

The doctors did not believe in talking with patients about their symptoms, which they assumed were rooted in some organic difficulty. The longest time I ever got was fifteen minutes during which the very charming young doc-tor pointed out that one must not hold the reins too tight in dealing with sex instinct. Nature, he said, must have its way.

The ministers from the neighboring village who conducted services might know something about religion, but certainly knew nothing about our problems. They did no visiting on the wards – which may not have been entirely their fault, as they probably received little encouragement to do so . . . another preached on the text, 'if thine eye offend thee, pluck it out'. I was afraid that one or two of my fellow patients might have been inclined to take the injunction literally.

(Boisen, 1936:5–6)

As he recovered, Boisen began to study his own illness and those of his fellow patients. This led to a research project in cooperation with medical colleagues (Boisen, 1936). Boisen invited theological students to come and work with him to help with the project, and as a contribution to their own training. He coined the phrase 'living human documents' for that research. He wanted religious leaders to learn about God from human beings, by applying techniques familiar from the critical study of biblical documents to them. From 1926, when the first group joined Boisen, until the present day generations of theological students and clergy in North America have undergone Clinical Pastoral Education (CPE). The students of all major Christian denominations, and some rabbinic students are required to do at least three months of full-time experience in a hospital, prison or community setting. Boisen also employed the clinical training methods used by physicians and surgeons and applied them to ministers. Trainees learnt their trade and won recognition for their expertise alongside other professions. Other countries in Europe, notably in Eire, and now in Asia and Africa have adopted similar methods in their training of ministers and laity. In the United Kingdom there are courses of this kind in London, at St George's and the Maud-sley Hospitals and in the Edinburgh hospitals (Foskett and Lyall, 1988). Recent publications in America record the significance of the CPE movement (Asquith,

1992; Hall, 1992). At its best it has helped establish and maintain constructive cooperation between pastors and other clinicians. In many places pastors now work within multidisciplinary teams, sometimes as the primary worker and often as the religious specialist or consultant (Foskett, 1984; Pruyser, 1984). This is a much more effective way of using different expertise than trying to teach medical and theological students something minimal and useful about each other's speciality.

There is also a theological significance to the development of clinical pastoral education. By coming as students, pastors are offered a model of discipleship which allows them to learn and not to arouse the anxieties of others already precariously established in the world of madness. Religion, as we have seen, raises questions and fears for other professionals, and the different assumptions which religious people bring to the understanding of madness can be a challenge to them. Clergy, anxious about their own competence, often underestimate the ambivalence they create in others. Consequently they can miss the opportunities which come from using their ignorance in the incarnate role of learner. Students on CPE courses are encouraged to make the most of just these opportunities. Current examples of experienced chaplains utilising the learner's approach in their own research are J. Browning (1986) and Borthwick (1988). In their studies of mental health and community care they encountered affirmation and encouragement from other professions, who wanted to share in the spiritual and religious care of people with mental illnesses. In Kent a project involving health, social services, churches and a university department in a rural and an urban area resulted in unexpected gains for everyone. The work and research revealed that:

> churches through individuals and their activities are involved in caring for those inside and outside its 'membership'; the different churches and Health and Social Services departments largely work in isolation from one another; churches and statutory agencies lack information about what resources are available and how to gain access to them.
>
> (Clark, 1989: iii)

At the end of the two-year project, Clark concluded that 'some churches are gaining that new sense of vision, which will enable them to reach out to the community and take their place alongside the statutory agencies' (ibid.: iii).

The path to such cooperation is rarely easy, and requires of the religious professional patience and perseverance. Their presence, more than their actions or expertise, will enable others to make the best use they can of any ambivalence they have about religion, and leave less of it resting upon clerical psyches (Carr, 1989).

There is a darker side to cooperation evidenced in the collusion, which allows one partner to dominate the other. When a fourteenth-century Pope put out a contract on his physician, religion was in the driving seat. Now Christians are likely to be ingratiating themselves with modern medicine men and women. The contemporary Christian healing movement, as well as reawakening the churches to this aspect of ministry, often uncritically adopts the curative stance of medicine. Illness is there to be fought and cured, and the battle, when it is won, reflects well upon the healer. Although there is much talk of causes and prevention, more important for healers is a steady supply of sick people to ensure their livelihood and reinforce their status (Busfield, 1986; Inglis, 1981; Pattison, 1989). Those who cannot dominate their rivals are likely to try and make them their friends. This kind of collusion is also apparent in the pastoral counselling movement, which grew from Boisen's initiative. Though a user of psychoanalytic ideas, he was adamant that his trainees should not become psychotherapists. The psychotherapeutic captivity of the pastoral counselling movement was anticipated by priest – psychiatrist Lambourne (1970), criticised by Oden (1984), and brought home to this author's discomfort by Pattison. In his study of pastoral care and liberation theology, he argues that hospital chaplains appeared to be oblivious of:

> the palpable structural evils which diminished all those living and working in psychiatric hospitals during the scandals of the 1970's. Few chaplains seem to have much understanding of the social and political structure of the institution in which they are working. Many speak warmly of being a part of the therapeutic team, and it does not seem to strike them that this might separate them from patients and give them a professional view of the world which might make them deaf to the stories of those who are powerless in the hospital.
>
> (Pattison, 1988:99)

In their uncertainties about their role, pastors can be flattered into adopting the methods and point of view of the powerful. The current trend in hospital chaplaincy is to be seduced by the delights of marketing and management (Sails, 1993). Obviously this will go some way towards saving jobs for chaplains, but at what cost to their souls?

INTERCOURSE

Conflict, cooperation and collusion typify the course of most human relationships which are of any substance. This reality should reinforce our determination to make the most and avoid the worst of what will always be our lot in reconciling Christianity and psychiatry. At their best these elements of the relationship can represent the foreplay essential to productive intercourse. For this we, like lovers, need the appropriate context and the right atmosphere. Fighting and cooperating, being seduced and colluding can all contribute to turning us on to one another. We need time and opportunity to identify what we have to give and what we want to receive, as well as what we fear and recoil from. We have to find ways to meet and court one another (see Bhugra, this volume). Starting with the least highly charged parts of our respective anatomies, and progressing towards those more erogenous zones wherever they may turn out to be. And if religion is psychiatry's last taboo, we should weigh carefully the consequences and our resources to meet them. The passive conflict referred to above, frustrating as it may seem, should warn us of the powerful forces from which our present impasse protects us. If we were to begin to explore each other's ideas and theories, as reason suggests we should, perhaps we will lay ourselves open to a revolution that neither psychiatry nor religion are ready to countenance. For Christians and mental health services minister to the victims of a crumbling, sinful and disease-obsessed society, seemingly mesmerised by its demise.

To stretch the analogy a little further, in families an impasse between the parents is often eased by the courage of the children, who have least to lose and most to gain by change. Clients and patients are not children but often their position in relation to religion and psychiatry is similar. They have least power and least to lose, what is more, they bear the cost of priests' and doctors' failure to relate effectively. They are the scapegoats, the sacrificial lambs dumb before their shearers, if they speak they are not listened to, because they are mad. Peter Campbell, of Survivors Speak Out, makes an impassioned plea for people like himself to be heard:

> From where I stand, psychiatry, community or otherwise, has a rather tired look. It certainly has some powerful equipment. But it does not appear to have the understanding or the imagination to successfully address the problems over which it claims special domination. The 'user movement' on the other hand, although undernourished, in terms of recognition and resources, seems to be breathing nicely. It is from this quarter that many of the good insights are now coming, not only in terms of alternative services, but in the exploration of the sensitive response to crisis, and, in particular, the positive revaluing of hitherto discarded personal experience.
>
> (Campbell, 1992:118)

We need to have courage, in the words of the sufferers, to find the reason and the strength to confront our 'madness' as well. To discover in it, as they have, signs not only of evils to be fought and beaten and ills to be cured, but good and creative things to be owned and cherished. That madness itself may be a way to our becoming the humanity we are destined to be. The expressed aims of community care as local and accessible, comprehensive, flexible, consumer-orientated, empowering of clients, focusing on strengths and skills, racially and culturally appropriate, incorporating natural community supports, and meeting special needs envisages a very productive intercourse between users and providers of services (see Bhugra *et al.*, 1995). In such a bonding patient and professional bring different things to one another and through their meeting make each other the richer. This remains the vision of the Richmond Fellowship's therapeutic communities (Gosling, 1979/80), and of many pastoral organisations like the Clinical Theology Association and the Westminster Pastoral Foundation. Here C. Jung's (1933; 1964) work on the importance of our shadows in the making and healing of minds and souls has contributed most to cementing productive relationships between patient and therapist, priest and counsellor. A collection of essays from pastors, theologians, psychologists and psychiatrists working in

Chicago (Browning *et al.*, 1990) broadens the intercourse to include philosophy and ethics. No attempt is made to paint a coherent and integrated picture, each author addresses issues of psychiatry, pastoral care and ethics from their faith and professional point of view (also see Fulford, this volume). In order that its power for good and ill could be opened to the widest debate:

> The practice of medicine needs connections to something like the practice of ministry, and the practice of ministry needs the mechanisms of something like the practice of medicine. Every aspect of the human environment dissolves into human functioning and permeates the whole.
>
> (Browning, 1986:12)

The coming of community care and psychiatry's exit from the asylums offer unique opportunities to Christians and those who contribute to and receive from the new mental health services. With sectorisation, key mental health workers are having to learn the skills and re-inhabit the persona of the curate of souls, the parish priest. Community liason officers have to unearth the knowledge which congregations have carried unconsciously for generations, and a new diaconate is consecrated amongst community psychiatric nurses. Short of finance and capital assets, health and social service authorities need places and spaces to launch and sustain their services. Churches fallen on hard times are looking to use their buildings more effectively. With visions as similar as asylum and sanctuary, sharing the same roof and floor can do much to nurture a healthy intercourse.

There is a negative side to intercourse, it can become a snare and a delusion in its corporate sterility. Marriage and the family are institutions which society uses for good and ill. Since Constantine and certainly as far as Margaret Thatcher both Christianity and psychiatry have been claimed by the State. Christianity has found it difficult to resist the seduction of governments and authorities, even in the extremes of their inhumanity and wickedness. The health service has striven and failed to maintain some independence from the State. The churches in the United Kingdom have distanced themselves from governments, criticising their policies and campaigning for those groups most likely to suffer madness and its attendant horrors. This has made the churches unpopular, and the State is quick to exploit that anxiety to bring them back in line. The *Faith in the City* report (Canterbury, 1985), which carried a political critique of society and advocated justice and not charity, has become, in the Church Urban Fund, yet another charitable exercise. Mental health professionals are compromised even more. They do not have the wealth of previous generations earning interest with the Church Commissioners. They have to do what the State or 40 per cent of the electorate want them to do. Those who suffer madness are an enormous drain upon the Chancellor's emptying coffers. It is a drain which many are keen to plug. Against such an evil, doctor and priest, mental health worker and pastor, patient and people of God must stand together or perish together.

CONCLUSION

The past and the present relationships between Christianity and psychiatry in the United Kingdom are frankly unencouraging of great hopes for the future. The institutions which each inhabit are beset with their own problems, and whatever the enlightened may aspire to, the reality is often a disappointment and sometimes a disaster. We are stiff-necked professions, unlikely to change because it makes sense. However, in as far as social and political pressures are forcing ministers and doctors out of their institutional ghettoes to go and work among the people, there are opportunities for change. Community care rarely looks like the Promised Land, but then neither did the original look that good to the Hebrews driven out of Eygpt. Moses, the leading professional in that exodus, had to be content with a sight of the promises his people were about to inherit. The same will be true for many who lead our mental health services and churches today. If that is the price of better mental health for the people, so be it. As long ago as 1936 Boisen believed that intercourse with the insane was an essential prerequisite 'to our building the city of brotherhood and cooperation where the jungle now stands and greed and ruthless competition rule' (Boisen, 1945:48). The time is ripe to help dislodge psychiatry's last taboo, to listen to the 'mad' speaking their mind, for God's sake and humanity's too.

REFERENCES

Allison, D. W. (1992) 'Communicating clinical pastoral assessment with health care team', *The Journal of Pastoral Care* 46(3): 273–80.
Asquith, G. H. (1992) *Vision From a Little Known Country*, Atlanta, GA: Journal of Pastoral Care Publications.
Bethlem Royal Hospital (1816) *Report to the General Court*.
Bhugra, D., Bridges, K. and Thompson, C. (1995) *Caring for a Community*, London: Gaskell.
Boisen, A. (1936) *The Exploration of the Inner World*, Philadelphia, PA: Harper & Row.
—— (1945) *Religion in Crisis and Custom*, New York: Harper & Row.
Borthwick, S. (1988) *Study of Mental Health and Chaplaincy*, unpublished paper.
Brierley, P. (1991) *United Kingdom Christian Handbook*, London: Marc.
Browning, D. S., Thomas, J., Evison, I. S. (eds) (1990) *Religious and Ethical Factors in Psychiatric Practice*, Chicago: Nelson Hall.
Browning, J. (1986) *Chaplaincy Modes in Mental Health*, Trent: RHA.
Busfield, J. (1986) *Managing Madness*, London: Unwin.
Campbell, P. (1992) 'A survivor's view of community psychiatry', *Journal of Mental Health* 1(2): 117–22.
—— (1993) 'Spiritual crisis', in *Open Mind*, London: MIND Publications.
Canterbury, Archbishop of (1985) *Faith in the City: Report of the Archbishop of Canterbury's Commission on Urban Priority Areas*, London: Church House.
Capps, D. (1993) *The Depleted Self: Sin in a Narcissistic Age*, Minneapolis: Fortress Press.
Carr, W. (1989) *Pastor as Theologian*, London: SPCK.
Clare, A. (1976) *Psychiatry in Dissent*, London: Tavistock.
Clark, E. (1989) *Commitment to Community?*, Council for Social Responsibility, 60, Marsham Street, Maidstone, ME14 1EW.

Cuppitt, D. (1986) *Life Lines*, London: SCM.

Fleischman, P. (1990) *The Healing Spirit*, London: SPCK.

Foskett, J. (1984) *Meaning in Madness*, London: SPCK.

Foskett, J. and Lyall, D. (1988) *Helping the Helpers*, London: SPCK.

Foucault, M. (1967) *Madness and Civilisation*, London: Tavistock.

Fowler, J. (1987) *Faith Development and Pastoral Care*, Minneapolis: Fortress Press.

Gelder, M., Gath, D. and Mayou, R. (1989) *Oxford Textbooks of Psychiatry*, Oxford: Oxford University Press.

Gosling, R. (1979/80) *Richmond Fellowship Annual Report*, 8 Addison Road, London.

Hall, C. (1992) *Head and Heart: Story of the CPE Movement*, Atlanta, GA: Journal of Pastoral Care Publications.

Halmos, P. (1965) *The Faith of the Counsellors*, London: Constable.

Hambidge, D. (1990) *Survey of Cross Training in Psychiatry and Religious Belief*, Christian Psychiatric Counselling, Ashtree House, The Moors, Branston Booth, Lincoln.

Department of Health (1993) *The Health of the Nation*, Key Area Mental Illness Handbook. Department of Health.

Hill, P., Murray, R. and Thorley, A. (eds) (1979) *The Essentials of Postgraduate Psychiatry*, London: Academic Press.

Houlden, J. L. (1991) *Bible and Belief*, London: SPCK.

Inglis, B. (1981) *The Diseases of Civilisation*, London: Hodder & Stoughton.

Jackson, M. (1992) 'The relationship between spiritual and psychotic experience', *Numinis*, newsletter of the Alister Hardy Centre, Westminster College, Oxford, No. 10.

Jacobs, M. (1988) *Towards the Fullness of Christ*, London: Darton, Longman & Todd.

James, W. (1902) *The Varieties of Religious Experience*, London: Longmans.

Jenkins, D. (1976) *Contradiction of Christianity*, London: SCM.

Jung, C. (1933) *Modern Man in Search of a Soul*, London: Routledge.

—— (1964) *Man and His Symbols*, London: Aldus Books.

Kung, H. (1986) *Religion: The Last Taboo*, Washington, DC: APA Press.

Lake, F. (1966) *Clinical Theology*, London: Darton, Longman & Todd.

Lambourne, R. (1970) 'With love to the USA', in M. Melinsky (ed.) *Religion and Medicine*, London: SCM.

McGlashan, R. (1989) 'The use of symbols in religion from the perspective of analytic psychology', *Religious Studies* 25: 501–20.

Maudsley, H. (1918) *Religion and Realities*, London: John Bale & Sons.

Moody, C. (1990) 'Folk religion and the diagnosis of mental illness', unpublished paper.

Neeleman, J. and King, M. B. (1993) 'Psychiatrists' religious attitudes in relation to their clinical practice: a survey of 231 psychiatrists', *Acta Psychiatrica, Scandinavica* 0:1–5.

Oden, T. (1984) *Care of Souls in the Classic Tradition*, Philadelphia, PA: Fortress Press.

Pattison, S. (1988) *A Critique of Pastoral Care*, London: SCM.

—— (1989) *Alive and Kicking*, London: SCM.

Post, F. (1989) 'Madness and creativity', *Maudsley Gazette* 35(3).

Pruyser, P. (1984) 'Religion in the psychiatric hospital', *Journal of Pastoral Care* 38:1.

Robinson, J. A. T. (1963) *Honest to God*, London: SCM.

Sails, A. (1993) *Health Care Chaplaincy Standards*, London: Hospital Chaplaincies' Council.

Sanders, E. P. (1987) *Jesus and Judaism*, London: SCM.

Solignac, P. (1976) *The Christian Neurosis*, London: SCM.

Szasz, T. (1974) *The Myth of Mental Illness*, New York: Harper & Row.

Weiss, F. S. (1991) 'Pastoral care planning: a process orientated approach to mental health ministry', *Journal of Pastoral Care* XLV(3): 268–78.

Winterson, J. (1985) *Oranges Are Not the Only Fruit*, London: Methuen.

Chapter 5

'The cracked crucible'
Judaism and mental health

Howard Cooper

WHAT IS MENTAL HEALTH?

There is a parable told by the great eighteenth-century Hasidic master Nachman of Bratslav. One day a king summoned his vizier and told him of a terrifying dream. He had dreamt that anyone who ate from the coming year's harvest would be struck with madness. What could be done?, the king asked in anguish. The vizier suggested that the best thing to do would be to set aside some wheat now, from the present harvest, so that at least the two of them would not need to eat of the blighted crop. But the king refused to separate himself from his people and said that he did not wish to remain lucid in the midst of a people gone mad.

'When the world is gripped by delirium,' he continued, 'it is senseless to watch from the outside. The mad will think that we are mad too. There is only one alternative. Let us also eat the wheat and become mad like the others. But before we eat it, let us each make a mark on our foreheads. Then whenever we look at one another in the future, we shall see the sign, and at least we shall know, you and I, that we are mad.'

There is a continuity between that dark and ambiguous rabbinic story and the suggestion some years ago by R. D. Laing and Aaron Esterson that schizophrenia could be considered a realistic response to our disordered civilisation. Both the Hasidic story and the contemporary 'anti-psychiatric' view call into question our traditional categories of madness and sanity, mental illness and mental health. And they in turn are not a million miles from Hollywood mogul Sam Goldwyn's possibly apocryphal, but, in any event, surrealist quip: 'Anyone who goes to a psychiatrist needs to have their head examined.'

But lest the reader think at this point that the subject of mental health is not being treated here with due seriousness, let it be said immediately that it is precisely because Judaism attempts to honour the uniqueness of each individual human being – created, as Genesis puts it, in the 'image and likeness of God' – that it is endlessly curious about how human beings actually think, feel and function; and consequently, within Judaic thought there is a constant preparedness to call into question received ideas, conventional notions, accepted ways of thinking and categorising.

Central to Jewish thought is an awareness of the dazzling complexity of the human being: the mysteries of life and death are a source of both boundless wonder and exploration, yet the fact that ultimately they remain mysteries ensures that all 'explanations' and 'interpretations' of human behaviour remain humbly within the realm of the provisional, of the temporary hypothesis which needs to be continually refined or re-visioned. In other words, Judaism is resistant to final solutions. It prefers the speculation and open-endedness of the question to the definitiveness and certainty of the answer.

It is within this context that Jewish attitudes to mental health and mental illness need to be seen.

HISTORICAL PERSPECTIVES

The biblical view

Although the conventional view is that, within the Bible, madness is a punishment for disobeying God's commandments, within its context (Deut. 28:28/34), it would seem that what the Bible calls 'madness' is actually an unobtainable despair brought about through loss. Similarly, the 'madness' which afflicts King Saul is described by the narrator as an 'evil spirit from the Lord' (1 Sam. 16:14; 19:9) and yet the behaviour described – sudden fits of paranoid terror, jealous rage and homicidal violence – are also shown to be a consequence of the insecurities attendant upon being Israel's ill-chosen first king, who knows he will be replaced by a more suitable figure.

That the man chosen to replace him, David, is both the object of Saul's violence as well as the person chosen to provide music therapy for the distressed king, is an irony that should not be lost to the attentive reader. We read that David's harp-playing both soothes the 'madness', yet also provokes it (1 Sam. 18:10); and we note that the storyteller chooses a word for Saul's 'raving' which is the same word used in different biblical contexts for 'prophesying'.

So it is that biblical thought subverts the traditional boundaries between sanity and madness – as anyone reading the prophetical literature contained within the book of Ezekiel could testify. A final irony within this context is the way in which David himself, precocious and wily as ever, later simulates insanity – 'scribbling on the doors of the gate and letting his spittle fall upon his beard' – in order to escape his enemy Achish (1 Sam. 21:11–16).

The rabbinic era

Within the Talmud, mention of mental illness is usually within a legal context. The word *shoteh* – which contains the idea of walking to and fro without purpose – was used by the rabbis to describe the mentally ill. This was not a clinical designation but a category based upon observed external behaviour. As the

Talmud puts it: 'Who is deemed a *shoteh*? One who goes out alone at night; who sleeps in the cemetery; who tears their clothes.' Later the Talmud adds: 'One who destroys all that is given to them' (*Hagigah* 3b).

The discussion continues by asking if all of these 'symptoms' had to be displayed in order to fall into this category, or whether any one form of behaviour from this list could justify the individual being deemed a *shoteh*; and, further, whether it was the simple act itself which rendered the person a *shoteh*, or the palpably disturbed manner in which the act was done which would then render it evident that the person was ill.

What primarily concerns the Talmud are the social-cum-legal implications of being a *shoteh*: they were not responsible for the damage they caused; nor for the shame they caused; and those who injured them had to bear the responsibility. They were not to marry; but (contrary to the Greek view) during periods of lucidity the individual was considered capable and responsible from every other point of view.

Although the Talmud mentions recognisable psychological conditions such as hysteria, phobias, and melancholia as well as what we might now term 'defence mechanisms' such as repression, sublimation and projection, rabbinic thinking assumed an inter-relationship between the physical, emotional and spiritual components of the individual.

So we find the third-century Babylonian rabbi Mar Samuel warning that 'a change in a person's usual life-habits is considered dangerous and a precipitant of illness' (*Baba Batra* 146a). And in line with current research which suggests that stress and depression can weaken the body's ability to fight illness, we have the statement that 'even if the body is strong, fright [i.e. stress/anxiety] crushes it' (*Baba Batra* 10a).

The rabbis of the Talmud even found a biblical precedent for the connection between anxiety and somatic complaints. Reading the verse from the book of Proverbs which states that 'worry in the heart of a person bows them down' (12:25), they commented: 'Worry can kill; therefore let not anxiety enter your heart, for it has slain many a person' (*Sanhedrin* 100b).

That this was not just rabbinic hyperbole is illustrated by a story in the Jerusalem Talmud: 'A man hated veal. Once without being aware of it, he ate some. Someone called out to him, "That was veal which you ate." He became nauseated, sickened, and died' (*Terumot* 8:46a).

As we will now see, until the advent of modern medicine – which began to observe the physical, emotional and spiritual spheres as relatively separate – Jewish thinking through the ages tended to follow this early rabbinic understanding, particularly in regard to the influence of the 'psyche' on the 'soma'.

The medieval period

Perhaps the pre-eminent exponent of Jewish attitudes to mental health in pre-modern times was the rabbi, codifier, philosopher and royal physician Moses Maimonides (1135–1204). Forced to flee Spain because of Moslem persecution, Maimonides lived for a while in Morocco, and then Palestine, before settling in Egypt, where he was eventually appointed court physician to Saladin's viceroy al-Fadil.

It was Maimonides' belief that the violation of moral principles contributed to illness, and that the 'abuse of passions such as anger, envy, hatred and lust, which in turn bring on a guilty conscience' were a primary factor in creating physical afflictions.[1] In his 'Treatise on Asthma' – prepared for his patient, the sultan – Maimonides suggests ways to reduce stress which he considers will help the sultan's asthmatic condition and improve his health. He advises him to avoid 'mental anguish, fear, mourning or distress', which create conditions in which a person 'cannot avoid falling ill'. In their place he counsels 'gaiety and liveliness', which 'have the opposite effect – they gladden the heart and stimulate circulation of the blood'.[2]

As diagnostically unsophisticated as this may seem, it is illustrative of Maimonides' conceptualisation of illness as having, in many cases, a psychosomatic basis. Within his medical writings he returns on many occasions to a consideration of what we would now describe as neurotic behaviour, advocating the treatment of mental disturbances as a priority in the treatment of any illness:

> When the patient is overpowered by imagination, prolonged meditation, or avoidance of social contact (which they never exhibited before), or when they avoid pleasant experiences which were in them before, the physician should do nothing before he improves the soul by removing the extreme emotions.[3]

Within his copious legal writings too, we find evidence of Maimonides' familiarity with a range of neurotic and psychotic behaviour. When he came to codify the qualifications for acting as a witness – one of which is sanity – we see him expanding upon the Talmudic discussion of the subject of the *shoteh* and attempting to resolve the questions left open in the previous debate:

> A *shoteh* is unfit to be a witness . . . . And not only an insane individual that walks naked, and breaks utensils, vessels, and throws stones, but rather all individuals whose minds have become deranged and their minds are found constantly confused/in error/entangled in regard to one matter – although they speak with relevance in other matters – they are unfit as witnesses and are counted among the insane (*shoteh*) . . . . This includes the extremely mentally disturbed who are unable to differentiate between things that conflict, contradict each other, and do not comprehend the subject matter as it is understood by the rest of the common people. Also the anxiously frightened, and those who are hurried/excited in their minds and those who are very crazy/confused are all counted as a *shoteh*. However this matter is dependent on the assessment of the judge/rabbi, because it is not possible to give an exact assessment of the mind in writing.[4]

By omitting the actual examples described in the Talmud, Maimonides is indicating that, in his opinion, they were examples of categories only. In his view, any one symptom that can be seen to fall into the same category renders that person a *shoteh*; but merely exhibiting that behaviour once is not sufficient to deem them 'insane' – it has to be their constant or regular pattern of behaviour. Maimonides' authority was such that he here articulates, within a legal context, what became – up until modern times – the normative Jewish position on the criteria for assessing 'mental illness'.

For many centuries, however, Maimonidean rationalism represented only one end of the spectrum of Jewish response to mental (and physical) health. Medieval medicine was an indiscriminate compound of science and superstition. Much of everyday popular Jewish folk religion involved a belief in the power of omens, magic, spirits, spells, potions, divination, amulets, astrology – a range of beliefs and practices which rabbinic authorities fought a losing battle to counter or contain. Many rabbis were themselves involved, seeing these activities as continuous with biblical and Talmudic precedents; others wavered between scepticism and a grudging regard for folk wisdom. An influential German medieval text captures something of this rabbinic ambivalence: 'One should not believe in superstitions, but still it is best to be heedful of them'.[5]

Although, like the psyches of many other peoples, the Jewish psyche too was often immersed in superstition, as we come nearer to our own times we begin to see occasions when a different form of understanding is present. Representative of this is a case which came to the nineteenth-century rabbi, Joshua Leib Diskin, concerning a pious Jewish woman who tasted tallow in whatever she ate. On hearing the problem, the rabbi reminded her that as a young girl she had served as a maid in an observant Jewish household. Once, when milking the cow by candlelight, the candle fell into the pail of milk. Although fearing the wrath of her mistress [the tallow being made of animal fat would contravene the dietary laws prohibiting the mixture of milk and meat products], she allowed the members of her family to drink the milk. The rabbi assured her that she had committed no wrong, for the small amount of tallow had become neutralised in the milk, which was therefore *kosher*. Her peace of mind was restored and the symptoms disappeared.[6]

This more 'psychological' approach to mental health takes us to the threshold of the psychoanalytic era.

THE EXAMINATION OF THE SOUL

Sigmund Freud coined the word 'psychoanalyse' to describe his work: 'psycho-analysis' – the examination of the soul. In his wise and important little book *Freud and Man's Soul* Bruno Bettelheim draws attention to the centrality of the soul in Freud's thinking. He maintains that erroneous or inadequate translations into English of the writings of the founder of psychoanalysis – as well as the need for acceptance from the medical establishment, particularly in the United States – have distorted a true understanding of Freud's intentions. What we have inherited in translation, Bettelheim characterises in this way:

> Abstract, depersonalized, highly theoretical, erudite and mechanized – in short, 'scientific' – statements about the strange and very complex workings

of our mind. Instead of instilling a deep feeling for what is most human in all of us, the translations attempt to lure the reader into developing a 'scientific' attitude toward man and his actions, a 'scientific' understanding of the unconscious and how it conditions much of our behaviour.[7]

Bettelheim maintains that Freud used the words 'psyche' and 'soul' in order to describe the essence of the human personality with words which deliberately lacked scientific exactitude and precision. Always to translate 'psyche' and *seele/ seelisch* as 'mind' or 'mental life' subverts Freud's intention. The German words are terms speaking 'for the ambiguity of the psyche itself, which reflects many different, warring levels of consciousness simultaneously'.[8]

Although he does not say so in these words, it seems that Bettelheim's revisionism is intent on restoring to us a more holistic and, dare one say it, 'Jewish' Freud. This century's revolution in the conception of the human personality after Freud stems from his emphasis on examining the neglected and hidden aspects of our souls and coming to understand something of the roles these unconscious forces play in our lives.

This can be seen as a secularisation of the traditional rabbinical quest for understanding and self-understanding. The rabbis of the Talmudic era had developed a proto-psychological notion of two opposing 'inclinations' (i.e. impulses/ drives) within human nature, the *yetzer tov* moving the individual towards good, the *yetzer ha-ra* moving one towards evil.

Roughly analogous to Freud's concept of 'id', the *yetzer ha-ra* was seen as corresponding to our natural appetites and passions, and especially our sexual impulses. Unfettered, the *yetzer ha-ra* could lead a person into a range of thoughts or actions deemed to be wrong or sinful. But this inclination was not intrinsically bad: it had to be controlled, but not completely suppressed, for – according to one famous rabbinic homily – 'were it not for the *yetzer ha-ra* no-one would ever take a spouse, have children, build a home, or engage in business'.[9]

Rabbinic realism here highlights the potentially creative dimension to sexuality; to the urge to possess one's own property – the acquisitive urge in us; and to the competitiveness necessary for personal and perhaps social survival. In this view the *yetzer ha-ra* is a vital life force within us that only becomes destructive ('evil') when it gets out of hand. Perhaps Freud was expressing this in his own secularised way when he aphoristically summarised the function and goal of psychoanalysis as being: 'where id was, there ego shall be'.[10]

Yet Freud was no crypto-rabbi. His concept of the 'soul' was not the traditional religious one – he considered religion to be a kind of collective delusion – for the psyche he was analysing had repressed and secret aspects that had nothing to do with the rabbinic belief in its purity or immortality.[11] Ironically it was C. G. Jung, the first Gentile allowed into Freud's original circle of seventeen fellow Jewish pioneers of psychoanalysis, who diagnosed the modern individual to be 'in search of a soul'.

Jung tells the story of a young Jewish woman, suffering from acute anxiety attacks, who came to him for a consultation. She was, he says (with a hint of condescension?), a 'well-adapted, Westernised Jewess, enlightened down to her bones'.[12] In the course of the conversation Jung found out that she came from a Hasidic family:

> Her grandfather had been a sort of wonder-rabbi – he had second sight – and her father had broken away from that mystic community, and she was completely sceptical and completely scientific in her outlook on life. She was highly intelligent, with that murderous kind of intellect that you very often find in Jews.
>
> So I thought, 'Aha! What does that mean with reference to her neurosis? Why does she suffer from such an abysmal fear?' And I said to her, 'Look here, I'm going to tell you something, and you will probably think it all foolishness, but you have been untrue to your God. Your grandfather led the right life, but you are worse than a heretic, you have forsaken the mystery of your race. You belong to a holy people, and what do you live? No wonder that you fear God, that you suffer from the fear of God'.[13]

Obviously this is not a conventional diagnosis but, according to Jung, it 'went through her like lightning'[14] and after a week of working with Jung her neurosis had vanished. (Those were the days.) Jung writes:

> It had no point in it any more, it had been based upon the mistake that she could live with her miserable intellect alone in a perfectly banal world, when in fact she was a child of God and should have lived the symbolic life, where she would have fulfilled the secret will in herself that was also in her family. She had forgotten all that, and was living, of course, in full contradiction to her whole natural system. Suddenly her life had a meaning, and she could live again.[15]

Although this story contains a rather typical idealisation by Jung of mythic living, he is pointing here towards a phenomenon that has wide ramifications for Jew and Gentile alike. For the consequences of living in a secular, post-religious age weigh heavily on many of us. The old certainties just do not hold any more. With the gradual abandonment of religious belief as the main source of personal and communal morality, there arose alternative moral sources, a situation which although it was in some ways liberating, was often deeply disorienting.

For many generations the Jewish people existed within the sphere of mythological truth: daily and seasonal life, story-telling and symbols, ritual practice and ethical action, celebration and mourning, history and legend and family and community were all bound up together to form the densely textured fabric of lives spent attentive to the inner rhythms of a religious and mythic tradition. These rhythms generated meaning for those who attended to them.

But nowadays very few Jews live within that myth any more. 'Myth' is here used in its original sense, where it represents something not opposed to reality but the most important form of collective thinking, a true revelation of reality in symbolic form. We Jews have largely lost that sense of being enfolded in a containing and sustaining myth – that whatever misfortunes threatened or transpired, God was in heaven and His people had a purpose and destiny on earth. The Enlightenment made severe inroads into this myth, and for many the Holocaust represents the radical break with the pieties and certainties of the past.

Present-day Western Jewish identity is fraught with ambiguity. As a minority in an open society which is experienced as both welcoming and threatening, contemporary Jews – whatever their degree of affiliation to, or distance from, the Jewish community – struggle with a series of tensions: between past and present; between tradition and modernity; between the individual and the community; and in particular, as we will now see, between the individual and the family. It is against this background that specific Jewish mental health problems need to be understood.

'THE CRACKED CRUCIBLE': JEWISH PSYCHOLOGICAL HEALTH TODAY

Modern Anglo – Jewish life contains some self-evident truths. The old stable pattern of family life – with an extended generational network spanning grandparents to grandchildren – is breaking down with a rapidity which leaves many bewildered and angry. Over the last decade the statistical litany has become familiar: one in three Jewish marriages end in divorce; nearly 20 per cent of Jewish children experience the breakdown of their parents' marriage; one in three Jews who marry, marry 'out'; less than half the Jews who marry do so in a synagogue; each year Jewish marriages are outstripped by Jewish burials; the annual birth rate is roughly two-thirds of the death rate. Overall, Anglo-Jewry is an ageing community shrinking numerically as the number of children born becomes insufficient to ensure the community's long-term continuity. This scenario makes us regretful about a past which seems beyond retrieval, confused about the present, and uncertain about the future.

These trends are unlikely to be reversed. From the ultra-Orthodox enclaves to the most assimilated suburban or rural milieux, all sections of Anglo-Jewry are subject to these pressures. Chief Rabbi Jonathan Sacks is by no means the only contemporary voice arguing for a return to traditional values in which 'the family is the crucible of the Jewish future'.[16]

Yet no amount of moral exhortation will change what is now happening within so many Anglo-Jewish families. The crucible is already cracked. What we are witnessing is the degeneration of the Jewish family as an incubator of purpose. The family as the social entity that embodied and enacted the collective ideals of the Jewish people is being replaced by a fragmented individualism.

Anglo-Jewish families are suffering from a psychic fatigue, where the natural stresses of family life become strains which threaten to lead to fracture. A gap has developed between the fantasy of what a Jewish family 'should' be and how we actually live our lives. The idyllic scenario of the joyful Friday night meal, with relaxed family members celebrating together in Sabbath peace, rarely happens in reality. Instead, there may be exhaustion, rows and recriminations as the week ends and the accumulated frustrations spill out There can be moments of respite, and some weeks are calmer than others, but then the bickering returns, or the angry silence, or the hurt withdrawal. Not all the time, and not all of this in every family. For, as Tolstoy wrote, 'all happy families resemble one another, but each unhappy family is unhappy in its own way'.[17]

In the past, through nurture and respect, work and discipline, education and celebration, the continuity of Jewish life was ensured through family life. But the idea of the family is now at war with the realities of emancipation and equality. For many Jews the family as traditionally conceived is no longer a source of nourishment and personal affirmation. For some it has begun to feel like a miniature totalitarian system. Once authoritarianism replaces tolerance and respect for differences, once the necessary adaptability feels too threatening, the family can no longer sustain its purpose.

So when we look at what is actually happening inside our families and to our families we see ourselves poised between evolution and disintegration. Reticence about personal matters is normative English behaviour, and in Anglo-Jewry this is combined with traditional Jewish self-deprecatory stoicism in the face of hardship: 'Don't worry about me . . . it's not so bad really . . . it could always be worse.' But in the privacy of their homes some Jewish families are carrying levels of pain which those outside the family may rarely see.

Doctors' surgeries are full of Jews with what are often, at root, psychosomatic complaints – a proliferation of backaches and chest pains and tension in the neck. But who is on our back? What is the source of our heartache? Who is the pain in the neck? Perhaps we do suspect sometimes that our heartburn doesn't come solely from the food we eat. And we know that the consulting rooms of psychiatrists and analysts and therapists are full of Jews who are depressed, Jews who are anxious, Jews who are neurotic, Jews with eating disorders . . . and it is no joke. The ill-health of British Jewry is not only a metaphor.

Non-Jews continually refer to the warmth and closeness of Jewish family life. We enjoy their feeling of our distinctive family life, for it corresponds to our own wishful thinking. That there are great strengths and much potential is indisputable. But the perception of outsiders does involve an idealisation, and one with which the Jewish community is eager to collude.

This idealisation leads inevitably to the marginalisation of those who do not fit the conventional picture: the divorced, the widowed, the unattached young and old, the outmarried, the infertile couples, the 5 per cent of the community who are not heterosexual – that whole plethora of groupings who are rendered invisible when 'the Jewish family' is lauded as the standard-bearers of 'authentic' Jewish living and the key to Jewish survival.

With the dissonance between the idea of the family and its reality becoming increasingly clear, our problem is to separate the life-affirming aspects of the family from the dead weight of the past. Of major relevance here is the new consciousness carried by Jewish women.

Male Anglo-Jewry is frightened of the power of women. Clearly, this is a phenomenon which is not confined to the Jewish community. But for religious and cultural and historical reasons, male fear of the creative and destructive potential of women has specific resonances in a Jewish context.

The lack of equality in the religious sphere does not need detailing here. Whatever the theoretical apologias given for their 'separate-but-equal' status, the experience of many contemporary Jewish woman is that they are marginalised by the male hegemony over Jewish religious practice. This spills over into the secular sphere and it also creeps into the dynamics of family life.

There is a historical dimension to this. Of necessity, many of the immigrant generation of Jewish women (who arrived in Britain in the twenty years on either side of 1900) worked outside the home. And although the tradition of the scholar – husband supported by his working wife is now to be found only in a few enclaves of Anglo-Jewry, it seems that the ethos of the Jewish working woman still predominates.

Yet the post-war generation of women, who along with their Gentile contemporaries in the emerging middle class tended to focus their energies on the home and the family, suffered the inevitable frustrations associated with this denial of their potential. The next generation of Jewish women have re-asserted their desire to be more than Jewish wives and Jewish mothers. In this they share in the contemporary re-evaluation in Western society of the role of women.

Nevertheless, in spite of the new ethos of liberation, the anger in Jewish women can often be immense (though camouflaged), as well as the hurt and sadness beneath it: about the lack of male support; or the inequalities and unfairness of traditional roles and expectations; or how their own mothers undermine(d) them through an unconscious envy of their daughters' freedoms and opportunities; or how their fathers were too busy to give them the necessary attention or feeling of feminine worth.

Some of this is, of course, shared with Gentile women, yet the anger in Jewish women at the repressions to which they are subjected – whether it be in the family or the community – is an inevitable consequence of a system of traditional values which seeks to assign a place to them without recognising and valuing their own autonomous desires. When the woman's strength, equality, authority, potency or sexuality are denied, she becomes – necessarily – destructive. Being rejected causes her to turn her energy into that which must destroy in order to create something new.

Conventionally, it is estimated that 70 per cent of patients with manic-depressive psychosis are women,[18] and in a 1983 study of Jews and mental health in Britain,[19] it was found that although rates of admission for Jews are not unusually high, Jews were low on schizophrenia but over-represented in manic-depression, the classic Jewish form of presenting distress. Jews in the United States have also been found to have significantly higher rates of major depression than Protestants or Catholics.[20] A recent study in London[21] highlighted a tendency for depressed Jewish patients to present predominantly hypochondriacal symptoms, a phenomenon which put them at risk of misdiagnosis and inappropriate treatment.

In an earlier cross-cultural study,[22] depression in Jews was linked to having a weak, non-assertive father; a loosening of ethnic or communal links; and a reduction in religious affiliation. Although Jews and Protestants did not differ in rates of hospital admission for depression, 'whereas depression in the Protestants was linked to inner-directed hostility around self-reproach and guilt, in Jews it brought out outer-directed hostility aimed at non-Jews'.[23]

The author of this study suggests that Jews may be carrying considerable repressed anger stemming from experiences of persecution and anti-semitism. My own clinical experience suggests, however, that persecutory feelings which originate within the patient's own parenting are often displaced into, or projected on to, such external figures, groups or issues. So, to give an obvious example, fantasies or dreams of Nazi persecutors may indeed be the residue of real trauma; or an anxiety based on an awareness of current manifestations of anti-semitism; but they may well turn out to be a distorted expression of an individual's private pathology cast in imagery culled from the collective historical memory of the Jewish people. For the mental health practitioner, the need to help the patient discriminate between – as well as trace possible connections between – individual and collective Jewish hurt is crucial, but sensitive, work.

Part of our problem is that anger is seen as a Gentile emotion. Historically, Jews saw themselves as the victims of that anger. And if Gentile anger wasn't directed outwards in the form of crusades and pogroms, then it was turned back inside their own families, where cruelty, violence and murder were felt to be the norm. Of course we would never have feelings like that – 'Jews aren't like that'.

It is hard to assess how much of this perception still prevails in the Jewish mind. Often we deflect our anger into irony or humour: 'Jews don't get angry – they have *broigus*.' (In every extended Jewish family there is someone who is *broigus* with another member of the family. *Broigus* is an untranslatable Yiddish word signifying smouldering disgruntlement where one feels slighted and offended by somebody's words or actions, usually years ago. And what makes matters worse is that they don't even know about it.)

And yet Jewish anger is all-pervasive, for anger is one response to fear. And we are a frightened community. Since the Holocaust, Jewish survival has not been able to be taken for granted. We glimpsed the abyss. We could have disappeared. Into nothing. A puff of smoke. The end.

Echoes of that trauma reverberate within us. We feel the fragility of Jewish continuity. And we feel it in our families. We feel that the continuity of the family is constantly under threat. A child leaving home; a youngster becoming less religiously observant – or more so; a student changing course in mid-stream away from what the family had hoped for; the choice of a different career from what had been expected; a change of career in mid-life; a non-Jewish partner; no partner at all.

On one level this is a long way from the Holocaust. But when we feel deep within us that survival and continuity hang on a thread, we react with defensive outrage to anything that hints at a departure from the behavioural straitjacket we feel we have to wear to maintain our sane survival. Our history has ensured that each generation will keep its anxious eye on its physical survival into the next generation.

Sometimes it is as if family members experience themselves as parts of a single body. In medieval literature, including Jewish texts, one of the most popular images used to describe the community was that of the human body.[24] So it is that mental health practitioners who work with Jewish clients will often hear this imagery emerging, especially when the family unit feels that it is under threat. Attacks on the 'wholeness' of the family 'body' can come from many quarters:

> Intermarriage, the break up of a marriage, or even a child leaving home, is experienced, by one or more members, as the amputation of part of the body . . . . For the family who are over-identified with each other, this may be felt to be more than a rejection of values, rather a rejection of everything they 'embody'.[25]

The atavistic impulse to keep the family together means that the necessary separation from parents by the next generation can become a deeply traumatic experience for all concerned. The over-enmeshment of Jewish families can mean that parents, while consciously wishing for their children's success and independence ('now they've gone we can take an extra holiday on what we save on phone bills'), may unconsciously fear or resent or envy that same independence. Feelings of emptiness or rejection or anger can be hard to acknowledge when one is supposed to want all the best for them.

A parent's difficulties in facing separation can lead to different forms of manipulative or controlling behaviour. This characteristic difficulty in Jewish families of parents letting go of their offspring means that the children in their turn may find separation difficult because of the guilt feelings it arouses.

It is not only that the child realises the parent's own unacknowledged need and feels called upon to continue to meet it. But if the child does nevertheless assert her or his independence, then they have to face the disappointment of the parent(s). This is hard enough when it is spoken about openly, even harder when nothing is said directly. Then the parent may rely on a range of sighs, innuendoes, or tones-of-voice that may have become so habitual that they constitute a way of life.

When children assert their own separate individuality there is a frightening awareness that has to be kept at bay – that separation involves destruction. (And has there not been enough enforced destruction of Jewish ties in the past?) In the absence of this awareness the child, now an adult, feels the need to continually pacify ('I wouldn't want to hurt them') and to 'make things good again' – that is, to keep the peace which is threatened by that assertive drive to grow up and be separate. When a parent cannot let go, the child can only break away – or become depressed.

Sometimes the anger at the smothering expectations of parents becomes directed by the child, or adolescent, or adult, against themselves. This leads to the depressions, the eating problems and disorders, the use and abuse of tranquillisers, alcohol or drugs, and the psychosomatic complaints that have become so prevalent in Anglo-Jewry. Self-destruction is the alternative to the destruction of the unconscious ties to parents.

Of course, these dynamics happen in non-Jewish families too. But our historical experience – the struggle for survival, the sacrifices made, the hopes invested in the next generation – means that the guilt-inducing, controlling Jewish parent is not only a stereotype. The wish to control is a defence against inner feelings of failure and worthlessness. And it is one response to our collective fear of helplessness and powerlessness.

Often in Anglo-Jewish families the pressures towards professional or business success – and academic success for the children – are inextricably intertwined with a deeply felt need for some kind of security in the face of the uncertainties of the world. In particular, the Holocaust has taught us that, for Jews, whatever the success we make of our lives, everything can be taken away in the twinkling of an eye. To live with this knowledge causes us too much anxiety to bear. We have to shut away our pain, our insecurity, our fears. And meanwhile our souls weep. For the deepest fear is about loss – loss of meaning.

THE QUEST FOR MEANING

Attempts to blot out the anguish in the souls of Anglo-Jewish families can take many forms. We are hungry for meaning. We nurture ourselves on our achievements and our activities and the distractions we invent. Predominantly though, salvation is sought in financial or material security: shares, insurance policies, investment in bricks and mortar, a proliferation of possessions, the latest fashions in clothes or cars or home computers, something to hold on to, physical and tangible when the inner world goes.

It is in paradoxical relation to this that we can also note how during this century Jews have been in the forefront of attempts to explore the psyche, to investigate the 'inner world', to help to find or create meaning in a world grown uncertain of meaning, or the sources of authority from which meaning could derive.

If Freud was the Jewish father of psychoanalysis, then Melanie Klein was its Jewish mother. These intellectual products of bourgeois Vienna, followed by their analytic disciples, have had an enormous impact on our capacity for introspection. As well as catalysing developments within the analytic tradition itself, these Jewish progenitors of psychoanalysis enabled succeeding generations to develop, adapt, and build upon the original insights, but to do so in some radically differing directions. Many of these developments illustrate the creative necessity for children to break away from parental *mores* and to move off – respectfully or defiantly – in directions where the 'parents' could not or would not go, even in directions that the 'parents' might condemn or feel betrayed by.

These Jewish 'children' form a roll-call of twentieth-century psychological innovators. Wilhelm Reich worked actively with the body and sexual energy, which led to the development of bioenergetic therapy by Alexander Lowen and

Stanley Keleman; Karen Horney and Erich Fromm developed the social and cultural dimensions of analytic understanding; Jacob Moreno created psycho-drama, Fritz Perls gestalt therapy, Arthur Janov primal therapy, Abraham Maslow transpersonal therapy, and Roberto Assagioli psychosynthesis. Holocaust survivors Bruno Bettelheim, Eugene Heimler and Viktor Frankl developed existential therapies devoted to helping people find a sense of meaning and purpose in their lives.

Many of these re-acknowledged the spiritual dimension in interpersonal work and in the psyche which Freud and Klein had disavowed.[26] Many of them too were drawing, unconsciously perhaps, on earlier rabbinic and Hasidic models of interpersonal work and intra-psychic understanding.[27] All of them, questing after meaning, saw 'mental' health as only part of that broad and richly textured tapestry which constitutes our human nature, impossible to fully comprehend and impossible to stop trying to comprehend.

And all of them might have relished this final enigmatic tale by the master story-teller and manic-depressive Rabbi Nachman of Bratslav, which raises questions about mental health, about those cared for, and about the carers – questions which, fittingly, the story refuses to resolve.

It is the tale of a prince who became mad and imagined he was a turkey. He took off his clothes, sat under the royal table and refused all food except oats and crumbs. The king, his father, brought all the doctors of the land to him, but none could cure him. At last a wise man came and undertook to cure the prince. Immediately the wise man took off his clothes and sat under the royal table next to the prince, and began to scratch amongst the oats and crumbs.

The prince asked him: 'Who are you and what are you doing here?' The wise man replied: 'And who are you and what are you doing here?' 'I am a turkey,' said the prince. 'And I am a turkey too,' rejoined the wise man. So the two turkeys sat there together till they grew accustomed to one another.

One day the wise man asked the king to hand him a vest. He put it on and said to the prince: 'Do you imagine that a turkey is not allowed to wear a vest? He is, and it doesn't make him less of a turkey.' The prince took his words to heart and consented to wear a vest also. After some days the wise man called for a pair of trousers and said 'Do you think that just because one is wearing trousers, a person cannot be a turkey?' The prince agreed with him and it went on like this until they were both fully dressed.

The wise man then asked for some human food to be brought from the table, and he said to the king's son: 'Do you think that just because one eats good food one cannot be a turkey?' After the prince began to eat like a human being, the wise man asked: 'Do you imagine that there is a law that a turkey is only to sit under the table? It is possible to be a turkey and to sit at the table itself.' The prince accepted this, stood up, and walked about thereafter like a human being, behaving like one in every respect. In this way, the wise man healed him.

CONCLUSIONS

Jews are, historically and existentially, iconoclasts. Perforce, we have grown into natural doubters of the world's certainties, underminers of received opinions and truths. We have a pious disbelief in truths too readily accepted, understanding too easily gained. Because we prefer the open-endedness of questions to the fixed formulations of answers, we retain an ambivalence about conventional notions about what constitutes mental health or mental illness.

Just as biblical thought subverted traditional boundaries between 'madness' and 'sanity', and later rabbinic thinking assumed a complex and fluid relationship between psyche and soma, so the psychological approach to mental phenomena of Freud and his analytic disciples undermined conventional notions concerning the aetiology of morality and sexuality. Yet side by side with this one can also observe the Judaic compassion towards – and attempts to understand – those individuals who suffer from emotional and psychological distress, whatever its provenance.

Contemporary psychological ailments and disease among Jews need to be viewed against the backdrop of those particular collective pressures which individual Jews experience – sometimes consciously, though mainly unconsciously – within modern society. We are, in today's jargon, an 'ethnic minority'; and at one and the same time we experience ourselves as both fully integrated into a multicultural society, and as potential victims. Memories of the Holocaust have both a painfully real, and an anxiety-provoking symbolic presence within the community. We live with a legacy of fear and anger. Much of this is somatised or projected.

We live too with an increasing dissonance between an idealised Jewish past of loving family security and values, and the fragmented individualism of contemporary Jewish family life. We feel that as a community we are poised between evolution and disintegration: perhaps manic-depression within the individual is a symbolic expression of this underlying collective tension. Perhaps too there is more than a figurative connection between the failure of the Jewish family to adequately 'feed' its members with a sense of identity and purpose, and the increasing incidence of eating disorders. Contemporary Jews are hungry for meaning – and frightened of that hunger, gnawing at their souls.

So, we fear for our continuity, and we fear a loss of meaning. The crucible of the Jewish family, formerly the incubator of purpose, the context in which the ideals of the Jewish people were embodied and which generated the nurturing environment enabling those ideas to be enacted within the wider society – this crucible is cracked. And, inevitably, when the psychic fatigue of the family becomes strains which lead to fracture, it is the individual who suffers: adult men and women, teenagers, children, unable to function without feeling varying degrees of psychological or somatic distress.

Yet, as Arthur Miller has one of his characters say, 'Jews have been acrobats since the beginning of the world'.[28] Our physical and emotional health has always balanced precariously between our dependence on the goodwill of others and our own capacities to generate meaning and understanding in our individual situations and collective settings. And part of our balancing exercise has been that alongside the ameliorating rigour of the scientific and medical approaches to mental phenomena, we Jews also approach the mysteries of the human mind and the complexities of the human personality through stories and parables, through metaphor, through whatever allows the ambiguities of human life room to breathe and the psychic scars of human life time to heal.

NOTES

1 *Mishneh Torah*, Laws of Human Tendencies, chapter 1.
2 Quoted in A. Stern, 'The psycho-biological effects of stress from a biblical, Talmudic and rabbinic perspective', *Journal of Psychology and Judaism* 13(3):177.
3 From Maimonides (1977) 'Essays in health', quoted in A. Amsel, *Judaism and Psychology*, New York: Feldheim, p. 70.
4 *Mishneh Torah*, Laws on Witnesses, chapter 9:9–10.
5 From the *Sefer Hachinuch*, quoted in J. Trachtenberg (1977) *Jewish Magic and Superstition: A Study in Folk Religion*, New York: Atheneum, p. 23.
6 Jacobs, L. (1973) *What Does Judaism Say About . . .*, Jerusalem: Keter Publishing House, p. 253 (article on psychoanalysis).
7 Bettelheim, B. (1982)*Freud and Man's Soul*, London: Collins, p. 5.
8 Ibid., p. 77.
9 *Genesis Rabbah*, 9:7, quoted in C.G. Montefiore and H. Loewe (1974) *A Rabbinic Anthology*, New York: Schocken, p. 305.
10 In Bettelheim's translation: 'Where it was, there should become I' (p. 61). Bettelheim comments: 'By this he did not mean that the I should eliminate the it or take over the it's place in our psyche, since . . . the it is the source of our vital energy, without which life itself could not continue' (pp. 61–2).
11 For an elaboration of the difference between heart and soul, cf. H. Cooper (ed.) (1988) *Soul Searching: Studies in Judaism and Psychotherapy*, London: SCM Press, p. xviii.
12 Jung, C. G. (1967/75) *Memories, Dreams, Reflections*, London: Collins, p. 161.
13 Jung, C. G. (1977) *Collected Works*, vol. 18, London: Routledge & Kegan Paul, paragraph 635, p. 279.
14 McGuire, W. and Hull, R. F. C. (1980) *C. G. Jung Speaking: Interviews and Encounters*, London: Picador, p. 327. Each of the works cited in Notes 12, 13, and 14 contains differently nuanced accounts of this case.
15 Jung (1977) op. cit., paragraph 636, p. 279.
16 Sacks, J. (1990) 'Women's role in our spiritual future', *Jewish Chronicle* February 23.
17 The opening sentence *of Anna Karenina* (author's translation).
18 Henderson, D. and Gillespie, W. H. (1969) *Textbook of Psychiatry*, Oxford: Oxford University Press, p. 213.
19 Cooklyn, R. S., Ravindran, A. and Carney, M. W. P. 'The patterns of mental disorder in Jewish and non-Jewish admissions to a district general hospital psychiatric unit: is manic-depressive illness a typically Jewish disorder?', *Psychological Medicine* 13:209–12.
20 Yeung, P. P. and Greenwald, S. 'Jewish Americans and mental health: results of the NIMH Epidemiologic Catchment Area Study', *Social Psychiatry and Psychiatric Epidemiology* 27:292–7.
21 Ball, R. A. and Clare, A. W. 'Symptoms and social adjustment in Jewish depressives', *British Journal of Psychiatry* 156:379–83. This paper includes a comprehensive bibliography of the relevant psychiatric literature.

22 Fernando, S. J. 'A cross-cultural study of some familial and social factors in depressive illness', *British Journal of Psychiatry* 127:45–53.

23 Dale, N. 'Jews, ethnicity and mental health', in H. Cooper, op. cit., p. 73. In this essay the author discusses the papers by Fernando and Cooklyn *et al.*

24 'Just as one would never think of deliberately injuring, or purposely neglecting, any limb of one's own body, so, too, every Jew must seek the well-being of all other members of the entity that is the Jewish people.' Quoted in A. Chill (1974) *The Mitzvot: The Commandments and their Rationale*, Jerusalem: Keter Brooks, p. 234.

25 Levens, M. (1983) 'Psychological conflicts in Jewish families', unpublished paper, p. 7.

26 See A. Pirani, 'Psychotherapy, women and the feminine in Judaism', in H. Cooper, op. cit., pp. 50–3.

27 Hoffman, E. (1981) *The Way of Splendour: Jewish Mysticism and Modern Psychology*, Boulder, CO: Shambala.

28 Gregory Solomon in A. Miller (1988) 'The price', in *Collected Plays: Two*, London: Metheun, p. 319.

Chapter 6

Psychosocial factors and the genesis of new African-American religious groups

Ezra E. H. Griffith and Khalipha M. Bility

INTRODUCTION

The psychosocial origin and evolution of black Christian groups have been neglected in studies of new religious groups, despite the significance of such groups in the black community. This chapter seeks to clarify the conditions that facilitate the emergence and development of new black Christian groups and to explain the characteristics that differentiate black from non-black groups. Data available about one well-known African-American movement are examined to test our ecological model of black church group development. This model suggests that black groups emerge under specific structural and psychosocial conditions and evolve in three distinct, yet overlapping phases. We posit that while all Christian groups share several fundamental characteristics, the attempt to produce a creative synergy between the quest for secular power in a white-dominated society and the struggle for spiritual or religious emancipation distinguishes black from non-black groups. We suggest that this framework is useful for understanding the roles of black groups as a psychological and healing resource in the black community.

Religious groups have captured the attention and interest of theologians, behavioural scientists, psychiatrists, and health practitioners for a long time. This has occurred particularly because such new religious groups often have been a crucible for examining the interactions of religion and healing (Galanter, 1989a; 1989b; Griffith and Mahy, 1984). By new religious groups, we refer objectively and without disparagement or praise to the emergence of a gestating or recently established religious group having some distinctive philosophy. We intend no reference to the normative religious groups that embrace the traditions and rituals of well-established churches. Furthermore, we agree with Washington (1973) that a new group may ultimately evolve to acquire the status of a sect and eventually even become an established church.

Despite a long and rich history of scholarship on new religious groups, African-American groups have received comparatively less attention in the literature. In fact, recent reviews about new religious groups once again did not adequately attend to black groups in the United States (Galanter, 1989b; Group for the Advancement of Psychiatry, 1992). This lack of attention creates a vacuum in our understanding of a very important aspect of the black experience, one we think deserves to be filled for scientific, health and social policy reasons. Moreover, the ubiquitous nature of black Christian groups, their influence on black religious traditions (Genovese, 1976), and the impact of the new group's activities on many aspects of black community life (Rohter, 1992) are reasons that warrant studies of new black groups. Also, the diversity of such black religious groups suggests the need for systematic study in relation to religious groups in other minority communities.

Historically, new black religious organisations have had considerable impact on the religious, political, socio-cultural, and psychological dimensions of black life in the New World (Baer, 1984; Williams, 1974). Over the years, this has been evident in examination of groups in the United States (Fauset, 1978; Sessions, 1989; Washington, 1973), such as the Universal Negro Improvement Association founded by Marcus Garvey in the 1930s; Daddy Grace's United House of Prayer for All People and Father Divine Kingdom in the 1940s; The Nation of Islam under the leadership of the Honourable Elijah Mohammed in the 1960s; and more recently, the Imani Temple organised in Washington, DC by the Reverend Stallings, a former Catholic priest. In the Caribbean and South America, the impact of such new groups has been witnessed through the Rastafari in Jamaica; Vodun in Haiti; the Spiritual Baptists in Barbados and Trinidad; Espiritismo in Puerto Rico; and Umbanda in Brazil (Glazier, 1983; Goodman *et al.*, 1982; Lovelace, 1988; Simpson, 1980).

We think the study of new and established religious groups provides a window of opportunity for understanding significant dimensions of black community life. The work by Griffith and colleagues on the Barbados Spiritual Baptists (1984; 1986) and black Churches in the United States (1980; 1981; 1984) concluded that in some cases black religious rituals and group membership may promote psychological well-being among members of the group. But we well recognise that these linkages to health are but one aspect of the functions of new black religious groups, which for years have contributed to community life in the areas already mentioned. Still, we shall insist that the connection to psychological well-being is not to be down-played or underestimated; these groups are as powerfully attractive through their religious dimension as through their promise of a new psychological state for their members.

In this present work, we wish to re-examine the socio-cultural conditions and psychological forces that facilitate the emergence of new black Christian movements. We do so by analysing psychiatric reports and historical data on the Father Divine Kingdom Group because the group embodies basic characteristics of a new black religious movement. Established in the Harlem community of New York City in the 1920s, the group flourished during the Depression of the 1930s. We think analysis of this group will help us understand how similar institutions emerge and evolve in the African-American community. We posit that the context of the interactions between blacks and whites form the bedrock for the development of important psychosocial conditions that then facilitate the evolution of a new black group.

We describe an explanatory model that is useful in understanding how the new black religious group is established, the factors that facilitate differentiation of the new group, and elements that mark the transition of the group to a specific movement with distinctive rituals and an idiosyncratic religious philosophy. Factors that favour or negate success of the new group are also examined. We think this model may be applicable to the understanding of contemporary black groups, such as Stallings' Imani Temple and other new religious groups throughout the United States. Over the last twenty-five to thirty years, socio-political developments in the United States and Britain, particularly regarding questions of racism and economic inequality, have had considerable impact on Afro-Caribbean culture in islands such as Barbados. We suggest, therefore, that this model may also be helpful in understanding the development of Afro-Caribbean movements like the Barbadian Spiritual Baptist Church.

MODEL OF DEVELOPMENT

The two dominant paradigms or models developed from research on new religious groups do not adequately portray the complex evolution of new black religious groups and their place in black community life (West, 1989). The 'Utopian' paradigm depicts groups as a congregation of kindred spirits searching for truth under benign guidance; whereas the 'Inferno' paradigm invokes images of a rebellious counterculture or satanic group on the path of self-destruction.

We think the development of black Christian groups reflects the commingling of a dynamic process in which the forms and functions of the religious movement are shaped by the group's internal needs and by external socio-cultural changes occurring in society, particularly within the black community. This mixture of internal and external processes may enable the group to establish a distinctive dogma that responds to the psychological, emotional and spiritual needs of its members.

The evolution of the group takes place in three relatively distinct, yet interactive, phases that are often initiated with the estrangement of a charismatic leader from a normative church to establish a new religious group. These phases, labelled predisposing, empowering, and operational, recapitulate the underlying socio-cultural conditions and psychological forces that blend together finally to determine the theological outlook and spiritual vision of the particular black Christian group. Furthermore, these phases should not be seen as rigidly separated, but as overlapping sequential stages along an evolutionary continuum. Although a complex array of reasons account for the development of any new black religious group, we think a central driving force is the adherents' socio-cultural preference and psychological need for belonging to a religious community that explicitly celebrates religious rituals and expressions of spirituality rooted in their black heritage. Membership in the group is nurtured through strong links between a sense of black identity and the possibilities of empowerment in religious and secular affairs. The predisposing phase is crucial for identifying the specific socio-cultural conditions favourable to group formation.

Predisposing phase

Human misery in its various forms – material deprivation, economic hardship, unemployment, poor housing – are important conditions that often characterise the predisposing phase. But these elements carry additional significance because they are perceived by disadvantaged blacks as being linked to their racial status. Our model depicts the significance of the powerlessness – racism nexus for understanding how emerging groups respond to both physical and psychological suffering. In this context the embryonic movement issues a call to power to improve life conditions and heal psychologically. But the call is also offered to improve the lot of blacks suffering acutely in a racist environment. For these reasons, the poorest segment of black society is often attracted to emergent black groups.

We postulate that poverty, in conjunction with the reality and perception of racial oppression, predispose black individuals and groups to accept new religions or ideas that they find compelling in light of their circumstances and conditions. Griffith and Mahy (1984) have demonstrated that this religious or spiritual quest for a more satisfying reality promising material well-being has the potential to heal psychological pains often associated with poverty. These healing effects may be mediated by the group's message of hope even when conditions of poverty remain intractable. Indeed, just the promise of material comfort and spiritual salvation may be important enough to the black individual's sense of well-being to overcome the frustrations of poverty – at least temporarily.

Simpson and Yinger (1972) have suggested that the desire for material progress and a heightened sense of personal self-esteem is a historic feature of successful black Christian groups. Although a new group may not offer practical and feasible solutions to the conditions of deprivation, its clear sympathetic identification with the sufferers helps to establish emotional ties to the new group. These ties symbolise a call to power in a context that is controlled by the group leader. The message, rituals, and songs developed by the new group often symbolise this emphatic identification with oppressive conditions in the temporal experiences of group members.

A significant step in the predisposing phase is the emergence of a charismatic individual who will generate considerable appeal among disadvantaged individuals. Initially, the leader is often an individual crying in the wilderness of desolation and racism, bearing witness to the fact that whatever the situation of scorn, poverty, rejection or powerlessness, the new group is a clear means for self-determination and ultimate redemption. The messenger and messages are personified in the group leader's call for secular power and spiritual emancipation in a setting controlled and defined by an autocratic leader.

While poor social situations are necessary conditions for creating a terrain that predisposes individuals to join a new group, a special individual must step forward to lead. One factor without the other may result in sustained hardship and likely failure. Charisma, narcissism, entrepreneurship, zeal and determination are often characteristic of these individuals who provide such leadership.

We are suggesting that the formation of the new African-American religious group requires more than the feelings of anomie that Levine (1979) described among members of white emerging groups. We think a unique characteristic of the new black movement is linked to black adherents' feelings about the race problem and the quest for alternative routes to empowerment outside the control of whites.

Often, the departure of the group leader from an established religious organisa-tion marks a critical period in the predisposing phase. Once independent of the established church, the leader often displays extraordinary capacities of entrepre-neurship and clever management that, once judiciously employed, lead naturally to the next stage of group development that is the empowering phase.

Empowering phase

Central to the empowering process is the creation of a context in which individual group members are socialised to practise the teachings and doctrines articulated by the movement's leader during the earlier predisposing phase. The group leader finds fault with existing social, political, economic and theological institutions. Typically, in relative obscurity, the group leader acquires a band of loyal followers who seek to build their lives outside of society's mainstream institutions that have apparently not responded to the needs of group members. The leader points out to would-be members that the old institutions have not served them well and simulta-neously urges their allegiance to the new group. Members are invited to relinquish conformity to society's norms and values that are in conflict with the group's.

Often, this journey is attended by hardships and pitfalls. However, leaders of the black group often interpret such difficulties as indicators of individuals who lack commitment or as obstacles created by an unenlightened humanity (Clark, 1965).

Successful group leaders exhort individuals to reframe their perceptions of the real conditions in which they live to fit the group's world view. This exhortation is intended to place the group at the centre of the individual's life. The leader must succeed in convincing a number of individuals that the new programme is viable and that collectively they are capable of succeeding. The group members must experience the acquisition of a new power that is often characterised by an epiphanous experience, psychological transformation, spiritual rebirth or special healing that may come soon after entry and acceptance into the group. Finally, new members who recall this special contact with the divine claim that they are better able to communicate about the group and the personal sense of security, hope, and happiness derived from group membership (Levine, 1981).

The group must also foster organisational coherence, as it tends to develop a family feeling and social structure. New groups that have these characterics tend to function increasingly and progressively better. The leader will, of course, rely on the adherents' improved ability to communicate as a cornerstone of the group's drive to recruit new members and foster solidarity within the group. Growth and expansion can lead to the third level of group formation, the operational phase.

Operational phase

The most significant task of the operational phase is to use the new group's resources to transform the group from a marginalised religion into an institution with some staying power. New Christian movements that successfully make this transition become a true social system, capable of making and enforcing rules and dispensing rewards and sanctions. This process is very critical for the survival of the group.

The confluence of godly ideals and the quest for earthly power in places owned by the new group is the hallmark of the operational phase. The transformation of conditions and situations of powerlessness to power requires that the group operationalise its programmes. The survival and viability of the group depend on how this is done within and outside the group, The group must demonstrate: efficacy of its programmes; ability to maximise social leverage of the group; potential for increasing the group's legitimacy, linkages and networks; capacity to build solidarity within the group; means of increasing organisational and financial resources; the development of skills that maximise the recruitment of new converts and the retention of old members. In this phase, communication with the public through the group's newspapers, radio programmes, or other media becomes prominent.

In return for substantive allegiance to the group, members are often provided with food, shelter, clothing, security, a social structure, a sharper sense of identity, and a simple, but coherent belief system. Social welfare and economic self-help are common aspects of black groups. All this is clouded in the mystery of the group's rituals and an intense emotional appeal that is sometimes incomprehensible to outsiders.

In essence, the operational phase seeks to create and provide the physical infrastructure, spiritual atmosphere, and emotional context for the movement's members to practise their beliefs and values, without hindrance from outsiders. Within the confines of an institution, the new group moves to overcome the constraints tending to circumscribe the practice of its values and beliefs. Particularly at this stage, the new movement may be the target of retaliation from the larger society.

Faced with internal and external threats to its very existence, there are several potential outcomes: the group sustains growth; it may become dormant but remain alive; or it may degenerate and finally die.

As we shall see, competing institutions may seek to destroy the new group through legal and/or illegal means. Nevertheless, it is hard to predict how long the initial operational phase lasts for any particular group.

THE FATHER DIVINE MOVEMENT

In 1876, Father Divine was born as George Baker to Gullah parents who were ex-slaves near Savannah, Georgia. He was raised in extreme poverty and amidst the broken dreams that plunged most blacks into the mire of misery in the wake of unrelenting oppression of the post-Reconstruction era. Religion was a potent solace and distraction from afflictions of body, mind and spirit. At this time, Mysticism and Pentecostal religion were taking root among blacks. Many responded to the union of religion and political process as an answer to their inhuman conditions (Parker, 1937).

In the early 1900s, George Baker left Georgia, following the Holiness and mystical route, only to return to Valdosta, Georgia as 'The Messenger' in 1913. Political and religious persecution forced him to flee from Georgia to Harlem, New York City. In Harlem, he began to respond to the yearnings among blacks for spiritual wholeness with ample food, shelter, and dignity here on earth. In Sayville, Long Island, he began to develop and operationalise a theology based on the doctrine that identification with the spirit of God required actual changes in the human conditions here on earth. He taught that one did not have to die in order to get to heaven.

By 1930, Father Divine had turned the corner from being a curiosity to becoming an institutionalised phenomenon controlling millions of dollars in real estate and a following estimated between two and twenty million on five continents. Lives were changed so radically until disciples could only understand themselves as being reborn in the 'Kingdom of God' (Hoshor, 1936).

It is impossible to know all the forces that moved this diminutive black man to become 'The Messenger' in Georgia and 'God among men' in Harlem. But it is clear that his fusion of a message of hope in visible action against poverty and religiosity seemed to satisfy many in the wake of despair and crisis in the human condition caused by the Great Depression of the 1930s.

Among the myriad and prominent storefront black religions of the early 1900s, Father Divine embodied the central theme of black religion, distinguished from white religious ethos: the need to create a black ethos that provided blacks with pride, integrity, freedom, and power to become dignified human beings here on earth.

Because Father Divine's Movement set in motion a synergy between religion and the complex social forces that created the environment in which new groups flourish, we will apply our model of new group development to his Kingdom Movement. The model attempts to illustrate how the group evolved from an obscure storefront revival meeting place into prominent healing communities known to the faithful as a 'Kingdom of Heaven'. The group became a means of protection – at least temporarily and imaginatively – from rejection and discrimination.

Predisposing conditions

The Depression of the 1930s had a great impact on the material well-being of everybody. However, its effects were most acute in the black community.

Between 1920 and 1940, Harlem was gradually becoming the centre of New York City's black community. The influx of blacks from the South, the vibrant Harlem Renaissance in the arts, the economic hardships caused by the Depression, and the continuing struggle for civil rights established a context that facilitated the evolution of black religious groups in Harlem. Gentrification in Harlem, Philadelphia, Detroit and many cities in the North created circumstances whereby new religious ideas and values flourished among poor blacks (Osofsky, 1963).

Harlem in the 1920s and 1930s was a community of economically depressed working people. The various ethnic communities in Harlem resembled hundreds of poor working communities, but with the added burden of the 'colour line' (DuBois, 1967). Nearly 42 per cent of working age black men were unemployed. As African-Americans gradually replaced whites as the majority population in Harlem, gentrification and economic opportunities decreased dramatically.

Both rental and residential housing were poor and overpriced. Often, the price of rental units increased upward of 30 per cent for black tenants in New York City. So ironic was the housing situation that Adam Clayton Powell noted: 'The worse the accommodation the poorer the people, and the higher the rent' (Schoener, 1968).

It was not uncommon for real estate firms to decrease actual property values, sometimes below 30 per cent of the original value in neighbourhoods that were becoming black. The resulting decrease in the tax base produced blatant inequalities in education and other social services. Population increase often exacerbated these inequalities.

As hundreds of thousands of blacks migrated from the South, the black population of New York City grew by 66 per cent between 1910 and 1920. This trend further deepened the employment crisis among blacks. In transforming the racial status quo in the North, the 'Great Migration' had two significant points of impact on the religious life of blacks in the urban North: the audience susceptible to joining religious movements, such as Father Divine's Peace Mission, grew significantly; and black migrants provided a reservoir of cultural beliefs, religious rituals, symbols and unique experiences that proved to be useful in organising new religious groups (DuBois, 1930).

Many migrants who came in search of greener pastures were disappointed with the conditions in the cities. Some experienced psychological and emotional dislocation as they made the transition from field to factory workers. In this context, Father Divine referred his followers for employment as waitresses, gardeners, cleaners, hairdressers, and maids. He established his reputation in the community for kindness and gentility, despite the fact that the actual number of jobs he provided was small.

Newcomers encountered life-styles in the North that were far different from their experiences in the rural South or in the Caribbean. The fusion of Caribbean, Southern and Northern cultures created a new, more aggressive and dynamic African-American community in the large, predominantly black neighbourhoods that were emerging in many Northern cities. In this new environment of cultural fluidity, religious doctrines became a force for continuity and stability. The symbols and rituals of the Father Divine Kingdom were readily acceptable to many emigrants from the South. For others, the Peace Mission was perhaps the most direct mechanism for boosting their self-esteem.

In the 1920s, the health status of blacks was poor due to many factors: inadequate and inaccessible health care, poor education, low income, racism and poverty. For example, the mortality rate in Harlem was 40 per cent higher than in the rest of New York City. The tuberculosis mortality rate (a major cause of death at the turn of the century) was 77 per 100,000 for whites compared to 300 per 100,000 for blacks. The black infant mortality rate was 124 per 1000 compared to 62 per 1000 for whites. Maternal mortality rate was twice as high for blacks, compared to whites (Schoener, 1968).

With death and illness ever present, healing was a favoured subject of the religious songs and rituals of Father Divine's Movement. Many of the songs and rituals of the group recalled past and present problems.

> Father's going to save this soul of mine:
> Yes, He is, I know He is.
> Father's going to heal this body of mine:
> Yes, He is, I know He is:
> Father's going to feed me all the time:
> Yes, He is, I know He is.
>
> (Cantril and Sherif, 1938)

Clearly, Father Divine exploited the conditions of the time to make his followers emotionally dependent. Faith in the power of Father Divine to provide food, shelter, and healing power provided hope among his followers for improving their life circumstances here on earth.

Father Divine's own childhood experiences in rural Georgia may have strengthened his conviction to lead a moral crusade. Condemning the established churches, Father Divine preached in 1930:

> Men have used religion to keep you in poverty! But I come to break this band and set the prisoner free . . . I have brought you down from the sky. We are not studying about a God in the sky. We are talking about a God here and now, a God that has been Personified and Materialized, a God that will free you from the segregations of the segregators.
>
> (Cantril and Sherif, 1938)

This radical confluence of religious and social reform doctrine subtly appealed to the important concerns and emotions of blacks alienated from the established church. His effectiveness in the use of language, the simplicity of this belief system, and his identification with racial progress generated greater enthusiasm for empowerment.

Empowerment in Father Divine's Kingdom

Empowerment in the Father Divine Kingdom was derived from individual and group phenomena. These twin processes consisted of two components: testimony and role modelling.

Testimony was a cathartic declaration of powerful and dramatic content. Our analysis of the content of these testimonies suggests that the individual's ego seemed to become undifferentiated as the individual expressed a strong desire to become one with Father Divine. Typically, testimony consisted of self-castigation for former sins of adultery, stealing, drunkenness, fornication and finally, thanking Father Divine for his divine power to heal. Catharsis was the effective physiological side of the moral and cognitive act of testifying. The free display of emotions, rhythmic swaying of the body, singing, dancing, praising Father Divine, and jerking seemed to signal the readiness of recruits to accept new behaviours and beliefs of the group. The core of this new belief system included sexual abstinence, a belief that heaven could be created here on earth, and that Father Divine was God, 'personified and materialised' (Bender and Spalding, 1940). Smoking and drinking were taboo. No medical or dental attention was allowed, because one was cured of all illness through the divine power of Father Divine. Husband and wife were separated, and children were removed from parental guidance and sometimes placed under the church's corporate care.

Role modelling was the second element defining the specific behaviour and dogma reinforced in the empowerment phase. Father Divine's exhortation, 'As you are, so am I' (Cantril and Sherif, 1938), expressed the essence of the second aspect of empowerment. Among the adherents, the desire to model belief in Father Divine elevated social status by proximity to God, meaning Father Divine.

The ethnocentric interpretation of the ideals of 'Omnipotence, Everlasting Peace, Race Pride, Self-determination and Racial Justice' was a major thrust of Father Divine's teachings. He taught that only those who followed him zealously could develop the power to become omnipotent and enjoy life eternal with him. His advocacy of this linear transference of power from God to Father Divine and then to his followers was largely accepted in the movement. In one sermon Father Divine admonished his followers:

> Peace everybody, I am unifying God and Man and unifying the heaven and earth as one man. Therefore I am limitless. Remember this is not confined to me as a person. It is converted into me as a person. It is a principle that is convertible into a person and it is just as operative for you as it is for me but remember you must bring your bodies into subjection. You will be expressers and manifestors and eventually the time will come when all mankind shall in reality be the Personification of this identical principle that I am advocating.
>
> (Bender and Yarrell, 1938)

While Father Divine did not claim divinity, he did not deny it. He contended: 'I teach that God has the right to manifest himself through any person or anything he may choose' (Cantril and Sherif, 1938). The practice of role modelling called for the psychic incorporation of the teachings of the group's 'messiahs' into practices of daily living. Role modelling deliberately applied permeated the lives of new members.

Operational phase

In the many branches of the organisation, called Kingdoms, individuals who claimed rebirth became 'angels'. The angels took on new names that were received by revelation, like Crystal Star, Job Patience, Faithful Mary (Cantril and Sherif, 1938). These names had both symbolic and ritual significance. They represented a conscious separation of the individual from the non-group community with concomitant connection to a new life. In exchange for total submission, all necessities of life were provided, everything from toothpaste to white clothes. Meals were served in communal style for all who visited the movement. In the Kingdoms, the angels gave everything over to Father Divine, including savings, insurance, personal belongings, and houses. Members were forbidden to read newspapers or magazines, except those published by Father Divine, or to listen to radio programmes, except Father Divine's broadcasts. Racial segregation was prohibited.

In the operational phase, the group developed a more explicit boundary and greater internal social cohesiveness, enforced rules and regulations, sanctioned loyalty, and punished deviance. Activities in the Kingdoms were designed to enable members to integrate the group's doctrine into daily living. In Father Divine's Peace Movement, the Kingdom provided a setting for worship without interference from the outside. Bender and Yarrell (1938) described the Kingdom as a place of contentment:

> At the Kingdoms he provides meals and lodging for any and all who come. No distinction is made between race, creed, or color – all are brothers and sisters in the faith. One is impressed when visiting his Kingdoms with the cleanliness, the abundance of food, the order, and the serenity and contentment of his followers.

The mechanisms for developing contentment and social cohesiveness within the Kingdom were twofold: denial or rejection of existing family ties and responsibilities; and integration into a new 'family' with Father Divine as head. Sexual continence played an important role in developing loyalty to Father Divine by outlawing intimate relationships between adults inside the Kingdom. The Kingdom became a surrogate family, while Divine urged his followers to:

> Wear the world as a loose garment. Relatives, kin, friends, and all that may have claims, must be relinquished, and you must deny them if you are anticipating inheriting life eternal. It is a matter of impossibility to have two families. If you have two families one is in adultery.
>
> (Bender and Yarrell, 1938)

Social cohesion fostered through obedience kept members engaged in the Kingdom. Fear, damnation, mental confusion, and alienation were said to result from deviations from group norms.

Within the Kingdoms, shared beliefs and social cohesiveness compelled behavioural conformity, apparently without physical coercion. Nevertheless, some social control seems to have been exercised since Father Divine controlled the 'context of communication' in the Kingdoms. This control was essential in order to prevent the expression, within the group, of perspectives contrary to Father Divine's.

While there seems to have been no evidence of physical coercion in the movement, one cannot minimise the potential coercive impact of a group able to restructure cognitively its members' views of the world around them and reorient their values. Bender and Spalding (1940) reported incidents of psychosocial disorders and a degree of well-being due to affiliation with the Father Divine movement.

Behavioural reinforcement obviously occurred both informally and through structured rituals. Meetings were developed to indoctrinate new converts, and the meeting places were designed to appear coherent and organised. Pictures of Father Divine were hung on the wall everywhere in the Kingdom.

Language, dress code, and leadership structure were very similar throughout 'heavens' in North America. By the mid-1930s, Father Divine had developed within the group a defined role and model for behaviour, values, speech patterns, and standards for right and wrong. A core group of disciples sought to model behaviour for the rest of the 'angels'.

The process of 'role-modelling' initiated in the empowerment phase reached maturity in the operational phase. Newcomers were encouraged to imitate the behaviour of individuals who had undergone the 'angelic' experience. Progress from simple imitation to emphatic identification and finally integration into the group was both individual and institutional. New members' full identification with the group peaked with a higher level of psychological and social integration. At this point, group membership and the personal life of the individual came together and emerged into a new start both in terms of social position and perception of self-worth (Larson, 1985).

CONCLUSION

We have attempted here to articulate a theory about the birth and early development of new African-American religious groups, emphasising first the elements that contribute to the gradual cultivation of a contextual terrain in which the new movement can take root. We have pointed out how a charismatic individual must then step forward and elaborate a philosophy of life and of hope that fits well with the terrain of need previously established. This philosophy must be naturally progressive and positive, but it must also take special cognisance of the experiences that African-Americans encounter daily in an environment plagued by racism and oppression. The most basic feature of the emerging black group is its ability to rely on race consciousness as the road to power in a society that restricts the pursuit of a meaningful life for black individuals.

We acknowledge several limitations in the exposition of our theory. We have relied on one Christian group that has been very successful. We are not sure, if at all, how our theory would fit those groups that have barely gotten off the ground. We have also paid attention to a major group led by men. At this time, we are not sure if groups led by black women have some unique elements that differentiate them from male-led groups. We have also specifically limited our attention to Christian movements, while being aware that non-Christian religious groups are alive and doing well both in the Caribbean and major urban areas of the United States. We think such groups appeal to new membership in fundamentally unique ways that contrast with techniques used by Christian groups, although some similarities between the two types of groups do exist.

Another important point to note is that the Father Divine Movement is practically unheard of today. So we cannot avoid the question as to what factors ultimately contribute to a group's demise, even after the group has been in existence for a long time. But we think it crucial to understand first how the new African-American religious group manages to make its initial embryonic steps. And we are obviously of the view that the integration of religion and psychological healing is a fundamental nexus in the African-American's use of a practical church group. Still, what maintains the new group or leads to its deterioration must be of interest to observers of these movements.

It would be useful in the future to apply our theory to a recently formed group such as Father Stallings' Imani Temple located in Washington, DC. Such a study could help answer questions about the elements that give birth to the group and what particular characterological features drive the group's leader to such impressive leadership activities. It is also possible that what is learned in the context of a religious movement might have some narrow application to understanding the birth and success of black, political, cult-like groups.

But that is a step in the future that must await better clarification of the black religious group. The tenacity of such groups in the African-American community reinforces the need to re-examine and reinterpret the legacy and spiritual foundation of the black experience in the Americas. Groups like the Imani Temple should also be closely studied on a longitudinal basis so that we can chart its development over decades.

REFERENCES

Baer, H. A. (1984) *The Black Spiritual Movement: A Religious Response to Racism*, Knoxville, TN: University of Tennessee Press.

Bender, L. and Spalding, M. (1940) 'Behavior problems in children from the homes of followers of Father Divine', *Journal of Nervous and Mental Disease* 89: 460–72.

Bender, L. and Yarrell, D. (1938) 'Psychoses among followers of Father Divine', *Journal of Nervous and Mental Disease* 87: 418–49.

Cantril, H. and Sherif, M. (1938) 'The Kingdom of Father Divine', *Journal of Abnormal and Social Psychology* 33: 141–67.

Clark, E. T. (1965) *The Small Sects in America*, Nashville, TN: Abingdon Press.

Dubois W. E. B. (1930) *The Negro Church*, Atlanta, GA: Atlanta University Press.

—— (1967) *The Philadelphia Negro*, New York: Schocken Books.

Fauset, A. H. (1978) *Black Gods of the Metropolis*, Philadelphia, PA: University of Pennsylvania Press.

Galanter, M. (1989a) *Cults: Faith, Healing and Coercion*, New York: Oxford University Press.

—— (ed.) (1989b) *Cults and New Religious Movements: A Report of the American Psychiatric Association Committee on Psychiatry and Religion*, Washington, DC: American Psychiatric Association.

Genovese, E. D. (1976) *Roll, Jordan Roll: The World the Slaves Made*, New York: Vintage Books.

Glazier, S.D. (1983) *Marchin' the Pilgrims Home: Leadership and Decision-Making in an Afro-Caribbean Faith*, Westport, CT: Greenwood Press.

Goodman, F. D., Henney, J. H. and Pressel, E. (1982) *Trance, Healing, and Hallucination*, Malabar, FL: Robert E. Krieger Publishing Company.

Griffith, E. E. H., English, T. and Mayfield, V. (1980) 'Possession, prayer, and testimony: therapeutic aspects of the Wednesday night meeting in a black church', *Psychiatry* 43: 120–8.

Griffith, E. E. H. and Mahy, G. E. (1984) 'Psychological benefits of Spiritual Baptist "Mourning"', *American Journal of Psychiatry* 141: 769–73.

Griffith, E. E. H., Mahy, G. E. and Young, J. L. (1986) 'Psychological benefits of Spiritual Baptist "Mourning" II: an empirical assessment', *American Journal of Psychiatry* 143: 226–9.

Griffith, E. E. H. and Mathewson, M. A. (1981) 'Communitas and charisma in a black church service', *Journal of the National Medical Association* 73: 1023–7.

Griffith, E. E. H., Young, J. L. and Smith, D. L. (1984) 'An analysis of the therapeutic elements in a black church service', *Hospital and Community Psychiatry* 35: 464–9.

Group for the Advancement of Psychiatry (1992) *Leaders and Followers: A Psychiatric Perspective on Religious Cults*, Washington, DC: American Psychiatric Press.

Hoshor, J. (1936) *God in the Rolls-Royce*, New York: Hillman Curl.

Larson, B. (1985) *Strange Cults in America*, Wheaton, IL: Tyndale House Publishers.

Levine, S. (1979) 'Roles of psychiatry in the phenomenon of cults', *Canadian Journal of Psychiatry* 26: 593–603.

—— (1981) 'Cults and mental health: clinical conclusions', *Canadian Journal of Psychiatry* 26: 534–9.

Lovelace, E. (1988) *The Wine of Astonishment*, London: Heinemann.

Osofsky, G. (1963) *Harlem: The Making of a Ghetto, 1890–1930*, New York: Harper & Row.

Parker, R. (1937) *The Incredible Messiah*, Boston: Little, Brown & Company.

Rohter, L. (1992) 'Sect's racketeering trial is set to open', *New York Times*, 6 January, p. A14.

Schoener, A. (1968) *Harlem on My Mind: Cultural Capital of Black America, 1990–1968*, New York: Random House.

Sessions, L. S. (1989) 'Black Catholics entangled in racial, religious conflict', *The Washington Post*, 3 August, p. A1.

Simpson, G. E. (1980) *Religious Cults of the Caribbean: Trinidad, Jamaica and Haiti*, 3rd edition, Rio Piedras, Puerto Rico: University of Puerto Rico.

Simpson, G. E. and Yinger, M. J. (1972) *Racial and Ethnic Minorities: An Analysis of Prejudice and Disrimination*, New York: Harper & Row.

Washington, J. R. (1973) *Black Sects and Cults*, New York: Anchor Press.

West, J. L. (1989) 'Persuasive techniques in contemporary cults: a public health approach', in M. Galanter (ed.) *Cults and New Religious Movements*, Washington, DC: American Psychiatric Association.

Williams, M. D. (1974) *Community in a Black Pentecostal Church*, Pittsburgh, PA: University of Pittsburgh Press.

Chapter 7

Hinduism and *Ayurveda*

Implications for managing mental health

Dinesh Bhugra

INTRODUCTION

In a book on religion and mental health, it is only right that one of the oldest religions, Hinduism, and its basic tenets are explored, and the implications for managing mental illness discussed. Hinduism as a religion has an incredible variety of expression, to the extent that it has been suggested that it is not possible to characterise it as a religion in the normal sense, since it is not a unitary concept nor a monolithic structure, but that it is rather the totality of the Indian way of life (Brockington, 1992). It will be fair to say that Hinduism does travel well and its symbols and motifs are seen outside India. What Brockington is implying is that the Indian way of thinking is inextricably linked with Hinduism, however, this also implies that the two can be equated, though this may not be always the case. From an Eurocentric viewpoint, Hinduism has been seen as a combination of innumerable subdivisions and subsections, and sub-subsections being a marked feature of the caste system (Beauchamp, 1906).

Dubois (1906) emphasises that the rule of all the Hindu princes and that of Mahomedans (sic) was, properly speaking, Brahminical rule. His imperial view of the ruled comes through his writing. This chapter does not purport to address the issue of colonialism and mental health (see Bhugra, 1993a). However, it must be emphasised that Hinduism has been seen as a positive and tolerant religion within a rigid prescriptive structure.

Certainly, there is no doctrine or ritual universal to the whole of Hinduism, and what is essential for one group need not be so for another. Furthermore, as Brockington (1992) points out, most people would accept that Hinduism is a definite and definable entity. A combination of beliefs, rituals, religious practice and minutiae of the activity form the religion. With Hinduism, where 40,000 gods and goddesses are available for prayer, and following the sheer volume of ritual and practice, it is an impossible task to offer an exhaustive description of the religion. One can, of course, look at the differences between various religions and try to make sense of Hinduism in that way, but any selective approach is doomed to failure when one is dealing with a vast religion like Hinduism. Brockington (1992) offers a way out by proposing that some internal and some external criteria can be laid down for Hinduism. The former can be a test of orthodoxy and the latter used for definition. The stereotypes of Hinduism, its rigidity of the caste system, and perceived obsessive behaviour can only add to the myths. Hinduism spread outside India, historically by cultural expansion to the Far East, but now Buddhism thrives there (see de Silva, this volume). The additional spread of Hinduism to the Caribbean and the Far East, like Fiji, was due to indentured labour. In addition, Westernised versions of Hinduism exist – the Hare Krishna cult being one such example (also see Barker, this volume). It is vital to consider the basic principles of Hinduism in relation to its practice. The reader is directed to various volumes that give excellent introductions to this topic (e.g., Brockington, 1992).

To a Hindu, religion is all-pervading, but that is not quite the same as being obsessively concerned about it. The practice of religion is internalised and it is neither extraneous nor imposed from outside.

BASIC PRINCIPLES

Castes

The most ancient and most ordinary classification divides Hindus into four *varnas* (Sanskrit equivalent of 'colour'). The first and the top of the hierarchy are *Brahmins* (the product of Lord Brahma – part of the Hindu trinity – arising from his forehead) who are responsible for priesthood and its various duties. The second rank belongs to *Kshtriyas* (arising from Brahma's arms, thereby indicating the warrior status) whose main function is to perform military service in all its branches. The third ranking is that of *Vaisyas*. They are the businessmen and the landlords (the product of Brahma's abdomen) and their main function is agriculture, trade and cattle breeding. The lowest rank of the hierarchy belongs to the *Sudras* (Mahatma Gandhi preferred the term *harijans* – the children of God). *Sudras* are said to have developed from the feet of Brahma and their main function is general servitude. Each of the main four castes is subdivided into many others, and the exact numbers are often difficult to enumerate. In some parts of India, especially in rural areas, the divisions within the castes and across the castes are very rigid and inter-caste marriages are frowned upon, even now. Dubois (1906) explains that it is easy to understand the allegorical significance of the origin of the castes in which one can distinctly trace the relative degrees of subordination of the different castes.

The caste system, as noted above, has a distinctive religious basis, in that *Dharma* and *Karma* go together. *Dharma*, though loosely translated, means religion – in Sanskritic terms – and covers a far wider span, incorporating not only the religious traditions but also social mores and requirements of law laid down by Manu (also see Doniger and Smith, 1991). *Karma*, on the other hand, represents literally action, but metaphorically denotes a wide-ranging combination of action and the belief that one's position in society and one's lot in this life are determined by one's actions in all previous lives. However, as Brockington (1992) cautions, the common view that belief in *Karma* is tantamount to fatalism rests on a misconception: one's present state is determined by one's own past activities, and one's future state is here and now, being determined by one's present actions, and so, basically, people can make themselves whatever they choose.

Vedas

Vedas are the source of all knowledge about Hinduism and have been considered the sole source of true religion. It is worth mentioning that the reading of *Vedas* was confined to the top three castes. Manu went as far as to recommend that if a *Sudra* hears Vedic words by accident, his ears should have molten lead poured into them as a punishment. As Brockington (1992) emphasises, in spite of the readings of *Vedas*, an accurate knowledge of it was lost at an early date and the works of medieval commentators give ample evidence of incomplete understanding, and the *Rgveda*, in particular, though handed down in the schools of reciters, remained unknown and uncharted territory to most philosophers and teachers.

Hinduism, as recorded in the four *Vedas*, is said to have originated with the Aryans settling into North India between 1500 and 1000 BC, although this has been questioned. The oldest of the four is *Rgveda*, with its obvious connections with the *Zoroastrian* influence. *Yajurveda, Samaveda* and *Atharvaveda* followed. The four *Vedas* are said to be the work of the God *Brahma* who wrote them with his own hand on leaves of gold. The myths of the origins of the religion and the writing of religious texts, as ever, are difficult to disentangle. Dubois (1906) alleges that the Brahmins invented (sic) the *Vedas* and the eighteen *Puranas*, the *Trimurti* (the Trinity of *Brahma, Vishnu* and *Mahesh*) and the monster fables connected with it, such as the *avtars* of Vishnu, the abominable *lingam* and the worship of the cow and other animals. Dubois' disapproval emerges in the tone of his writing, and he goes on to accuse the Brahmins of all these sacrilegious innovations very gradually. Brockington (1992), while discussing cow-worship, suggests that veneration of the cow has not only connections with the doctrine of non-violence but is also a reflection of the economic importance of the cow at an early period as a source of milk and related products. Many originally sensible hygienic practices were given religious status in order to enhance their observance. The use of cow dung and urine as purificatory materials has a practical as well as a religious aspect. The recommended use of the right hand for eating and the left hand for cleaning oneself after defaecation, can be seen as some safeguard against faeces-borne diseases. The problem, however, according to Brockington (1992), is that such practices, once given religious status, became fossilised into meaningless rituals.

The causes of ill-health, as perceived by the ancient communities, were external or internal. The former included climate changes, eating wrong or excessive food, poisoning and supernatural causes. These causes included the wrath of supernatural powers, sorcery and the evil eye. The management of illness therefore covered a wide range of treatments such as prayers, sacrifices, propitiation of spirits and gods, magic amulets, charms and medicines.

The impact of the Hindu religion also needs to be seen across a longitudinal time scale. Referring to the Indus civilisation (3250–2750 BC), Raina (1990) argues that the religious beliefs inferred from the excavations represent two types of images – representing the likeness of the object (iconic) and symbolic. The most remarkable object is that of Pasupati, which has three faces, three eyes, and two horns and is sitting on a throne-like structure. This image is that of Siva, who is stated to have composed the first work of medicine and is also the founder of the Sidhic system of medicine. The hymns of the *Rgveda* suggest that Harappans in the ancient civilisation were well-organised, wealthy people who had nutritious diets and who took considerable care in matters of personal hygiene and sanitation. The rulers of the Indus valley civilisation had an organised system. The presence of medicine pots, some drugs and weights suggests a carefully devised system of pharmacy. Since both secular and magico-religious medicines were used, Raina (1990) assumes that the physicians were priest – physicians. In the latter periods of *Rgveda* (around 2500 BC), the medicinal hymns and knowledge were also attributed to Brahma, Vishnu and Siva. Asvins – twin brothers who were physicians – were described in *Rgveda*. It is reported that the success gained by Asvins raised them in the estimation of all. Unlike gods, they are human – although they are described along with the gods. They are described as handsome, wearing garlands of lotus flowers, swift-handed, rescuers, and fond of honey and *soma*. In addition to providing rejuvenation, they are also responsible for restoring eyesight, deliveries, correcting weaknesses and providing artificial limbs. The Asvins are credited with writing abstracts of treatment, a treatise on medicine and other works and in addition to being healers, they are also identified in cosmic terms – as moisture and light, heaven and earth, and day and night. Sarasvati is the first female physician, but she is also the goddess of knowledge and wisdom. She belongs to the group of gods and goddesses associated with procreation, and is said to have propounded formulae for the cure of sterility in women and seminal insufficiency in men (Raina, 1990). Another goddess, Shivali, has been written about as either an obstetrician or a birth attendant and people would pray to her to prevent miscarriages. She too is bestowed with divine status.

In *Atharvaveda*, maladies due to supernatural agencies are listed and along with incantations, invocations and exorcisms, drugs too are recommended. In this era, great emphasis was placed on marital harmony, as well as harmony between body and mind, between mind and knowledge, between neighbours as well as with strangers. This could be seen as the existential balance in a broad systems analysis.

The *Rgveda* recognises thirty-three gods connected with heaven, earth and the waters of the air. The essential ingredients of the sacrifice were fire and *soma*, which were accorded high prestige. The hymns of *Rgveda* were probably composed in the Brahmavata region (probably modern Haryana) and the 1028 hymns composed in stanzas, often grouped in threes, were composed in fifteen different metres. The collection is divided into ten books, and the hymns appear addressed to different gods in order of diminishing importance. *Agni*, the god of fire, is invoked in some 200 hymns. In the Hindu scriptures, *Ramayana* and *Mahabharata, Agni* appears time and again and represents not only cremation and destruction but also the heat of sexual desire, thereby helping emperors to impregnate their wives. Often the image portrayed is that, during the *yajna, Agni* appears with a bowl full of *kshir* (rice cooked in milk). The role of *Agni* is identified with the householder and also as sacrificial fire. *Agni* is said to drive away diseases, purify, reduce high temperatures, cure indigestion and, using one of its seven tongues, able to eat various demons. *Indra* was the most popular and was the dominant deity of the region between Earth and Heaven. His virtues and functions are described at some length in the *Rgveda. Samaveda*, on the other hand, comprises a handbook of the chants. The *Yajurveda* is a compilation of ritual material drawn from Rgvedic hymns. *Atharvaveda*, like *Rgveda*, is a collection of complete hymns. The pantheon of the *Rgveda* is preserved in the *Atharvaveda* and the latter consists of a diverse compilation of spells for every purpose. The older *Upanisads*, according to Brockington (1992), can be regarded as a natural continuation of the creation hymns in the tenth book of the *Rgveda* and of certain cosmological hymns of the *Atharvaveda*. These date from the eighth century BC and are properly Vedic. Most of the *Upanisads* are in dialogue form and contained within are occasionally great sets of debates. In addition to the nature of *Brahman*, the *Upanisads* also demonstrate a tendency towards inwardness fostered by dissatisfaction with the externals of the religion – the concept of the *atman*, the permanent soul, often equated with *prana* or breath. These are the main preoccupations, and yogis often use these principles not only for meditation but also for taking control of the body – a method often used in India for managing anxiety (also in Buddhism, see de Silva, this volume).

The word *Ayurveda* (knowledge of long life) first appears in the medical *samhitas*. Generally, it is considered as an *upveda* (a subdivision) of the *Atharvaveda*. The divine origin of *Ayurveda* is emphasised in all ancient medical treatises. Since *atman* is not born and does not die, it is eternal and indestructible. Beyond the senses are the objects, beyond which is the *manas* (mind); beyond the great is the unmanifest; beyond the unmanifest is the *purusa*, beyond which there is nothing. This idea of nothingness beyond a great soul, or self, in a way encourages Hindus to think of control being within and yet without. This can enable one to take charge of one's actions and destiny without being too fatalistic.

A work of encyclopaedic scope, *Manavadharma Sastra* or *Manusmrti*, consists of 2685 verses on various topics. *Manusmrti* remains a pivotal text of the dominant form of Hinduism as it emerged historically and at least in part in reaction to its religious and ideological predecessors and competitors (Doniger and Smith, 1991). As these authors suggest, no modern study of Hindu family life, psychology, concepts of the body, sex, relationships between humans and animals, attitudes to money and material possessions, politics, law, caste, purification and pollution, ritual social practice and ideals and world renunciation and worldly goals, can ignore Manu. The true authorship of this volume is not clear, although attributed to Manu, it was probably composed by various gurus, and this was not only a text by the *Brahmins* but also for the *Brahmins*. In Vedic texts, social ideology was fixated on food. The doctrine of *ahimsa* (non-violence) encouraged individuals to challenge the Vedic text which encouraged that those more powerful and higher on the food chain (humans) consume those weaker and below (animals). Vegetarianism, though the standard practice amongst the *Brahmins*, had a limited place among the *Kshtriyas* who were encouraged to hunt, and the *Sudras* who were supposed to deal with dead animals. Its rationale is linked with the doctrine of non-violence. Since the *Vedas* were established quite early on as unquestionable revelation, they are seen as the source of all knowledge and as the canonical touchstone for all subsequent 'orthodox' truth claims. Manu deals with the laws of *Karma* and creation of various classes of beings and restriction of food, and punishments for various acts of violence, theft and injury to humans and animals. The discussion of good and evil is an important aspect of the writings of Manu (for details see Doniger and Smith, 1991). *Manusmrti* not only advises kings about justice but also outlines the roles of householders and their behaviour. There is advice about choosing a wife and about the role of women and their dependence. The individual is advised to concentrate his mind (because) 'a man should see everything, including what is real and unreal, in the self, for if he sees everything in the self he will not set his mind on what is wrong'.

Ayurveda

The traditional Ayurvedic texts, which deal with the Indian method of medicine, have been dated several centuries BC (Bhugra, 1992). The *Rgveda* is among the world's oldest books and contains descriptions of surgical procedures (Balodhi, 1984). Of the original eight texts, *Caraka Samhita* deals with medical diagnoses and management, and *Sushruta Samhita* with surgical procedures and texts. *Atharva-Veda* mentions mental illnesses, largely as a result of divine curses. *Sushruta* states that the original *Samhita* was in 1000 chapters and 10,000 verses but, because of the poor intellect and short life-span of human beings, these 1000 chapters were recast into eight divisions, and of these, one division dealt with illnesses of body and mind. The eight divisions were as follows: *salya tantra* (surgery); *salakya* (minor surgery); *kayachiktisa* (medicine); *bhuta vidya* (demonology); *kumara bhartya* (paediatrics); *agada tantra* (toxicology); *rasayana* (tonics and vitalisation) and *vajakarana tantra* (aphrodisiacs). Of the eight divisions, *Salya tantra* deals with the description and uses of surgical instruments and appliances, preparation and properties of cautery, removal of external substances, e.g. grass, wood, stones, and of internal substances manufactured by the body, e.g. pus, blood. *Salakya tantra* deals with diseases of the eyes, nose and ear. *Kayachiktisa* deals with internal medicine. *Bhuta vidya* dictates the rules to be observed in performing various religious procedures, offering sacrifices to gods and conciliating planetary influences in order to deal with possessions by any of the eight possible sources. The other *tantras* are self-explanatory. As noted above, for centuries valuable knowledge was passed on through verses for easy memorisation and transmission. However, because original texts were not always strictly followed, newer components were added, which makes it difficult to differentiate between the original and subsequent materials.

Siddha system of medicine is practised in some parts of the Indian subcontinent and, as noted elsewhere, Siva is the first teacher of this system. The five components are: *janamja* (from previous birth); *ausidhija* (medicine can make the body healthy); *mantraja* (mind can be made peaceful through *mantra*); *tapaja* (attaining perfection through prayers, and getting rid of unclean elements); and *samadhi* (through meditation merging oneself with supreme being). The aim of the *siddha* is to achieve the state of imperishable body (Raina, 1990). In the Siddha system, great attention is paid to the biochemical nature of a living cell and to processes of degeneration and regeneration. This was to be attained through yoga, personal discipline and drugs. The aim was to use drugs which, unlike herbs, could be kept stored for a longer period. They also focused on metals and elements (minerals) which could be used to prolong life and maintain the body as healthy, vigorous and youthful through *kayakalpa* (changing the body), and to prevent death.

Ayurvedic *samhitas* observe fine arts, dance and music to be an essential part of life. The effects of music on digestion of food and the descriptions of *rasas* (sentiments) are of great value to mental health professionals (see Raina, 1991).

Caraka Samhita is the foremost text of the ancient Indian medical system. The spiritual and possession explanations of mental illness in the *Atharva-Veda* were not displaced by the subsequent development of medical humeral system, but came to rest together in concepts and in management. The Hindus class schools of thought as *shastras* or systems, and each have a common body of doctrines (*sutras*), explanation (*bhashya*) and commentary (*teeka*) (Balodhi, 1983). *Caraka* emphasised that the mind has two purposes: atomic and indivisible unity (*Caraka Samhita*, vol. III, p. 975). The functions of the mind are direction of the senses, control of itself, reasoning and deliberation. Beyond this is the field of intellect. Man is composed of twenty-four elements: mind plus ten organs (five each cognitive and conative), five sense objects and eight *prakriti*, or evolutes of nature.

Theories of *Ayurveda*

Caraka advanced a holistic view of life, and included not only the physical aspects but also social, ethical and spiritual aspects of health and disease. *Caraka* did not consider the laws of *Karma* to be immutable and allowed a limited amount of freedom to human efforts. The 'cognitive triad' for well-being was desire for self-preservation, desire for wealth and desire for a happy future. Any consequences of ordinary or non-moral actions can be averted by the exercise of human intelligence, wisdom, well-balanced conduct and appropriate medical treatment.

Caraka's observation was of the human body being an aggregate volume of cells – where growth depends upon *karma, vayu* (air, but can be equated with bio-energy) and *svabhava* (personal nature or habits). *Ayu* (life) is a combination of *shareera* (body), *indriya* (senses), *satva* (psyche) and *atma* (soul). *Manas* (mind) has three operational qualities (*satwik, rajas* and *tamas*). These qualities are often, to this day, used in typologies, e.g. of food or personality. *Satva* includes self-control, knowledge of the self and an ability to discriminate (i.e. make thought-out choices). *Rajas* is indicated by violence, despotic envy and authoritarianism. *Tamas* reflects dullness and inaction.

The Ayurvedic theory of *dosas* may have developed independently, or possibly the Hindu system may have travelled westwards (Davis and Deb Sikdar, 1960). Obeyesekere (1982) has proposed that the Ayurvedic principles are derived from the superimposition of metaphysical ideas upon concepts of physiological function and dysfunction. The descriptions of constitution and personality types according to *Caraka* have been described elsewhere (see Bhugra, 1992, for a review). The basic doctrine included five *bhutas* (the basic elements of the universe); the *tridosa* (three humours) and the seven *dhatus* (basic components of the body). The five elements are ether (*ksa*), wind (*vayu*), water (*āp*), earth (*prithvi*) and fire (*agni*) (Obeyesekere, 1976). The Buddhist tradition adds consciousness (*cetana*) (Filliozat, 1964) to this list.

Bhutas were known by different names such as *bhuta, grahasattva, vayu, raksa, gandharva, pisacha*, etc. The stronger *grahas* were called *maha grahas*. These *grahas* enter the body unnoticed, as an image enters into a mirror. The persons attacked with *grahas* do not recollect such incidences after the fits. Various *tantric* practices were common which would affect the person such as *sammohana, prasvapna, sam vanana anjanaprayoga* and *antardhna. Mantras, yogas* and *mulas* (roots) were used for these. The people proficient in this study were called *narendra*. The *tridosic* theory was responsible for maintaining the good health of the individual.

Physical health of the individual is maintained when the three humours are in perfect harmony. When these are upset, they become *dosas* or troubles of the organism. The three humours are fundamental to body functioning. The universal element of wind appears in the body as a humour and illnesses result due to disequilibrium of these conditions (Obeyesekere, 1976).

The belief that certain illnesses are related to the seasons is also linked to the *prakriti* (the constitution) of the individual. The most notorious disease related to heat, according to Obeyesekere, was smallpox and this, along with mumps and measles, the Ayurvedic physicians found difficult to allay or control. Hence the interpretation of these diseases became strongly associated with religion and ritual – a metamedical interpretation of illness and its cure. If an illness was caused by the anger of one of the humours, the metamedical view postulated that the anger (*kopa*) of the relevant deity was responsible through stimulation of the appropriate humour. The rituals included worshipping the goddess Sheetla and tying sacred threads around a *peepul* tree and offering prayers and sweets. In Tamilnadu and Sri Lanka, for example, the goddess *pattini* was seen as responsible for fire and droughts. When gods intervened with her and the rain came from the heavens the people offered milk in new pots to the goddess. Thus, fire was opposed by water, and drought (depletion of fertility) was corrected by milk (fertility), which is also a soothing, cooling and cold substance. For a detailed discussion of this and other symbolisms, the reader is directed to Obeyesekere (1976).

Classification of illnesses

In addition to the beliefs described above, the concepts of *jadu tona* in North India and various other forms of sorcery exist in South India. *Tona* includes an earthen pot full of food with a lit *deeya* (oil lamp), red thread and rice that is always left at a crossing. The first person to come across it is expected to take the evil. To avoid or cast away the evil eye, red chili powder is thrown on an open fire along with incantations. In Sri Lanka, five *bhutas* are used in sorcery and ash melon fruits are used for the purpose. Religious specialists may prescribe Ayurvedic medicines along with their medico-religious curing techniques, though Ayurvedic physicians are less likely to offer supernatural cures.

The most important concept which links the Ayurvedic and religious traditions is to do with *dosa* (literal meaning, fault or trouble). In Sinhalese sub-culture, the *dosa* also refers to the troubles caused by actions of supernatural beings. According to Obeyesekere (1976), these are *preta* (meaning ancestral spirit), *yaksa* (demons), *asvha* and *katavaha* (effects by gods), *huniyan* (caused by sorcery), *graha* (misfortunes), and *karma* (due to bad karma). Ayurvedic and supernatural theories are linked by the external and internal aetiological theories of causation of illness. The three *dhatus* of *vayu, pitta* and *kapha*, and three types of *prakriti* (constitution), along with different varieties of food, thus give a range of diseases (see Bhugra, 1992, for further details). *Vayu* or *vat* is responsible for movement: coordinator of external and internal movements; adjusting the movements to suit environment. *Pitta* appears to be the thermal regulating device keeping heat at the optimum level in order to regulate the body's metabolism. *Kapha* is the main ground substance of all the constituents of the human body.

The diseases in *Ayurveda* are divided into those of *sirir* (body) and *manasa* (mind). These can be endogenous (*nij*) or exogenous (*agantuk*). They are further subdivided into seven subdivisions – three in endogenous and four in exogenous categories, viz. inherited from parents (*adibalpravarta*), congenital from the womb (*janambalpravata*), psychosomatic disease and disorders due to metabolic or nutritional factors (*doshbal pravarta*), injury from physical, chemical and biological sources (*samghatbal pravarta*); disease due to climate and seasons (*kalbal pravarta*); supernatural causes (*devyabalpravarta*) and natural causes like hunger, thirst, fatigue (*swabhavabal pravarta*) etc. *Sushruta* classified these in three groups, viz. those with source in oneself (*adhyatmic*) including *adibal, janambal* and *doshbal pravarta*; sources in the creatures and physical elements of the world (*adhibhantika*) including *samghatbal pravarta*; and, finally, supernatural and natural factors (*adhidavik*), which include *kalbal, devbal* and *swabhavbal pravartes* (Raina, 1990). *Sushruta* argues that *dosas* are the root of all diseases.

Internal diseases were of the two basic types, those that included and manifested symptoms of *yaksma* (consumption) and *takmān* (fever) and those that included *āmīvā*, tetanus, ascites, insanity, worms, urine retention and constipation. External afflictions involved broken bones, flesh wounds, loss of hair and various types of skin disorders. A third category of morbid bodily conditions resulted from different types of poison. Poison had both visible and invisible causes. The long and renowned tradition of toxicology in Indian medicine is well known.

Management

Unlike the Egyptian and Mesopotamian systems, the Indian diagnosis did not include divination. Determination of cause of one's affliction was accomplished by isolating and identifying dominant and recurring symptoms, many of which were considered to be separate demonic entities. Since the emphasis was on the absence of disease-causing agents, there were many sound states (Zysk, 1991). Elimination of morbid bodily conditions was the domain of a healer who was male and whose professional craft was the curing of the sick by the removal of disease demons and the repair of injuries. A Vedic healer possessed only a superficial notion of human anatomy and, since they were not necessarily of *Brahmin* class, they could not perform sacrificial rituals. The evidence suggests that in the Vedic period the purpose of learning about bodily parts was religious rather than scientific, although the anatomical information offered in the religious documents approaches scientific precision.

In the *Rgveda*, *soma* is the juice of a milky climbing plant extracted and fermented to form a beverage liked by the gods and priests (Mukhopadhyaya, 1922/1974). The soma-oblations are directed to be made three times a day to *Agni, Indra* and the *Rishis. Soma* juice is an immortal draught and medicine for a sick man, and all the gods drank it. According to Mukhopadhyaya, *soma* also refers to the moon and is also a god, though in some contexts *soma* is seen as *amrit* (nectar) (equivalent to the Greek ambrosia) and refers also to drink. Thus, the relationship between religion, medicine and gods becomes increasingly strong.

The Ayurvedic *samhitas* make a special reference to the qualities of the student who should be given instructions in *Ayurveda* along with the qualities of the teacher of *Ayurveda* who takes pupils in front of *agni* (fire) as a witness. The students need to be well behaved, brave, clean in habit, modest, possessed of bodily strength, firmness, intelligence, good memory, a desire to learn and achieve success, honest, cheerful and able to bear pain and trouble. The students were to give up lust, anger, avarice, folly, vanity, pride, envy, rudeness, deception and idleness. They were to treat poor people, ascetics and orphans and those travelling long distances free and as their friends.

However, the importance and role of food need to be described here, albeit briefly. The wind in the body (*vata*) is often related to different kinds of diet and dietary patterns, and the juice of food (*vasa*) produces blood (*rakta*) which produces *mansa* (flesh). From flesh arises fat (*medas*) which produces bone (*asthi*) which gives rise to marrow (*majja*) which eventually produces semen (*sukra*). Individual personality characteristics and the seasonal variation affect all these processes. Thus, semen is said to be the most highly refined element in the body – 'the vital juice' toning the whole organism (Das Gupta, 1922; Filliozat, 1964).

In general, insanity is said to be the result of an inappropriate diet; disrespect towards the gods, teachers and the twice-born (the *brahmin*); mental shock due to excessive fear or joy and faulty bodily activity. The descriptions of various illnesses have appeared elsewhere (Bhugra, 1992). Suffice it to say that the diagnostic systems did involve collecting both subjective and objective information.

PRACTICAL IMPLICATIONS

In *Ayurveda*, the four major components of any therapeutic regimen had to include the physician, the drugs and the attendants along with the patient. In addition to drugs, various *yajnas* with specific offerings to *Agni* were recommended. In exogenous type of mental disorders psychotherapy was used quite extensively. Talismans and charms were often employed together with religious discourses and prayers. The relatives and friends were advised and taught to calm the patient by religious and moral discourses. Guilt emanating from Karmic deeds was treated by culturally determined observances, for example, religious rituals and dietary restrictions.

The treatment was directed towards removing the cause or repairing the tissue and building the resistance of the body. In addition to relieving the symptoms, treatment was offered to bring about the proper balance of *dosas*. Some special therapeutic procedures were developed over the years such as the purificatory fivefold procedure – the *pancha-karma* in *Ayurveda* – a similar procedure in yoga but without the use of drugs, and *kaya-kalpan* in *Siddha*. In addition to cleaning the body and building resistance, there are other procedures such as vitalisation (*rasayana*) and virilification (*vajikarna*). Their aims are to replenish the worn-out tissues of the body, strengthening vitality and combating infirmities of old age and promoting long life (Raina, 1991).

Surya and Jayaram (1964) have criticised Indian psychiatrists as products of Western learning with the usage of foreign words and concepts. This legacy of colonialism needs to be taken into consideration when ascertaining the client – therapist interactions. British colonial rule had led to a destruction of the traditional Ayurvedic system of medicine, certainly in urban areas, and through identification with rulers' acceptance of the Western system occurred the further detriment of the Ayurvedic practice. With the introduction of mental asylums, the emphasis shifted to containment, thereby medicalisation of mental illness developed further with little emphasis on psychotherapeutic interactions (Lloyd and Bhugra, 1993).

In traditional societies, with emphasis on therapeutic relationships using the bridge of religion and religious values, the preachers and the religious leaders offer 'group' therapy using parables, stories and models from the scriptures. Within such gatherings, possession states occur frequently and are accepted as a way of expressing distress. The failure of Western psychotherapy in India (Neki, 1975) is due to various reasons – of these, non-reliance on ego-psychology is only one, and illiteracy, poverty and lack of cultural relevance are others. Neki (1973) had gone on to develop themes of *guru-chela* (teacher – pupil) relationship in the context of psychotherapy. This meant that the therapist had to be more active and directive and the patient had to follow certain rules implicit in the traditions of the religion. Often role models from scriptures have been used to put the patient's suffering in context by suggesting that if god incarnates had to suffer, the suffering of humans is relatively insignificant. In the West, psychotherapy is the cultural undertaking to meet the deficits of the Western way of life and to cope with negative psychological implications of its premises. The cosmic existential and religious values are vital in determining the success or failure of psychotherapy but these are virtually never assessed. Cultural differences in cognitive and linguistic styles are also important in the acceptance or rejection of psychotherapy.

The implications of the knowledge of *Ayurveda* in managing patients in modern-day clinical practice are important. The origins of symptoms of burning in parts of or the whole body can be traced to folk beliefs derived from Ayurvedic systems in which 'burning' of the body is a main component of the diseases described.

As Obeyesekere (1976) emphasised, *Ayurveda* is more than a system of physical medicine because its underlying ideas have permeated religion and ritual. As noted earlier, semen is virtually the essence of life and any loss is obviously of great importance (see Bhugra and Buchanan, 1989; Bhugra and de Silva, 1993, for further discussion of semen loss anxiety). However, it is worth emphasising here that the Indian *dhat* syndrome constitutes a distinct clinical entity where nocturnal emissions lead to severe anxiety, hypochondriasis and often sexual impotence. The patients attribute their distress to an excessive loss of semen and appear tense, preoccupied, seeking a cure for the imaginary loss of semen with urine. Bottero (1991) suggested that any Ayurvedic physician is likely to have 15 to 20 per cent of his consultations related to semen loss anxiety (also see Paris, 1992). Malhotra and Wig (1975), using a case vignette of nocturnal emission, interviewed 110 respondents from four socio-economic classes. Their sample acknowledged that semen loss is harmful and the preservation of semen was seen as a guarantee of health and longevity. There were differences across social classes – the lower classes being in favour of medical intervention. Avoidance of certain kinds of food was seen as extremely important. In addition to the personality and the seasons, which affect the individual's health and functioning, food is a very important factor indeed (see above). De Silva and Dissanayake (1989) assessed a group of thirty-eight males attending a university clinic in Sri Lanka and observed that, though the four groups of complaints recorded were to do with physical symptoms with or without mental symptoms and sexual dysfunction and anxiety, especially about the sexual functioning, the underlying theme was that of semen loss, which they called 'the loss of semen syndrome'. The Ayurvedic physicians in India and Sri Lanka promote and perpetuate these myths through hoardings, the press and other advertisements. In India, huge hoardings display pictures of these *hakims* and *vaids* in masculine garb with turbans and gun-belts and they sell their medicines in different categories of platinum, gold, silver, etc., and charge accordingly. Thus, these culturally held cognitions are transmitted powerfully.

The medical hymns of the *Atharvaveda* indicate that therapy was carried out by means of specialised healing rites, in the course of which *mantras* or charms from the sacred text were recited and various activities characteristic of the healing seance were performed (Zysk, 1991). The recounting of mythological events pertaining mostly to diseases and plants was central. This recitation was a ritual and this Atharvavedic medical charm presents a mythology specific to the function of healing. Divinities of the traditional Vedic pantheon are mentioned, usually as subordinates to the dominant Atharvavedic deity, often because their characteristics resemble those of the gods being addressed. As Zysk (1991) points out, the existence of a medical mythology, pointing to a particular Vedic tradition, had the principal function of restoring members of the society to physical and mental wholesomeness and of maintaining them in this condition through specialised rituals. Its practitioners were not a part of the priestly, sacrificial tradition, but were able to borrow elements freely from it to accomplish their tasks. Zysk argues that evidence from the medical mythology of *Atharvaveda* suggests a conscious effort by followers of this tradition to combine aspects of priestly and medical traditions, perhaps to authorise the latter in a society dominated by the former, and to make the healers equivalent to the sacrificial priests, at least within the arena of medical ritual.

The use of charms is not uncommon and these are worn for many reasons, such as immunity from diseases, protection from the evil eye, from malignant stars, from accidents and for good luck. Among the believers, there is a common belief that the protection provided by the amulets is for the body and not for the welfare of the soul. Thus, *sanyasis* will not wear amulets. Amulets may be cylindrical, worn on the arm or around the neck and made of iron, copper, knotted thread, or wish threads. For mental disorder, the amulet should be made of *palan* root (*Butea frondosa*), against witchcraft, made from the bark of the *gua babla* and *nagdona* leaf, and against evil spirits, from *mantras* and rotten wood struck by lightning.

Shamans or medicine men may be both priests and shamans. Various rituals have different meanings and often shamans are invited to help get rid of evil spirits. Such a spirit is invited to leave by simple rituals, initially. If these fail, elaborate rituals are then carried out. For protection against diseases, several other practices are encouraged. Some of the simple ones include decorating the front door with mango leaves, but other rituals are more complex.

The Hindu scriptures are often used as models for psychotherapy in modern India. The concepts of *guru-chela* had been derived from the *Bhagvadgita*. Parables and stories are used to show the universality of human suffering and to facilitate rapport between therapist and patient. Group therapy using the reading of the *shastras* has been described (Unnikrishnan, 1966). Recent work has demonstrated the efficacy of using *Agnihotra* (a Vedic ritual of lighting a fire and offering prayers) in cases of alcohol and drug addiction (Golechha *et al.*, 1991).

Yoga and meditation have been used frequently in managing anxiety (Vahia *et al.*, 1966, 1973), and developing optimum body functioning and social and environmental integration (Vahia, 1969).

Faith and the power of suggestion are important therapeutic factors frequently employed in the religious temples (Somasundaram, 1973). Satyanand (1961) emphasised: 'Religion is a pattern of ego-feeling, and ego-boundaries are given specific functions. A particular self-concept, namely, "Who am I?" is its main assumption.' The therapeutic value of religious sentiment needs to be reestablished. A combined approach using psychiatric and spiritual insights is effective in managing certain patients (Stringham, 1969).

It is important to emphasise that this has been a brief introduction to a complex religion. The traditional beliefs about origins of illness, its course, prognosis and treatment are seen wherever Hindus live. However, it raises a very interesting issue about the impact of the therapist's culture on the therapist – patient interaction. Furthermore, if a therapist from one culture is trained in another culture and then returns to the original culture, how are these dilemmas resolved? It is certainly possible that a modicum of culture shock will occur, but with the clinical skills, cultural sensitivity and practical training it should be possible to minimise such shocks (see Bhugra, 1993b, for further discussion of some of these issues).

The basic knowledge of the system will enable the therapist to be of maximum assistance to those who may need help in managing their distress and stress. The practical implications discussed above offer only a limited glimpse into using Hindu beliefs of religion in the management of some psychiatric conditions.

REFERENCES

Balodhi, J. P. (1983) 'Methodology of shastra in India', *The Vedic Path* xiv: 21–6.
—— (1984) 'Phenomenology of aggression in ancient Indian thought: an analysis of Rig Veda', *The Vedic Path* xiv: 14–20.
Beauchamp, H. K. (1906) Introduction, in A. J. Dubois, *Hindu Manners, Customs and Ceremonies*, Delhi: Oxford University Press.
Bhugra, D. (1992) 'Psychiatry in ancient Indian texts: a review', *History of Psychiatry* 3: 167–86.
—— (1993a) 'Colonial psyche: British influence on Indian psychiatry', unpublished manuscript.
Bhugra, D. (1993b) 'Influence of culture on presentation and management of patients', in D. Bhugra and J. Leff (eds) *Principles of Social Psychiatry*, Oxford: Blackwell.
—— and Buchanan, A. (1989) 'Impotence in ancient Indian texts', *Sexual and Marital Therapy* 7: 87–92.
Bhugra, D. and de Silva, P. (1993) 'Sexual dysfunction across cultures', *International Review of Psychiatry* 5: 243–52.
Bottero, A. (1991) 'Consumption by semen loss in India and elsewhere', *Culture, Medicine and Psychiatry* 15: 303–20.
Brockington, J. L. (1992) *The Sacred Thread: A Short History of Hinduism*, New Delhi: Oxford University Press.
Caraka Samhita (1949) six volumes. Jamnagar: Shree Gulab Kunerba Ayurvedic Society.
Das Gupta, S. N. (1922) *A History of Indian Philosophy*, 2 vols, Cambridge: Cambridge University Press.

Davis, R. and Deb Sikdar, B. (1960) 'Body fluids 500 BC', *Indian Journal of Psychiatry* (ii): 6–9.

de Silva, P. and Dissanayake, S. A. W. (1989) 'The loss of semen syndrome in Sri Lanka', *Sexual and Marital Therapy* 4: 195–204.

Doniger, W. and Smith, B. (1991) *The Laws of Manu*, New Delhi: Penguin.

Dubois, A. J. (1906) *Hindu Manners, Customs and Ceremonies*, Delhi: Oxford University Press.

Filliozat, J. (1964) *The Classical Doctrine of Indian Medicine*, trans. D. R. Channa, Delhi: Munshiram Manoharlal.

Golechha, G. R., Sethi, I. C. and Deshpande, U. R. (1991) '*Agnihotra* in the treatment of alcoholism', *Indian Journal of Psychiatry*, 33: 20–6.

Lloyd, K. and Bhugra, D. (1993) 'Cross-cultural aspects of psychotherapy', *International Review of Psychiatry* 5: 291–304.

Malhotra, H. K. and Wig, N. N. (1975) 'Dhat syndrome: a culture-bound neurosis of the Orient', *Archives of Sexual Behaviour*, 4: 519–28.

Mukhopadhyaya, G. N. (1922/1974) *History of Indian Medicine*, vols 1 and 2, New Delhi: Oriental Books Reprint Corp.

Neki, J. S. (1973) 'Guru-Chela relationship: the possibility of a therapeutic paradigm', *American Journal of Orthopsychiatry* 3: 755–66.

—— (1975) 'Psychotherapy in India: past, present and future', *American Journal of Psychotherapy* 29: 92–100.

Obeyesekere, G. (1976) 'The impact of Ayurvedic ideas on the culture and the individual in Sri Lanka', in A. D. Leslie (ed.) *Asian Medical Systems*, Berkeley, CA: University of California Press.

—— (1982) 'Science and psychological medicine in the Ayurvedic tradition', in A. J. Marsella and G. M. White (eds) *Cultural Conceptions of Mental Health and Therapy*, Dordrecht: A. Reidel.

Paris, J. (1992) 'Dhat: the semen loss anxiety syndrome', *Transcultural Psychiatric Research Review* 29: 109–18.

Raina, B. N. (1990) *Health Science in Ancient India*, New Delhi: Commonwealth Publishers.

—— (1991) *Health Science: March Through Centuries*, New Delhi: Commonwealth Publishers.

Satyanand, D. (1961) 'A comparative study of scientific and religious psychotherapy with a special study of the role of the commonest Shivite symbolic model vs total psychoanalysis', *Indian Journal of Psychiatry* 3: 261–73.

Somasundaram, O. (1973) 'Religious treatment of mental illness in Tamil Nadu', *Indian Journal of Psychiatry* 15: 38–48.

Stringham, J. A. (1969) 'Resentment (Bitterness, hostility and hate) symptoms and treatment', *Indian Journal of Psychiatry* 11: 15–22.

Surya, N. and Jayaram, S. (1964) 'Some basic considerations in the practice of psychotherapy in the Indian setting', *Indian Journal of Psychiatry* 6: 153–6.

Unnikrishnan, K. P. (1966) 'Research in Ajurvedic psychiatry', *Indian Journal of Psychiatry* 8: 56–9.

Vahia, N. S. (1969) 'A therapy based upon some concepts prevalent in India', *Indian Journal of Psychiatry* 9: 7–14.

Vahia, N. S., Doongaji, D. R., Jeste, D. V., Kapoor, S. N., Ardhapurkar, I. and Ravindra, Nath S. (1973) 'Further experience with the therapy based upon concepts of Patanjali in the treatment of psychiatric disorders', *Indian Journal of Psychiatry*, 15: 32–7.

Vahia, N. S., Vinekar, S. L. and Doongaji, D. R. (1966) 'Some ancient Indian concepts in the treatment of psychiatry disorders', *British Journal of Psychiatry* 122: 1089–96.

Zysk, K. G. (1991) *Asceticism and Healing in Ancient India: Medicine in the Buddhist Monastery*, Delhi: Oxford University Press.

Chapter 8

Buddhist psychology and implications for treatment

Padmal de Silva

INTRODUCTION

Buddhism originated in Northern India several centuries before the Christian era. As a religion and a philosophical system, it grew in influence quite rapidly, and spread both to the south and to the far east. This growth and expansion also led to the development of various schools and sects which, while retaining a core set of teachings, differed from one another in details of practice and theory. The focus of this chapter is on Early Buddhism, also known as Therav¡da Buddhism. The main texts of early Buddhism are called the canon, and are in the Pali language. The Pali canon was put together at a council of monks shortly after the Buddha's death and was committed to writing in Sri Lanka in the first century BC (Saddhatissa, 1976). It consists of three parts, known as the 'three baskets' (*Tipiṭaka*). These are the *Vinaya Piṭaka*, containing the rules of discipline for the monks; the *Sutta Piṭaka*, containing discourses of the Buddha on various occasions; and the *Abhidhamma Piṭaka*, containing philosophical and psychological analyses that were finalised in their present form about 250 BC, later than the material in the other two parts.

The main teachings of the Buddha are contained in the Four Noble Truths (Rahula, 1959; Saddhatissa, 1971):

1 Life is marked by 'suffering' and is unsatisfactory (*dukkha*).
2 The cause (*samudaya*) of this suffering is desire, or craving.
3 This 'suffering' can be ended (*nirodha*) via the cessation of desire or craving: this is the state of *Nibbana*.
4 There is a way (*magga*) to achieve this cessation, which is the Noble Eightfold Path.

The Noble Eightfold Path is also called the Middle Path, as it avoids the extremes of a sensuous and luxurious life on the one hand and a life marked by self-mortification on the other. The Middle Path is described as consisting of eight aspects: right understanding, right thought, right speech, right action, right livelihood, right effort, right mindfulness, and right concentration. The individual who undertakes a life based on this path, renouncing worldly attachments, hopes eventually to attain the *arahant* state, which may be described as a state of perfection. This marks the attainment of *Nibbāna*. The attainment of the *arahant* state requires not only disciplined living, but also concerted meditative efforts (Katz, 1982).

The other main teachings of the Buddha include the negation of a permanent and unchanging soul (*anatta*) and the notion of the impermanence of things (*anicca*). Buddhism also excludes the notion of a God; there is no supreme being who rules and controls everything. Each individual is his or her own master, and determines his or her own life and fate.

For the laity, the vast majority of people who did not renounce worldly life to devote themselves to the immediate quest for *Nibbāna*, the Buddha provided a sound, pragmatic social ethic (Premasiri, 1991; Tachibana, 1926). They were expected to lead a life of restraint and moderation, respecting the rights of others and being dutiful to those around them. Such a restrained and dutiful life was not only considered to be an essential prerequisite for one's ultimate religious aim, but was valued as an end in itself. For example, the Buddha advised his lay followers to abstain from alcoholic beverages because indulgence in them could lead to demonstrable ill effects, such as loss of wealth, proneness to socially embarrassing behaviour, unnecessary quarrels, disrepute, ill health, and eventual mental derangement. This pragmatic approach is a prominent feature of the ethics of Buddhism (de Silva, 1983).

BUDDHIST PSYCHOLOGY

Buddhism has a rich and sophisticated psychology, which has been studied in some detail in recent years (e.g. de Silva, 1990a; Kalupahana, 1987; Pio, 1988).

Some parts of the canonical texts, as well as later texts, are examples of explicit psychological theorising, whereas most of the others include psychological ideas and much material of psychological relevance. For example, the *Abhidhamma Pitaka* contains a highly systematised psychological account of human behaviour and mind (see Narada, 1968); the English translation of one of the *Abhidhamma* books, the *Dhammasann ganiī*, in fact bears the title *A Buddhist Manual of Psychological Ethics*. The practice of Buddhism, as a religion and a way of life, involves much in terms of psychological change. The ultimate religious goal of the *arahant* state reflects and requires major psychological changes. In addition, as can be seen from the previous section, the path towards the achievement of this goal, the Noble Eightfold Path, also involves steps, many of which can only be described as psychological (Katz, 1982) (also see Majjhima Nikiya 1882–1902).

While the rapid popularisation of Zen Buddhism in the West no doubt provided a special impetus for the relatively recent interest in the study of Buddhist psychology (Hirai, 1974; Maupin, 1962; Sekida, 1975; Shapiro, 1978), quite independent of this several scholars had begun to appreciate, and to examine closely, the psychological aspects of Buddhism. An early example of these early studies into aspects of the psychology of Buddhism is Jayasuriya's *The Psychology and Philosophy of Buddhism* (1963). This and other descriptive–expository studies were soon followed by publications which concentrated on specific aspects of Buddhist psychology and which attempted to compare them with modern psychological notions and/or to analyse Buddhist concepts in terms of theoretical frameworks derived from Western psychology. For example, Govinda (1969) analysed the basic principles and factors of consciousness as found in the *Abhidhamma Piṭaka*, and Johansson in 1965 offered an analysis of some fundamental psychological concepts of Buddhism (*citta, mano* and *viññāna*, all of which refer to different aspects of 'mind') using a psychosemantic paradigm. He subsequently undertook a similar exercise for the concept of *Nibbāna* (Johansson, 1969), and attempted to elucidate it using the semantic differential paradigm of Osgood. Joy Manne-Lewis (1986) has discussed the Buddhist concept of enlightenment, or perfection, in terms of the concepts of Western psychology. She argues that the Buddhist psychology of enlightenment provides a paradigm for a challenging new model that has relevance to modern psychology. In this discussion, two basic Buddhist psychological concepts, *saññā* and *sankhāra*, which respectively refer broadly to the perceptual and recognising functions in the texts, are seen as parallel to aspects of George Kelly's personal construct theory. To quote: '*Saññā* may be [seen as] the process of forming elementary and basic constructs and hypotheses: *sankhara* is that of putting these together, concretizing them, in Kelly's terminology, into testable predictions' (p. 130). Manne-Lewis also offers a Kellyan interpretation of the cognitive aspects of the state of enlightenment: 'All personal constructs have been eradicated, and there is a perfect correspondence between the mind of the perceiver and the phenomena perceived' (p. 136). Kalupahana (1987) has provided probably the most detailed discussion of the psychological concepts of Buddhism. In his work, he draws illuminating parallels with the psychology of William James. One of the parallels particularly highlighted by Kalupahana is the notion of the stream of thought or consciousness. Kalupahana's analysis also emphasises the close links between the philosophy of Buddhism and its psychological notions.

BUDDHISM AND PSYCHOLOGICAL THERAPY

Although studies such as the above are of much academic interest, it is the examination of the psychology of Buddhism from a therapeutic point of view that offers potentially valuable and exciting practical possibilities. The potential value of Buddhism for psychological therapy and mental health has been commented on by many authors (e.g. de Silva, 1984; 1985; 1986; 1990a; 1990b; Goleman, 1976, 1981; Mikulas, 1981, 1991). In the remainder of this chapter, several topics falling within this area will be discussed.

This discussion will focus, as noted earlier, on Early, or Theravāda, Buddhism. Many of the general points that will be made, however, are equally applicable to other schools and forms of Buddhism. It is perhaps worth noting that there is already a rapidly growing literature on other schools of Buddhism, especially Zen, from the standpoint of psychological therapy (e.g. de Martino, 1983;

Reynolds, 1980; Shapiro, 1978; Suzuki, 1970) and several relevant discussions are provided in a volume recently edited by Maurits Kwee (1990).

Meditation

One major aspect of Buddhist psychological practice that has already entered modern psychological therapy is meditation. In the Buddhist texts, meditation is given pride of place as an essential aspect of the individual's religious endeavour. The aim of this endeavour, as mentioned above, is to reach a state of perfection, and personal development is an essential part of this quest. Whereas restrained and disciplined conduct is part of this training and preparation, meditation is considered a crucial ingredient. It is worth noting that the Pali word for meditation is *bhāvanā*, which literally means development or cultivation. In Buddhism, meditative efforts are seen primarily as a means of personal development.

In Buddhism, the individual's emancipation (i.e. the attainment of the state of perfection) is to be achieved through his or her own effort and striving. Neither the Buddha nor anyone else can do this for him/her; the Buddha can show the way, but the rest is essentially up to the individual. There is, of course, a role for a teacher, under whose guidance a disciple will learn to meditate and who will help with difficulties that may arise, but the actual work of meditation is to be practised and developed by the person himself/herself.

Two forms of meditation are described in the canonical texts, *samatha* (tranquillity), and *vipassanā* (insight). For the sake of completeness, a brief account is given below of what these two forms of meditation consist of (for a detailed discussion, see Sole-Leris, 1986; also see Nyanaponika, 1962).

The word *samatha* means tranquillity or serenity. *Samatha* meditation is aimed at reaching states of consciousness characterised by progressively greater levels of tranquillity and stillness. It has two aspects: the achievement of the highest possible degree of concentration and the progressive calming of all mental processes. This is done through increasingly concentrated focusing of attention, where the mind withdraws progressively from all external and internal stimuli. In the end, states of pure and undistracted consciousness can be achieved. The *samatha* meditation procedure starts with efforts at concentrating the mind on specific objects and progresses systematically through a series of states of mental absorption, called *jhāna*.

Vipassanā, or insight, meditation also starts with concentration exercises using appropriate objects to focus on. In this procedure, however, once a certain level of concentration is achieved, so that undistracted mindfulness can be maintained, one goes on to examine with steady, careful attention, all sensory and mental processes. One becomes a detached observer of one's own activity. The aim is to achieve total and immediate awareness of all phenomena. This leads, it is claimed, eventually to the full and clear perception of the impermanence of all things and beings.

It is held that *samatha* meditation by itself cannot lead to enlightenment or perfection; *vipassanā* meditation is needed to attain this goal. Whereas the former leads to temporarily altered states of consciousness, the latter leads to enduring and thoroughgoing change in the person's consciousness and paves the way for achievement of the *arahant* state.

The relevance of the claims made in Buddhism for meditation to improve mental health in general, and for psychological therapy in particular, should be obvious. The meditative experiences of both types, when properly carried out and developed, could be expected to lead to greater ability to concentrate, greater freedom from distraction, greater tolerance of change and turmoil around oneself, greater ability to be unaffected by such change and turmoil, and sharper awareness of and greater alertness to one's own responses, both physical and mental. It would also lead, more generally, to greater calmness or tranquillity. Although the ultimate goal of perfection requires a long series of regular training periods of systematic meditation, along with major restraint in conduct, the more mundane benefits of meditation should be available to serious and persistent practitioners.

From a therapeutic perspective, this means that Buddhist meditation techniques can be useful as an instrument for achieving certain psychological benefits. Primarily, meditation would have a role as a stress-reduction strategy, comparable to the more modern techniques of relaxation (Benson, 1975; Carrington, 1982; Goleman, 1976). In fact, there is a substantial and growing literature in present-day clinical psychology and psychiatry that shows that meditation does in fact produce beneficial effects in this way (see Carrington, 1982, 1984; Shapiro, 1982). Studies of the physiological changes that accompany meditation have shown several changes to occur that together indicate a state of calmness or relaxation (Woolfolk, 1975). These include: reduction in oxygen consumption, lowered heart rate, decreased breathing rate and blood pressure, reduction in serum lactic acid levels, and increased skin resistance and changes in blood flow. These peripheral changes are generally compatible with decreased arousal in the sympathetic nervous system. There are also central changes, as shown by brain wave patterns. The amalgam of these physiological changes related to meditation has been called the 'relaxation response' (Benson, 1975). This kind of evidence clearly establishes the role of meditation as a relaxation strategy.

Meditation techniques have been used systematically for numerous clinical problems, and recent work has moved towards the scientific evaluation of the efficacy of these techniques. Indeed, if meditation is to establish itself as a viable and worthwhile stress-control strategy in modern mental health care, the only way this can be achieved is through subjecting it to such systematic evaluation (Woolfolk and Franks, 1984). The available data show that, when systematically carried out, meditation has definite value for certain problems with certain client populations. The problems for which meditation has been used in clinical settings include general stress and tension, general anxiety, test anxiety, drug abuse, alcohol abuse, and sleep problems (Carrington, 1982, 1984; Kabat-Zinn *et al.*, 1992; Shapiro and Walsh, 1984). Some impressive recent research has also shown the usefulness of mindfulness meditation (a form of *vipassanā* meditation) training for the self-regulation of chronic pain (Kabat-Zinn, 1982; Kabat-Zinn *et al.*, 1985). It is interesting that the early Buddhist texts contain specific references to the value of this form of meditation for the control of pain (e.g. *Saṃyutta Nikāya*, vol. 4). Similarly, the Buddha also recommended meditation as a means of achieving trouble-free sleep (*Vinaya Piṭaka*, vol. 1).

It is perhaps worth dwelling briefly, at this point, on the use of mindfulness meditation for pain control. Kabat-Zinn *et al.* (1985) report that ninety chronic patients who were trained in mindfulness meditation in a ten-week stress-reduction programme showed significant improvement in pain and related symptoms. A control group of patients who did not receive meditation training did not show such improvement. The authors explain their rationale for selecting this strategy for the treatment of pain as follows:

> In the case of pain perception, the cultivation of detached observation of the pain experience may be achieved by paying careful attention and distinguishing as *separate* events the actual primary sensations as they occur from moment to moment and any accompanying thoughts about pain.
>
> (Kabat-Zinn *et al.*, 1985, p. 165, emphasis added)

It is this detached observation of sensations that mindfulness meditation, as described in the Buddhist texts, helps one to develop. This makes such meditation a strategy particularly well suited to pain control. It is significant that the references to pain control by mindfulness meditation in the original Buddhist texts appear to make this very point. Several relevant examples are discussed in de Silva (1990b). A notable account is that of the monk Anuruddha, who fell quite ill. When some visiting monks asked him about his pain, his reply was that the pain-generating bodily sensations could not perturb him, as his mind was firmly grounded in mindfulness. The implication here is that meditation can reduce, or 'block out', the mental aspect of the pain – that is, although the physical sensations of pain may remain, vulnerability to subjectively felt pain is reduced. This account is from the *Saṃyutta Nikāya*, which appears to maintain this position quite explicitly in a different passage (*Saṃyutta Nikāya*, vol. 4).

It has also been suggested that meditation can have a useful function as an integrated part of a dynamic psychotherapeutic approach. Referring specifically to Buddhist mindfulness meditation, Kutz *et al.* (1985) discuss several ways in which such a combined approach would help. For example, the kind of psychological content that meditation of this type produces could provide useful raw material for psychotherapy sessions. With certain kinds of clients such meditation could also help by enhancing their ability to discern and discuss their negative emotions. Kutz *et al.* also argue that, if a client engages in regular meditation, this would in effect be like extending therapy beyond the formal sessions with the psychotherapist, thus leading to both intensification and condensation of therapy. They stress that the combination of dynamic psychotherapy and mindfulness meditation is 'technically compatible and mutually reinforcing' (p. 6). As both dynamic psychotherapy and meditation are ways of achieving personal psychological change and development, this proposed role for meditation in a modern psychotherapeutic context is not surprising (Watts, 1963).

It must be stressed, however, that meditation techniques are not to be taken as a panacea for all psychological disorders. They were intended in early Buddhism for self-development, and the texts refer, as seen above, to their additional beneficial effects in certain contexts and conditions. The point here is that the nature of the meditational endeavour and its results as part of a Buddhist's self-development suggest a useful role for it in therapy for certain psychological disorders, especially stress-related ones, and for the psychological aspects of certain physical conditions. The available clinical literature shows that this is often the case. Further studies, especially systematic and rigorously controlled trials, will in the future shed more light on what specific uses meditation can have in clinical therapeutic settings.

Other strategies for behaviour change

There is a second aspect of Buddhist psychology that is of particular relevance from a therapeutic perspective. The literature of Early Buddhism contains a wealth of behaviour change strategies, which can only be described as behavioural, used and recommended by the Buddha and his disciples. This is an aspect of Buddhism that had been neglected by modern scholars until very recently. It is only in the past few years that these behavioural strategies have been highlighted and discussed (e.g. de Silva, 1984, 1985, 1986, 1990b). These strategies are remarkably similar to several of the established techniques of modern behaviour therapy. Thus, Buddhism can be said to have a clear affinity to present-day behavioural psychology. The ways in which the overall approach of behaviour modification and that of Buddhism may be said to be broadly similar have been discussed by Mikulas in two important papers (1978, 1981). Some areas of similarity highlighted by Mikulas include: the rejection of the notion of an unchanging self or soul, focus on observable phenomena, emphasis on testability, stress on techniques for awareness of certain bodily responses, emphasis on the here and now, and wide and public dissemination of teachings and techniques. Given this broad similarity, and the general empiricist/experientialist attitude of Buddhism as exemplified by the *Kālāma Sutta* (*Anguttara Nikāya*, vol. 1), in which the Buddha advises a group of inquirers not to accept anything on hearsay, authority, or pure argument, but to accept only what is empirically and experientially verifiable, it is not surprising that specific behavioural techniques were used and recommended in Early Buddhism. It is also entirely in keeping with the social ethic of Buddhism, which recognises the importance of behaviours conducive to one's own and others' well-being as a goal in its own right. When and where specific behaviour changes are required, both in oneself and in others, these are to be effected using specific techniques

The *behavioural* nature of these strategies needs to be stressed. When a certain response needs to be altered, an attempt is made to change it at a behavioural level – that is, directly, by operating on the behaviour itself, and not indirectly, via other means. This is precisely the approach of modern behaviour therapy (e.g. Wolpe, 1958, 1991). Behaviour therapy distinguishes itself from other therapeutic approaches by concentrating on the problem behaviour directly. There is no attempt to change the target response indirectly, either through the exploration of assumed unconscious factors or through pharmacological substances acting via the nervous system. The problem behaviour itself is operated upon. The same applies to the behavioural strategies found in Early Buddhist literature. This is not to suggest that this is the only means of behaviour change accepted or recommended in Buddhism. In fact, major behaviour changes are expected to occur through personal development, including restrained conduct and systematic meditation training. On the other hand, quite independent of this overall personal development, the Buddha and his disciples did not hesitate to resort to, and advocate, direct and behavioural ways of changing responses where needed.

The range of behavioural strategies found in the literature of Early Buddhism is impressive (de Silva, 1984; 1990b). These techniques include the following:

fear reduction by graded exposure and reciprocal inhibition
using rewards to promote desirable behaviour
modelling to induce behaviour change
stimulus control to eliminate undesirable behaviour
use of aversion to eliminate undesirable behaviour
training in social skills
self-monitoring
control of intrusive thoughts by distraction, switching/stopping, incompatible thoughts, and prolonged exposure
intense, covert focusing on the unpleasant aspects of a stimulus or the unpleasant
pleasant consequences of a response, to reduce attachment to the former and eliminate the latter
hierarchical approach to the development of positive feelings towards others use of cues in behavioural control
use of response cost to aid elimination of undesirable behaviour
use of a family member in carrying out a behavioural change programme cognitive – behavioural methods (e.g. for grief)

Details of these, including references to the original texts, have been cited elsewhere and will not be repeated here (de Silva, 1984; 1985; 1986; 1990b). It will be useful, however, to provide an example of this behavioural approach in Buddhism and to highlight its similarity to modern parallels.

For the control of unwanted, intrusive cognitions, which particularly hinder meditative efforts and can therefore be a major problem for a Buddhist, several strategies are recommended. These include: switching to an opposite or incompatible thought, ignoring the thought and distracting oneself, and concentrating intensely on the thought (for a fuller account, see de Silva, 1985). As can be seen, all of these bear close similarity to techniques used in modern behaviour therapy for the problem of intrusive cognitions, especially obsessions. The first (switching to an opposite, incompatible thought) is basically no different from the thought-switching or thought-substitution technique described by Beech and Vaughan (1979), de Silva and Rachman (1992), Marks (1981), Rachman and Hodgson (1980), and others. In this technique, the client is trained to switch to thinking a thought different from the unwanted intrusion. The Buddhist technique has the added refinement that the thoughts to be switched to should be both incompatible with the original one and wholly acceptable in their own right. For example, if the unwanted cognition is associated with lust, one should think of something promoting lustlessness; if it is associated with malice or hatred, one should think of something promoting loving kindness. The second Buddhist technique mentioned above (ignoring and distraction) is essentially similar to the distraction techniques advocated by modern therapists (e.g. Rachman, 1978; Wolpe, 1991). The client is instructed to engage his or her attention on a different stimulus or activity. The Buddhist texts also offer suggestions as to what distractions might be usefully employed; these include both physical and cognitive ones. For instance, one might recall a passage one has learned, concentrate on actual concrete objects, or undertake unrelated physical activity. The third technique (concentration on the intruding thought) is similar to the modern technique of satiation/habituation training (e.g. Rachman, 1978; Rachman and Hodgson, 1980). Present-day therapists may instruct the client to expose him/herself to the thought repeatedly and/or for prolonged periods of time. The Buddhist texts advise one to face the unwanted thought directly and continuously, concentrating on that thought and nothing else. Similar comparisons can be made between most of the other behavioural strategies found in the Buddhist texts and those established in present-day behaviour therapy for similar purposes.

The importance of the presence of these behavioural techniques in the Buddhist texts is manifold. First, it highlights the fact that Buddhism has something to offer in the area of day-to-day management of behavioural problems, often as a goal in its own right, for the individual's own and his/her fellow beings' benefit and happiness. These techniques are applicable irrespective of whether or not one has committed oneself to a life devoted to the goal of personal development. Second, these techniques are well defined, easy to use, and – above all – empirically testable. Indeed, the Buddhist approach is one of testing various strategies until an effective one is found. The Buddha's advice to the K&l&mas on the importance of not accepting any view on the basis of hearsay or authority, but only on empirical grounds, reflects this approach. The Buddha's own quest for enlightenment followed this path; having tried out various methods and teachings available at the time, he rejected each of them as they failed to lead to his goal and eventually developed his own path (Saddhatissa, 1976). Third, the techniques are for use on oneself as well as for influencing the behaviour of others; examples are found of both types of uses.

IMPLICATIONS FOR PRESENT-DAY THERAPY

In terms of present-day psychological therapy, the relevance of this aspect of Buddhism should be clear. A range of well-defined techniques is available for use with common behavioural problems. The fact that many of these are similar to modern behaviour therapeutic techniques in remarkable ways implies that their validity and utility are already established, as many of the latter have been subjected to rigorous clinical and experimental investigation (Rachman and Wilson, 1980). Those Buddhist strategies that so far have no counterpart in modern behaviour modification should be tested empirically. If evidence is then found for considering them to be clinically useful, they can be fruitfully incorporated into the repertoire of techniques available to the present-day practitioner.

It can also be argued that these techniques will have particular value in the practice of therapy with Buddhist client groups. A problem that arises in using techniques derived from Western science with client populations of different cultural backgrounds is that the techniques offered may seem alien to the indigenous population. Thus, they may not be readily accepted or, if accepted, compliance with instructions may be poor. These cultural difficulties in therapy and counselling have been fully recognised in recent years (e.g. d'Ardenne and Mahtani, 1989). On the other hand, if the techniques that are used and offered, although they are part of a Western psychological system, are shown to be similar to ideas and practices that have been accepted historically by the indigenous culture, then they would have a greater chance of gaining compliance and success. Singh and Oberhummer (1980) have described how a behaviour therapy programme was successfully devised for a Hindu patient that included the Hindu religious concept of *karma yoga*. Similarly, therapeutic packages that include traditional Zen practices have been used successfully with neurotic patients in Japan (Kishimoto, 1985; see also Reynolds, 1980). It is likely that modern behaviour therapeutic strategies will be more readily acceptable to Buddhist client groups if their similarities with those found in the Early Buddhist literature, and the use of the same or similar techniques by the Buddha and his early disciples, are highlighted. The use of meditation techniques as a stress-reduction strategy with Buddhist groups in several places provides an example of this phenomenon. A case in point is the use of Buddhist meditation in a psychiatric setting in Kandy, Sri Lanka (de Silva and Samarasinghe, 1985).

A further possible use of Buddhist psychology for therapeutic purposes lies in the area of prophylaxis, both with Buddhist client groups and with others. For example, training in meditation, leading to greater ability to achieve calmness and tranquillity, can help enhance an individual's tolerance of the numerous inevitable stresses in modern life. It may be possible, in other words, to achieve a degree of immunity against the psychological effects of stress and frustration (see Meichenbaum, 1985, on stress-inoculation training). Further, training in mindfulness meditation can enable a person to develop the ability to be alert to, and to recognise, his or her own thoughts, feelings, anxieties, and worries as they arise, and to exercise some control over them. The facility and skill in self-monitoring that can be acquired with the aid of mindfulness meditation can provide a valuable means of self-control. The overall self-development that Buddhism encourages and recommends also has much to offer for preventive purposes. For example, if people begin to learn not to develop intense attachments to material things and to those around them, they may be less vulnerable to psychological distress and disorders arising from loss, including abnormal and debilitating grief reactions. This is not to suggest that the total renunciation of all worldly comforts and attachments should be the goal of every person. Indeed, very few in today's world will want to renounce all material things and devote themselves to the attainment of personal perfection. The Buddha himself recognised that the majority of people would remain lay persons, with normal household duties and day-to-day activities and pursuits, and that only a relatively small number would renounce lay life completely; hence the prominence given in Buddhism to lay ethics (Tachibana, 1926). On the other hand, some of the meditation exercises and other personal development strategies found in Buddhism can potentially enable a person to develop an outlook on life and patterns of response that will help him/her to cope with the problems of living with greater calmness and assurance and with reduced vulnerability to common psychological disorders. This kind of primary prevention is worth exploring seriously.

CONCLUSIONS

To recapitulate, there are several ways in which Buddhist psychology has implications for present-day therapeutic practice. First, Buddhist meditation techniques have already begun to be used, and shown to be effective, for certain clinical problems. This practice is growing and is being investigated clinically and experimentally. Second, Buddhism possesses an array of behaviour change strategies, most of which bear striking resemblance to modern behaviour modification techniques. Highlighting these similarities when such techniques are used with Buddhist client groups is likely to enhance compliance in therapy. Those other behavioural techniques found in the Buddhist literature that so far have no modern parallels should be tested empirically. Third, there is potential for the use of Buddhist techniques for psychological prophylaxis. In sum, then, Buddhist psychology has a clear contribution to make to the practice of psychological therapy in today's world. Some use of it is already being made; there is room for a greater role.

REFERENCES

Anguttara Nikāya (1885–1900) 4 vols, R. Morris and E. Hardy (eds), London: Pali Text Society.

Beech, H. R. and Vaughan, M. (1979) *Behavioural Treatment of Obsessional States*, Chichester: John Wiley.

Benson, H. (1975) *The Relaxation Response*, New York: Morrow.

Carrington, P. (1982) 'Meditation techniques in clinical practice', in L. E. Abt and I. R. Stuart (eds) *The Newer Therapies: A Sourcebook*, New York: Van Nostrand.

—— (1984) 'Modern forms of meditation', in R. L. Woolfolk and M. Lehrer (eds) *Principles and Practice of Stress Management*, New York: Guilford.

d'Ardenne, P. and Mahtani, A. (1989) *Transcultural Counselling in Action*, London: Sage.

de Martino, R. J. (1983) 'The human situation and Zen Buddhism', in N. Katz (ed.) *Buddhist and Western Psychology*, Boulder, CO: Prajna.

de Silva, P. (1983) 'The Buddhist attitude to alcoholism', in G. Edwards, A. Arif. and J. Jaffe (eds) *Drug Use and Misuse: Cultural Perspectives*, London: Croom Helm.

—— (1984) 'Buddhism and behaviour modification', *Behaviour Research and Therapy* 22: 661–78.

—— (1985) 'Early Buddhist and modern behavioral strategies for the control of unwanted intrusive cognitions', *Psychological Record* 35: 437–43.

—— (1986) 'Buddhism and behaviour change: implications for therapy', in G. Claxton (ed.) *Beyond Therapy: The Impact of Eastern Religions on Psychological Theory and Practice*, London: Wisdom.

—— (1990a) 'Buddhist psychology: a review of theory and practice', *Current Psychology: Research and Reviews* 9: 236–54.

—— (1990b) 'Self-control strategies in Early Buddhism', in J. Crook and D. Fontan (eds) *Space in Mind: East-West Psychology and Contemporary Buddhism*, Shaftesbury: Element Press.

de Silva, P. and Rachman, S. (1992) *Obsessive – Compulsive Disorder: The Facts*, Oxford: Oxford University Press.

de Silva, P. and Samarasinghe, D. (1985) 'Behavior therapy in Sri Lanka', *Journal of Behavior Therapy and Experimental Psychiatry* 16: 95–100.

Goleman, D. (1976) 'Meditation and consciousness: an Asian approach to mental health', *American Journal of Psychotherapy* 30: 41–54.

—— (1981) 'Buddhist and Western psychology: some commonalities and differences', *Journal of Transpersonal Psychology* 13: 125–36.

Govinda, A. (1969) *The Psychological Attitude of Early Buddhist Philosophy*, London: Rider.

Hirai, T. (1974) *Psychophysiology of Zen*, Tokyo: Igaku Shain.

Jayasuriya, W. F. (1963) *The Psychology and Philosophy of Buddhism*, Colombo: YMBA Press.

Johansson, R. E. A. (1965) *Citta, mano, viññāṇa*: a psychosemantic investigation', *University of Ceylon Review* 23: 165–215.

—— (1969) *The Psychology of Nirvana*, London: Allen & Unwin.

Kabat-Zinn, J. (1982) 'An outpatient programme in behavioral medicine for chronic pain patients based on the practice of mindfulness mediation: theoretical considerations and preliminary results', *General Hospital Psychiatry* 4: 33–47.

Kabat-Zinn, J., Lipworth, L. and Burney, R. (1985) 'The clinical use of mindfulness meditation for the self-regulation of chronic pain', *Journal of Behavioral Medicine* 8: 163–90.

Kabat-Zinn, J., Massion, A. O., Kristeller, J., Peterson, L. G., Fletcher, K., Pbert, L., Linderking, C. O. and Santorelli, S. F. (1992) 'Effectiveness of a meditation-based stress reduction program in the treatment of anxiety disorders', *American Journal of Psychiatry* 149: 936–43.

Kalupahana, D. (1987) *The Principles of Buddhist Psychology*, Albany: State University of New York Press.

Katz, N. (1982) *Buddhist Images of Human Perfection*, Delhi: Motilal Banarsidas.

Kishimoto, K. (1985) 'Self-awakening psychotherapy for neurosis: attaching importance to Oriental thought, especially Buddhist thought', *Psychologia* 28: 90–100.

Kutz, I., Borysenko, J. Z. and Benson, H. (1985) 'Meditation and psychotherapy: a rationale for the integration of dynamic psychotherapy, the relaxation response, and mindfulness meditation', *American Journal of Psychiatry* 142: 1–8.

Kwee, M. (ed.) (1990) *Psychotherapy, Meditation and Health*, Amsterdam: East-West Publishers.

Majjhima Nikāya (1888–1902) 3 vols., V. Treckner and R. Chalmers (eds), London: Pali Text Society.

Manne-Lewis, J. (1986) 'Buddhist psychology: a paradigm for the psychology of enlightenment', in G. Claxton (ed.) *Beyond Therapy: The Impact of Eastern Religions on Psychological Theory and Practice*, London: Wisdom.

Marks, I. M. (1981) *Cure and Care of Neuroses*, New York: John Wiley.

Maupin, E. (1962) 'Zen Buddhism: a psychological review', *Journal of Consultation and Psychology* 26: 367–75.

Meichenbaum, D. (1985) *Stress Inoculation*, New York: Pergamon.

Mikulas, W. L. (1978) 'The four Noble Truths of Buddhism related to behavior therapy', *Psychological Record* 28: 59–67.

—— (1981) 'Buddhism and behavior modification', *Psychological Record* 31: 331–42.

—— (1991) 'Eastern and Western psychology: issues and domains for integration', *Journal of Integrative and Eclectic Psychotherapy* 10: 229–40.

Narada Thera (1968) *A Manual of Abhidhamma*, Kandy, Sri Lanka: Buddhist Publications Society.

Nyanaponika Thera (1962) *The Heart of the Buddhist Meditation*, London: Rider.

Pio, E. (1988) *Buddhist Psychology: A Modern Perspective*, New Delhi: Abhinav Publications.

Premasiri, P. D. (1991) 'Ethics', *Encyclopaedia of Buddhism*, vol. 5, Colombo: Department of Buddhist Affairs.

Rachman, S. (1978) 'An anatomy of obsessions', *Behavior Analysis and Modification* 2: 253–78.

Rachman, S. and Hodgson, R. (1980) *Obsessions and Compulsions*, Englewood Cliffs, NJ: Prentice Hall.

Rachman, S. and Wilson, G. T. (1980) *The Effects of Psychological Therapy*, 2nd edition, Oxford: Pergamon.

Rahula, W. (1959) *What the Buddha Taught*, New York: Grove.

Reynolds, D. K. (1980) *The Quiet Therapies*, Honolulu: University of Hawaii Press.

Saddhatissa, H. (1971) *The Buddha's Way*, London: Allen & Unwin.

—— (1976) *The Life of the Buddha*, London: Unwin Paperbacks.

SamyuttaNikāya (1884–1898) 5 vols., L. Peer (ed.), London: Pali Text Society.

Sekida, K. (1975) *Zen Training*, New York: Weatherhill.

Shapiro, D. H. (1978) *Precision Nirvana*, Englewood Cliffs, NJ: Prentice Hall.

—— (1982) 'Overview: clinical and physiological comparison of meditation with other self-control strategies', *American Journal of Psychiatry* 139: 267–74.

Shapiro, D. H. and Walsh, R. N. (eds) (1984) *Meditation: Classic and Contemporary Perspectives*, New York: Aldine.

Singh, R. and Oberhummer, I. (1980) 'Behavior therapy within a setting of karma yoga', *Journal of Behavior Therapy and Experimental Psychiatry* 11: 135–41.

Sole-Leris, A. (1986) *Tranquility and Insight*, London: Rider.

Suzuki, D. T. (1970) *Zen Mind, Beginner's Mind*, New York: Weatherhill.

Tachibana, S. (1926) *The Ethics of Buddhism*, London: Curzon.

VinayaPitaka (1879–1883) 4 vols., H. Oldenberg (ed.), London: Pali Text Society.

Watts, A. (1963) *Psychotherapy East and West*, New York: New American Library.

Wolpe, J. R. (1958) *Psychotherapy by Reciprocal Inhibition*, Stanford, CA: Stanford University Press.

—— (1991) *The Practice of Behavior Therapy*, 4th edition, New York: Pergamon.

Woolfolk, R. L. (1975) 'Psychophysiological correlates of meditation', *Archives of General Psychiatry* 32: 1326–33.

Woolfolk, R. L. and Franks, C. H. (1984) 'Meditation and behavior therapy', in D. H. Shapiro and R. N. Walsh (eds) *Meditation: Classic and Contemporary Perspectives*, New York: Aldine.

Chapter 9

New religions and mental health

Eileen Barker

A sociologist of religion is taking quite a risk when she agrees to write about mental health – and, in one sense, this is not a risk that I intend to take – I have no expertise in the fields of psychiatry, psychotherapy, psychiatric social work or even professional counselling. To write about new religions *and* mental health is still to take a risk, but not quite such a big one. Having studied new religious movements (NRMs) for about quarter of a century, I do know something about the movements – but it is about the *relationship* between them and mental health that I am going to risk writing, in the hope that others who know more about mental health, but less about NRMs, may be alerted to some of the ways in which mental health might be affected (for better or worse) by direct (or indirect) association with one or other of the movements. What I shall attempt to do is to introduce some of the situations – the beliefs, practices, organisations and processes – that might be of relevance to mental health practitioners as they try to unravel the influences affecting any particular individual or group of individuals with whom they are concerned.

Perhaps one should start by asking 'what is a new religion?' I believe that too precise a definition is constraining and unnecessary for our present purposes; several of the movements about which we shall be talking are not obviously new or religious. Generally speaking, however, I shall be referring to movements that are new in so far as they have become visible in their present form since the Second World War – thus, although Krishna devotees trace their origins back through the sixteenth-century monk, Chaitanya Mahaprabhu, ISKCON (the International Society for Krishna Consciousness) was not founded until the 1960s when His Divine Grace A. C. Bhaktivedanta Swami Prabhupada went to the United States. Some of the movements, such as ISKCON or the Unification Church, would be religious according to almost any definition, but there are the Raëlians (members of a flying saucer movement that expects the Elohim, 'our fathers from space', to come to earth) who say that they belong to an atheistic religion; and there are several movements, many associated with the New Age or the so-called Human Potential movement, who deny that they are in any way religious. These may, however, be included in so far as they help their follow- ers to search for, discover and develop 'the god within' or to get in contact with cosmic forces, or explore 'the spiritual'; indeed, any movement that offers in some way to provide answers to some of the ultimate questions about 'meaning' and 'the purpose of life' that have traditionally been addressed by mainstream religions would be included in this broad understanding of the term 'NRM'.

To illustrate rather than to define: among the better-known NRMs are the Brahma Kumaris, the Church of Scientology, the Divine Light Mission (now known as Elan Vital), *est* (Erhard Seminar Training, now known as the Landmark Forum), the Family (originally known as the Children of God), ISKCON (the Hare Krishna), Rajneeshism (now known as Oslo International), Sahaja Yoga, the Soka Gakkai, Transcendental Meditation, the Unification Church (known as the Moonies) and the Way International. One might also include Neo-Paganism, Occultism, Wicca (or witchcraft) and several movements that are within mainstream traditions, such as part of the House Church (Restoration) movement from within Protestant traditions, and Folkolare, the Neo-Catechumenates, Communione e Liberazione and perhaps even Opus Dei from within the Roman Catholic tradition.

All of these movements have been termed destructive cults by members of the so-called anti-cult movement – a group of individuals and organisations devoted to exposing what they perceive to be the dangers, wickednesses and/or heresies of the movements. Although sociologists of religion employ the concept of the 'cult' in a technical way (often to distinguish a particular kind of movement from a 'sect'), the word 'cult', as it is used in the media and in popular parlance, has come to mean a religious (or 'pseudo-religious') group about which the speaker or writer is denoting a negative evaluation. As it does not seem to me to be particularly useful, apart from reasons of rhetoric, to beg the question as to whether or not a movement is destructive or worthy of negative evaluation by the mere labelling of it as such, I prefer to use the term employed most frequently by my fellow sociologists of religion: new religious movement or NRM.

This dislike of *a priori* assumptions about the movements rests partly on what is perhaps the most important point to be made about NRMs: one cannot generalise about them. The only statement that can be made which applies to all of them is that they have been called an NRM or 'cult' at some point; any other generalisation is well nigh certain to be refuted by one of their number. While nineteenth-century sects such as the Jehovah's Witnesses, Christian Science, the Mormons, Seventh-day Adventists and the Christadelphians all came, more or less directly, from the Judaeo-Christian tradition, the present wave of NRMs draws not only from Hindu, Buddhist, Shinto, Islamic, Jain, Zoroastrian, Celtic and other Pagan traditions, but also from Marxism, psychoanalysis, astrology, science fiction and all manner of further ancient and modern philosophies and ideologies.

So far as practices are concerned, some NRMs (such as ISKCON or the Aetherius Society) partake in elaborate ritual, others (such as the Unification Church) have relatively little in the way of day-to-day ritual. Life styles vary from working full-time for the movement and living in one of its communities (as with members of the Family) to having ordinary jobs in the wider community and living by oneself or with non-members (as with many Human Potential practitioners). Attitudes towards women, the family and children vary. Some movements (such as Rajneeshism) have encouraged free sex, others (such as the Brahma Kumaris) place a high value on celibacy. Some movements (such as the Church of Scientology) have a highly structured organisation, others (such as Elan Vital or most New Age groups) exhibit little formal structure. Methods of collecting money include tithing, donations from members, collecting contributions from strangers for literature, plants, candles or 'missionary work', and a wide variety of business enterprises for which members may supply non-unionised labour.

As the danger of generalisation is such an important point, let me elaborate briefly with a few examples from the range of beliefs to be found within NRMs. Some belief systems are elaborated in detail – an example would be Unification theology as it is contained in the *Divine Principles* (Kwak, 1980), which is centred around a strong belief in God and which has its own cosmology, theodicy, eschatology, soteriology, Christology and biblically-based interpretation of history. Unificationists are, furthermore, privy to certain additional revelations, most of which centre on the Reverend Sun Myung Moon as the Messiah, and the role that he and his family are playing in the restoration of the Kingdom of Heaven on earth (Barker, 1991). The Family has its beliefs disseminated through 'Mo letters', cartoon strips, which, during his lifetime, were written or approved of by the founder and Endtime prophet, 'Moses' David Berg, which provide Father David's interpretations of the Bible. The Mo letters that are distributed to outsiders contain child-like drawings of happy people in heaven – with, always, the sun shining; DO letters (for disciples only) contain details of the coming apocalypse and instructions on how to behave: how to bring up children and, at one time, how attractive young women should go about their task of 'flirty fishing' – a method of recruitment and/or fundraising, discontinued in 1987, which involved sexual relationships as an illustration of the extent to which Jesus (and members of the Family) loved the potential convert or donor.

Known to his followers as Osho after his return to India and following his expulsion from the USA when a series of crimes had been exposed in his 64,000-acre Oregon estate, Rajneeshpuram, Bhagwan Rajneesh consistently instructed his followers, or sannyasins, to reject all philosophies and beliefs, including those which he himself had taught them. Members of the Church Universal and Triumphant study the messages that have been received by their leader, Elizabeth Clare Prophet, from 'Ascended Masters' such as Jesus, the Buddha and, especially, St. Germain. Members of the Church of Scientology are strongly opposed to many of the practices of conventional psychiatry and psychology; they spend long hours studying the works of L. Ron Hubbard, a science fiction writer who invented the technique of Dianetics, a kind of therapy ('auditing') which, they claim, enables them to overcome mental blockages from the past. 'Premies', as the followers of the erstwhile boy guru, Maharajji, were once known, learned little in the way of theology but became enlightened through taking the 'Knowledge', which consists of techniques enabling initiates to turn their senses within and thereby to perceive Divine Light, hear Divine Music, taste Divine Nectar and feel the 'primordial vibration' of the Holy Name. Members of the Aetherius Society believe not only that they can receive thousands of Prayer Hours of spiritual energy beamed from a giant spacecraft, but also that energy invoked through a Buddhist Mantra and Christian prayer can be stored in a special Spiritual Energy Battery so that it is ready for use when it is most needed. Members of the Eternal Flame Foundation believe that 'death of the physical body is an imposition of limitation no longer acceptable to those of us who have awakened to spiritual immortality'. Indeed, after one of their leaders had come to the understanding that Jesus was speaking of physical, not spiritual, immortality, the group has been teaching the way to achieve eternal (physical) life on this earth.

Some of us may believe that people who hold some of these beliefs must be crazy – literally so. How, we might ask, could any except the mentally deluded believe that they are going to live for ever? That, by chanting some weird mumbo-jumbo, we can store spiritual energy from outer space? That a chubby little boy can give us instant enlightenment and perfect Knowledge? That holding two tin cans attached by wire to a flickering needle can get rid of all our hangups from this world and the last, so that we can eventually become a free-floating Thetan, able to defy the laws of gravity? That by jumping up and down, by exploring freely our own sexuality and by denouncing all the constraints of society, we can become totally free and realise our real selves? That, by working round the clock for a Korean who has been imprisoned on a number of occasions, we are working to restore the Kingdom of Heaven on earth? And that by going through a ceremony with a marriage partner which this messiah has chosen, we shall be able to give birth to children free of the fallen nature that has been responsible for the sins of the world ever since Adam and Eve disobeyed God's command in the Garden of Eden? Or that the world is to come to an end – on, say, the first day of the first month of the year 2000?

Could any sane, normal person believe such things? A brief examination of history and anthropology shows us all too clearly that the majority of the people who have lived on this planet have and do hold some very strange beliefs. Indeed, to some people, the belief that the wine that the priest offers communicants is really the blood of a man who was killed two thousand years ago, having been born as the result of a deity impregnating a virgin, seems a very questionable one.

Be that as it may, the point that is being made is that those concerned with the diagnosis of mental illness would be well advised to ensure that 'strange beliefs' should not be taken by themselves as being an indicator that a person is mentally ill – unless one is willing to risk applying the same standard to far more people than those who happen to be members of an NRM, and unless one can come up with a convincing criterion for judging what are 'normal' or healthy beliefs – an exercise that history (and a number of contemporary events) can show us is fraught with dangers.[1]

But even if we agree that disagreements about the truth of beliefs which cannot be empirically refuted will always remain with us, and that it is unhelpful to label others as mentally ill solely on the grounds that they persist in their beliefs despite the fact that others disagree with them, questions about mental health may still arise over 'reality testing'. Just as there is well-documented evidence that psychiatry was used to certify as insane those dissidents who could not accept the 'reality' of Marxist-Leninism, so, in the United States and elsewhere, individuals who hold to unconventional beliefs have been 'medicalized' on the grounds that, by accepting the beliefs of an NRM, they are incapable of testing reality and/or they are in an advanced state of 'dissociation' – even when neurological and psychological tests have revealed no abnormality and others (including other psychiatrists) have assessed their behaviour to be perfectly rational (Coleman, 1985).[2]

I certainly do not want to suggest that there are not people who are crazy and are incapable of 'reality testing'; nor is it being denied that there are some people who believe that they are Napoleon or Jesus because they are mentally ill. What may appear difficult to assess, however, is the sanity of people who have seen visions, heard voices or had unusual experiences which might be called religious or spiritual and that would seem to be inexplicable according to canons of 'ordinary' experience. Yet work by David Hay and his associates at the Alister Hardy Research Centre, and others such as Andrew Greeley in the United States, suggests that not only may a third or more of the population have such experiences, but that the people who have them tend to be, according to a number of independent variables, slightly more well adjusted and mentally healthy than the population as a whole (Hay, 1982).

Before leaving the realm of beliefs, it might be pertinent to make one more point. Not only has a significant proportion of the population had experiences that cannot be explained by science or even 'common sense', but many of these experiences have been significant events, affecting the lives of the recipients in one way or another – yet quite frequently they have not told anyone about their experience, because they were afraid of being thought of as mentally ill (ibid.: 6). The point is that in modern Western society there are few social contexts within which it is safe to confess to having such experiences and, unlike the situation in the majority of societies, modern Western culture offers no clear explanation for such experiences – except in situations such as those provided by certain of the new religions.

Two points follow from this: first, the NRM may provide a haven within which people are given permission to lead a religious and/or spiritual life – something that many feel the traditional churches no longer offer. Second, there being no single interpretation of such experiences sanctioned by society, the door is left wide open for a wide variety of interpretations.

In making this point, it is assumed that one can make a clear analytical and, indeed, actual distinction between an objective experience and a subjective interpretation of that experience. Two potential mistakes can occur with the frequent blurring of this distinction. First, the individuals who have had the experiences may not be believed or may be thought to be mentally ill when they say that they have experienced something out of the ordinary; second, the experiencers may be unaware of the extent to which others have interpreted their experience for them – they may have had a genuine experience, but whether it was because Jesus or the anti-Christ was contacting them or because their imagination had been triggered by an event or a book they read in childhood is another question. It is also possible that the movement will have played a role in preparing them for a particular kind of experience and in shaping the form the experience takes. Just as the Freudian analyst's patients will have Freudian dreams and the Jungian's patients will have Jungian experiences, so it seems, it is Catholics, rather than Hindus or Muslims who tend to have visions of the Blessed Virgin Mary, and believers in reincarnation rather than Catholics, who report experiences of former lives.[3]

In NRMs, one can frequently observe both subtle and not-so-subtle interpretations of experiences being offered in order to justify and/or reinforce a group's position. Sometimes the experience has been induced by the NRM itself through a variety of techniques such as hyperventilation or certain meditation practices. Sometimes the movement overtly eschews any involvement in the production of the experience. Thus, at a Unification workshop, potential converts are likely to be told that it is up to them themselves to find out whether Unification theology is true – the potential convert is told not to accept the Unificationists' word for it, but to ask God for confirmation. The next morning at breakfast potential converts may be asked to describe their dreams. I have witnessed an impressive array of what might have appeared to be 'ordinary' dreams being interpreted in ways that confirm a particular group's ideology. And if the potential convert refuses to admit to having dreamt at all, then members of the movement may well relate how they had a dream about the potential convert and are thereby able to convey a special message to him or her.

It is possible that mental health practitioners may spend time denying the objective experience (which the experiencers are convinced they really *have experienced*) when actually what would be more productive would be to help the 'patient' to recognise that there may be no necessary connection between the experience and the interpretation. For example, if ex-members still believe that their erstwhile guru has a powerful influence over their lives, with the belief system that they think they have abandoned continuing to be used to interpret headaches and stomach cramps as the result of the guru's attention and displeasure being focused on them, then pointing out that there could be a number of other explanations for the discomfort, including their own fear, may not immediately convince them, but it could be a first step in freeing them from the association that has been planted in their minds.

A different kind of assumed causal connection may act to deter people leaving a movement: within certain NRMs, for example, stories are told of the terrible events that have happened to defectors – how a particular apostate had a serious car accident shortly after leaving, or how another fell down a cliff and broke his leg, or yet another developed a fatal cancer. Here again, the antidote is not to deny that the misfortune occurred but to help those who have to come to see the world in a particular way to question the inevitability of the meaning that has come to be associated with the event or experience.

Of course, the consequence of attaching an unproven meaning to one's experiences need not be destructive. A non-scientific world view (even an unscientific world view) can be perfectly benign; it may even be beneficial for members who may claim – and many do – that their new understanding of how they or society or God works has changed their lives radically for the better. Many have reported that they suffered from all kinds of stress-related illnesses (asthma, migraines, stomach cramps) or even that they were suicidal – until they joined a particular NRM.

One of the most popular images of NRMs involves the 'brainwashing thesis'. But it is not only from the mass media or the general public that one can hear accusations that NRMs employ irresistible and irreversible techniques of 'brainwashing' or 'mind control'; there have been and still are a few psychiatrists and psychologists who promote such ideas – and who have offered their services as 'expert witnesses' in a considerable number of court cases. Space does not permit me to go into the detail that this position deserves, but it ought to be stressed that scholars who have actually studied the movements have not unearthed any evidence that sinister new techniques are used that have not some counterpart in the 'ordinary' world; no processes have been observed in an NRM that one might not find in a convent, a monastery, a boarding school – or the US marines. Unlike the situation with Korean prisoners of war or those subjected to Chinese 'Thought Reform' (Lifton, 1961), NRMs almost never use physical coercion to get or to keep their members (Synanon and the Peoples Temple are two of a few possible exceptions). What influence the movements do use is nearly always at the level of 'meaning' rather than by affecting the brain directly (through drugs, diet, lack of sleep etc.), although such circumstances may on occasion contribute to 'meaning-through-the-mind' influences.

None of this is to deny that several of the NRMs put pressure on their members and potential converts: some use emotional blackmail, some 'lovebomb', some induce feelings of guilt – and so on. However, the fact – and it is a fact – remains that the overwhelming majority of people subjected to such pressures are perfectly capable of saying 'no'. None of the better-known movements which have been accused of having an irresistible hold over potential and actual members has had success in recruiting more than a tiny proportion of those whom they subject to their 'techniques'. In 1979, when brainwashing accusations against the Unification Church were at their height, of the thousand or so persons in the London area who had shown sufficient interest to agree to go on a residential Unification workshop, over 90 per cent rejected the invitation to become Unificationists – and the majority of those who did join the movement left of their own free will within a comparatively short time (Barker, 1984a). Similar findings have been recorded in other studies of NRMs (Bird and Reimer, 1983; Galanter, 1982, 1989). In other words, the so-called mind-control techniques would seem to be remarkably ineffective – certainly a lot less effective than those used by many of the 'old religious movements' into which most of us were born. It seems, rather, that there is something about the particular individuals which makes them decide that they want to be members – for a short time at least – and which separates them from the majority who say no.

It has been claimed that the distinction between those who join and those who resist the overtures of NRMs is that the joiners are, according to a number of criteria, particularly vulnerable; they were, it is asserted, already mentally maladjusted in some way. When this hypothesis has been investigated, however, the evidence seems to be slight. The use of a whole battery of tests and control groups indicates that the psychological well-being of the membership of NRMs falls well within the normal distribution of a population matched for age and social background – so long, of course, as one does not tautologically take membership of an NRM to be an index of mental illness (Barker, 1989).

Let me stress, it is not being claimed that people with mental health problems cannot be found in NRMs – they can be. Sometimes problems are exacerbated, sometimes they are improved, sometimes they remain as they were before (Barker, 1989). Investigations of cases in which ex-members are found to be suffering from mental illness are often those in which there was a history of mental disturbance *before* the person joined (Barker, 1984b; Richardson *et al.*, 1986). Ex-members who are most likely to say that they were subjected to mental pressures are those who have been 'deprogrammed' or subjected to the pressures of the anti-cult movement to interpret their 'cult experience' in such a way (Lewis, 1986; Solomon, 1981; Wright, 1987).

That said, one can certainly find cases of members of NRMs who are terrified by the thought of what members of the movement or non-empirical powers may do to them for their actual or imagined sins. It is not unusual for religions to induce feelings of guilt, and several new religions also blackmail members who may have confessed to past wrong-doing – or been persuaded to take part in actions that they now regret. It is also the case that some NRMs foster feelings of dependency upon the movement – the member may come to be dependent not merely for material goods, but also for receiving God's love, for friendship, or even for his or her sense of identity. The 'outside' world may be painted in black terms, with non-members being defined as evil, dangerous and/or satanic, thus reinforcing dependency on the group (Barker, 1992). Charismatic leaders, claiming either to have a special hot-line to God or actually to be God, may demand unquestioning obedience to their commands, which are not subject to the constraints of either tradition or rational rules (Barker, 1994). Some movements develop special concepts and their exclusive language can contribute still further to the isolation of those using it. In those NRMs that are geographically or, more importantly, socially cut off from the rest of the world, alternative definitions and under-standings of reality may become increasingly difficult for the member to envisage. Outsiders too may help to strengthen the 'them/us' divide by reinforcing the movement's definition of them as enemies to be shunned (Wallis, 1976).

The tendency that non-members have to blame NRMs for a whole range of problems is understandable: it absolves everyone else from blame, and, at least in the short term, it provides a useful scapegoat as a way of resolving – or hiding – more serious underlying causes of mental breakdown. In fact, it may be that an NRM is performing a function that neither the family of origin nor society seems to be able to offer the convert. A medical doctor, Saul Levine (1984), describes how he studied over 800 young people who had joined an NRM. The vast majority of the members had, Levine concluded, joined their movement because, to at least some extent, they had felt the need to get away from an over-protective or over-expectant family which had not let them grow up in the way they wanted. They had found it easier to move into an alternative 'family' for a year or two in order to develop themselves in a protective environment and to give them time to renegotiate their relationship with their parents. Once this was done and the parents had learned to relate to their children as independent adults, the son or daughter no longer needed the protection of the NRM and moved out into the wider society.

Many of the stresses found in NRMs are similar to those found within older religions (also see chapter 6) – guilt, fear, a them/us approach to the world so that alternative edifices may crumble. But new religions, due to the very fact that they are new, with – at least to start with – a first-generation membership, are prone to exhibit some characteristics that distinguish them from the older religions. First, the fact that the membership is more likely to be 'born again' than 'born into' the movement means that there is frequently a degree of enthusiasm and commitment often lacking in mainstream traditions. Converts are more likely to be idealistically motivated and more prepared to sacrifice themselves for God or the cause. This intensity of belief and practice can be experienced as liberating and wonderful – or it may result in people finding themselves in difficult situations because they have not fully thought through the consequences of their situation. They may, for example, find themselves giving up their money, their careers, and, perhaps most seriously, cutting off ties with their family and erstwhile friends. In some movements, long hours of work, poor diet and/or emotional exhaustion may result in 'burn-out', leaving the member in a vulnerable state, and without the support that he or she might have expected from the wider society – some NRMs (and some older movements) exhibit a deep suspicion of, or even denounce, traditional medicine and several communal groups have not kept up insurance or social security payments for their members.

Another characteristic of NRMs is the unaccountability of the leadership. If priests in the Church of England or the Roman Catholic Church start to make undue demands upon their flock, they are usually answerable to a higher temporal authority (although there have been many reports of malpractice, such as the sexual abuse of boys by Catholic priests, that have been covered up for years). It is, furthermore, difficult for members to question the beliefs and practices of some of the movements or their leadership without being made to feel disloyal to the group – or to God. An ethos which demands unconditional surrender or belief without question can lead individual members to feel that they are the only ones to have doubts and that what is assumed to be the general consensus within the movement is right – or God's unquestionable Word.

Sometimes it is forgotten that new religions cannot remain new religions indefinitely; they inevitably change with the passage of time. Thinking about demographic factors alone suggests that a movement with a membership of young adults with little or no responsibilities is unlikely to be the same as one with a membership of middle-aged parents. Another inescapable fact is that founders die – although it does, of course, remain to be seen whether the leaders of the Eternal Flame Foundation follow this heretofore mortal pattern (see Griffith and Bility, this volume).

The intensity of belonging and the cutting off from the rest of the world that occur in some NRMs may result in quite severe problems when people leave their movement. Not only may they have difficulties in accounting for the gap in their curriculum vitae in a society that tends to be suspicious of anyone who has 'spent time' in a cult, but it is likely that their peers have advanced in their careers, their bank balance is at best low, and, most difficult of all, they may have problems in relating to non-members, particularly those of the opposite sex. If they have been in a highly structured, authoritarian movement, they may have difficulty in making even comparatively simple decisions, let alone important ones. In many ways, the loss of the companionship and identity provided by the group can be similar to the feelings of helplessness and hopelessness experienced with the death of a partner on the one hand, or release from a 'total institution' (such as prison, mental hospital or the armed forces) on the other (Goffman, 1968).

Perhaps one of the greatest difficulties that ex-members of NRMs have is the inability of those who have not been members to allow them to tell their own story. Everyone seems to be an instant expert on what life in an NRM is like – and will often insist on defining the ex-member's experiences in their terms rather than his or her own. Ex-members are likely to have ambivalent feelings about their time in the movement and it is important for their 're-entry' that they should be able both to come to terms with things that they disliked and, perhaps, now wish they had not been associated with, and to acknowledge the more positive aspects of their experiences. They need to be able to incorporate their NRM life into their past rather than being made to deny it and pretend that they are starting a new life from the point they were at when they had entered the movement.

At several points in this chapter it has been suggested that outsiders play or have played an important and often unrecognised role in the shaping of the mental health of members of NRMs. Before concluding, it should be mentioned that quite often it is members of the family or close friends of someone who joins an NRM who are in more need of help than the convert, who is likely to be delighted with his or her new-found faith. Parents may suffer extreme anxiety through ignorance and fear and possibly feelings of guilt which may or may not be warranted; a partner may feel as though a third party has come between them; siblings not infrequently feel that their brother or sister has deserted them and/or that their parents are now preoccupied with the convert.

It has, of course, been impossible in this short space to offer more than a few comments that might be of use to those concerned with mental health. The one important message that cannot be over-emphasised, however, is that one cannot generalise about either NRMs or about the individuals who join and leave them, or about the families and friends who may be affected or thought to be affected in one way or the other by the movements. Those wishing to find out more about a particular movement or about a particular group of movements can contact INFORM (Information Network Focus on Religious Movements), a charity that was founded in 1988 with the support of the government to provide information that is as accurate and up-to-date as possible about NRMs.[4] INFORM not only deals with telephone and postal enquiries, but it puts on seminars and conferences, provides support groups for friends and relatives of members of NRMs and for ex-members. It has been training a small group of professional counsellors about NRM-related problems for a number of years and can put enquirers in touch with a wide range of experts including academics who have studied particular movements, lawyers, doctors, specialist agencies and various other people and/or organisations with relevant professional and/or personal experience of the movements.

In conclusion, it should be stressed that NRMs have no unknown magic powers. They may have more than their fair share of rogues – and saints – but the ways in which members of the movements treat themselves and others are not new ways. The fact that they are religious movements means that pronouncements from leaders and commitment to the beliefs and practices may have a more powerful effect than would be the case in secular organisations (Durkheim, 1915); and the fact that they are new means that there tends to be an intensity and enthusiasm frequently lacking in more established religions. But although the processes associated with NRMs may be quantitatively more powerful and intense than in other situations, they are the same kinds of processes, with similar effects as those to be found in other areas of society. The mental health of some members and some of their friends may be adversely affected by some of the movements, that of some others may be improved and that of yet others may remain relatively unaffected. What experience does show is that confrontational reactions to the movements, based on ignorance and/or fear, can exacerbate matters, possibly making the member more fanatic and creating a situation in which it becomes increasingly difficult for problems to be resolved. Finally, if somewhat obviously, it should always be recognised that mental health problems which arise when someone is directly or indirectly connected with an NRM are not necessarily problems that have arisen because of the NRM. Equally, it should always be recognised that they might be. To repeat, each NRM and each person should be approached as individual entities, taking into account the more general social context within which each functions.

NOTES

1 There have been a number of interesting attempts to define 'genuine' religion in the United States' Supreme Court and in other countries. Of special interest at the present time is the drafting of new Constitutions and laws with respect to the differences between established and new religions in Eastern Europe and the former USSR.
2 Recent work into allegations about ritual child abuse and satanic practices has revealed the crucial role that professionals such as police, social workers and mental health specialists can play in creating a 'reality' through questioning and/or therapy (Richardson *et al.*, 1991).
3 Actually, a surprising number of Catholics report that they believe in reincarnation.
4 INFORM, Houghton Street, London WC2A 2AE, Telephone: 0171 955 7654.

REFERENCES

Barker, E. (1984a) *The Making of a Moonie: Brainwashing or Choice?*, Oxford: Basil Blackwell; reprinted by Gregg Revivals, Aldershot (1993).
—— (ed.) (1984b) *Of Gods and Men: New Religious Movements in the West*, Macon, GA: Mercer University Press.
—— (1989) *New Religious Movements: A Practical Introduction*, London: HMSO.
—— (1991) 'La rivelazione della Chiesa dell' Unificazione del reverendo Moon', in M. Introvigne (ed.) *Le Nuove Rivelazioni*, Turin: CESNUR, Editrice Elle Di Co.
—— (1992) 'Authority and dependence in new religious movements', in B. R. Wilson (ed.) *Religion: Contemporary Issues. The All Souls Seminars in the Sociology of Religion*, London: Bellew.
—— (1994) 'Charismatization: the social production of "an ethos propitious to the mobilization of sentiments"', in E. Barker, J. T. Beckford and K. Dobbelaere (eds) *Secularization, Rationalism and Sectarianism*, Oxford: Clarendon Press.
Bird, F. and Reimer, W. (1983) 'Participation rates in new religious movements and parareligious movements', in E. Barker (ed.) *Of Gods and Men: New Religious Movements in the West*, Macon, GA: Mercer University Press.
Coleman, L. (1985) 'Using psychiatry to fight "cults": three case histories', in B. K. Kilbourne (ed.) *Scientific Research and New Religions: Divergent Perspectives*, San Francisco: American Association for the Advancement of Sciences, Pacific Division.
Durkheim, E. (1915) *The Elementary Forms of the Religious Life*, London: Allen & Unwin.
Galanter, M. (1982) 'Charismatic religious sects and psychiatry: an overview', *American Journal of Psychiatry*, 139(12): 1539–49.
—— (1989) *Cults: Faith, Healing, and Coercion*, New York and Oxford: Oxford University Press.
Goffman, E. (1968) *Asylums: Essays on the Social Situation of Mental Patients and Other Inmates*, Harmondsworth: Penguin.
Hay, D. (1982) *Exploring Inner Space: Scientists and Religious Experience*, Harmondsworth: Penguin.
Kwak, C. H. (1980) *Outline of the Principle: Level 4*, New York: Holy Spirit Association for the Unification of World Christianity.
Levine, S. (1984) *Radical Departures: Desperate Detours to Growing Up*, San Diego and London: Harcourt Brace Jovanovich.
Lewis, J. R. (1986) 'Restructuring the "cult" experience: post-involvement attitudes as a function of mode of exit and post-involvement socialization', *Sociological Analysis* 47(2): 151–9.

Lifton, R. J. (1961) *Thought Reform: A Psychiatric Study of 'Brainwashing' in China*, London: Gollancz.

Richardson, J. T., Best, J. and Bromley, D. (eds) (1991) *The Satanism Scare*, New York: De Gruyter.

Richardson, J. T., van der Lans, J. and Derks, F. (1986) 'Leaving and labelling: voluntary and coerced disaffiliation from religious social movements', *Research in Social Movements, Conflicts and Change* 9: 97–126.

Solomon, T. (1981) 'Integrating the "Moonie" experience: a survey of ex-members of the Unification Church', in T. Robbins and D. Anthony (eds) *In Gods We Trust: New Patterns of Religious Pluralism in America*, New Brunswick and London: Transaction.

Wallis, R. (1976) *The Road to Total Freedom: A Sociological Analysis of Scientology*, London: Heinemann.

Wright, S. (1987) *Leaving Cults: The Dynamics of Defection*, Washington, DC: Society for the Scientific Study of Religion.

Chapter 10

Islamic communities and mental health

Aziz Esmail

I

Wittgenstein said of his philosophy that it ought, ideally, to be treated as a ladder that one discards after having climbed it. I have an overwhelming temptation to do the same with the subject on which I have been asked to speak.[1] To speak on 'Islam and mental health' is an undertaking beset with such pitfalls that it forces one to ask whether one must attempt it at all. Nevertheless, the issues which are likely to be illuminated in the very course of showing up the deficiencies of the topic are so important, that it is worth following this road, and starting with a title even if only to undo it in the end. For at the end of this journey with a false start, I expect that we shall arrive at significant insights into the field of mental health and its relationship to the life of a community. I shall use the question of Islam and mental health, therefore, as a challenge to show why, put in this way, it highlights significant problems in our conception of mental health. In short, the topic is for me a flawed means to a valid end. But the very fact that it is flawed gives me an opportunity to make corrections to it, so as to carve out a path to the desired destination. Thus, in part (but only in part) through a sleight of hand, I arrive at the reassuring conclusion that the issue on which I have been asked to speak is, after all, a welcome means to a welcome end.

What is the basis of my hesitation over the subject? I should like to answer indirectly, by pointing out two models of mental health and illness that exist in the field of psychiatry.[2] I may speak of these models as characterised by blindness to culture in the one case, and blindness induced by culture in the other. The medical model is at best oblivious, and at worst antagonistic, to the idea of cultural influence in the genesis, phenomenology, and treatment of mental ill-health. We must remember that modern medicine is not only founded – at least to a large extent – on science, but aspires to strengthen this foundation wherever it may be found to be tenuous or insecure. This is as it should be. There is no hope for mankind in its war against disease if we turn our backs on modern science. Whatever more is needed besides science in the promotion of human welfare and happiness, we certainly do not need anything less than the knowledge and means that science has placed at our disposal. Even more fundamentally important is an ethos, a culture enabling continuing scientific discovery, and a scientific outlook on life.

In speaking of a medical model as 'blind to culture', I am not, therefore, arguing even remotely against the supreme value of modern science. I have in mind, rather, an outlook that limits the understanding and treatment of psychological distress to the methods and insights of physical science. Paradoxical as it may seem, psychiatry is no less prone (and sometimes, indeed, more so) to this bias than other branches of therapeutics based on modern science. This is because it is among the youngest of the offspring of modern medicine, one of the most hybrid among them, and therefore, in a professional world where sovereign status attaches to scientific standing, the most anxious to prove its scientific credentials. Odd as it may now seem, this hankering for a scientific paradigm was prominent in the whole enterprise of psychoanalysis, a subject which has since come under sustained fire from medical researchers, experimental psychologists, and philosophers of science alike, for the notorious resistance of its claims to controlled observation or experimental verification. But Freud himself had no doubts that his ideas would one day be securely anchored in the findings of neurology and physiology. Indeed, his very first sketch of a framework for his early intuitions of concepts like libido, repression, the unconscious, etc. – which were later to become fundamental to the mature product of his thought – were governed entirely by a speculative neurology.[3]

The course of clinical theory and practice, in so far as it concerns mental ill-health, has proceeded, over the last hundred years, along several parallel or divergent tracks. They all share, however, a certain myopia, an inadequate appreciation of the role of community and culture both in the way that mental distress is conceptualised and labelled by the patient, and in the process of healing and recuperation. Ostensibly, psychoanalysis was deeply interested in culture. Freud's own forays into the spheres of art (witness his reflections on Leonardo da Vinci), or primitive institutions (in 'Totem and taboo'), or religion (in 'The future of an illusion'), were emulated by generations of disciples. But this interest was both fragmentary, single works or concepts being torn out of their historical and social context in the process, and reductive, as it treated the mind as an at once universal and individual phenomenon, independent of history or culture. Behaviourism, for its part, hostile to the whole world view of psychoanalysis, viewed the organism as a product of stimulus and response mechanisms in its interactions with the environment. In this case, the severely empirical bent of its theory precludes the complexities and blurring of contours that would result from any broadening of the 'environment' beyond sources of pleasurable or painful stimuli. The whole field of experimental psychology, whether based on behaviourist or (more recently) cognitive foundations, is self-debarred – by its own methodological scruples – from systematic interest in an environmental context like that of religious culture.

Yet another trend in modern psychiatry has been the search for the biochemical determinants of mood or emotion. This search has led, in some instances, to profoundly significant findings. Because this trend was a conscious departure from the *woolliness* and scientific shortcomings of psychoanalytic or humanistic psychologies, and because (especially in the USA) this opposition corresponded to professional cleavages – between medical and non-medical professionals, and between biologically and psychoanalytically oriented doctors – biological psychiatry has kept clear of anything that might deflect it from the straight road of science to the murky swamps of culture or religion. These areas have alarming associations owing to the wildly inspired and muddle-headed zealots who have at times set up lodgings there. Besides, how can the methods of biochemistry even remotely apply to culture, and to what end?

Nor was the exclusion of culture and community from the horizons of traditional psychiatry due solely to the constraints of theory. The institution and practice of therapy impose their own boundaries to what might be imagined and understood within their terms. The therapist sees the patient, in most cases, either in a consulting room, or in a group of individuals with matching forms of distress, or else in hospitals, which are special rather than natural communities. (They involve interaction between individuals only in restricted, transient, and narrowly defined roles.) Thus, the natural communities in which individuals live form at best the invisible essence of the patient facing the doctor. Where the fabric of community life is especially robust, due to metaphysical, ethical, and ritual commonalities – as is the case, notably, with Islamic culture – the invisibility, to the doctor, of this all too important dimension of the person requiring help represents a serious lacuna in the doctor's conception of the patient.

In recent decades, some psychiatrists have made a serious attempt to integrate the phenomenon of culture into the conceptual and practical structure of psychiatry. Arthur Kleinman, for example, the Harvard psychiatrist and anthropologist, has made an important distinction between disease and illness, a distinction that applies to all ill-health, whether physical or mental. Disease is a biological fact, amenable (and most successfully so) to investigation and treatment by the methods of medical science. Illness is the cultural act of giving the suffering or state caused by the disease, a meaning and a value. It is, in a word, a cultural interpretation.[4] Modern scientific medicine encompasses both aspects. It diagnoses and treats disease, but it does more. It also imposes its own philosophical picture of illness on the disease. Even the proposition that illness is no more than disease – that biology is all – is, of course, a cultural (one might say a philosophical) statement, rather than a statement of biology.

The tenets of cultural anthropology, when applied to medicine, may be summed up as follows. While explanations of disease in traditional systems of medicine may be judged, correctly, to be wrong, the same cannot be said about interpretations of illness. Western medicine cannot, therefore, legitimately claim to be superior, in its entirety, to its traditional counterparts. Every culture has its own construction or interpretation of illness. Each makes sense within the universe of meanings that constitutes the culture in question. By this account, the Western interpretation of illness as nothing more than a pathology affecting an individual organism is not inherently more 'correct' than its interpretation, say, as a God-ordained punishment for wrongdoing; or (as in certain tribal societies) as the sign of a disharmony in the group; or (as in possession cults) of the usurpation of the afflicted personality by an ancestral or evil spirit. Western medicine, by this account, has exploited its successes in the scientific understanding of disease to claim hegemony for ideas which belong to Western culture rather than science. Medical anthropology seeks to uncover this Western ethnocentrism, and so to combat its arrogance.

Despite the genuine broadening of horizons that this focus on culture has helped to bring about in our understanding of therapy, it rests on several assumptions which have often gone unnoticed. These assumptions call for a critique. One such premise is that we can properly speak of more or less bounded units called 'cultures', and that the members who belong to these 'cultures' might be expected to share, in varying degrees of purity, the features unique to the culture or society in question. In consequence, medical anthropology is partial to differences rather than similarities between cultures. Its underlying premises influence it – indeed, oblige it – to seek out and emphasise the respects in which each culture constructs its unique universe of meanings. In short, medical anthropology revels in difference, diversity, and plurality of cultures.

II

So much for the philosophical considerations. I would now like to explore what implications they have for mental health. The philosophical points I have just made are supremely relevant here. The very supposition that 'Islam' has a peculiar significance for mental health is something that we must question. For, what lurks behind this supposition is the very model of culture, in the sense just defined – i.e., as an identifiable essence, separate and self-contained – which I consider to be defective. It is this model that leads one, unconsciously, to expect that 'Islam' will contain, inherently within itself, a picture of mental health differing, in interesting or significant respects, from comparable pictures in the 'West'. And that a mental health practitioner working with 'ethnic' communities, with Muslims among them, would do well to learn something about what Islam means, and how it conditions the experience of the Muslim client or patient.

How far is this true? I shall argue, further below, that the Islamic paradigm does indeed offer a vision of community, self, and self-realisation which differs, in significant respects from the dominant philosophy of the modern West. But we must view this paradigm historically. The circumstances surrounding the rise of Islam differed strikingly from those which had to do with the rise of Christianity. The political and social evolution of the two faiths likewise differed. (The presence of an ecclesiastical institution in Christian history, and its absence in Islamic history, is a case in point. It bred contrasting attitudes to the demarcation of the sacred and profane in human culture.) Again, the post-industrial history of the West has brought into being fundamental assumptions about self and society

– about the individual and his relations with family and community – contrary to those obtaining in Muslim cultures conscious of their formative traditions.

What difference does it make, practically, whether we treat these paradigms historically or not? One obvious difference is that if, say, practitioners of mental health in the West were to come to see their models of mind, self and society as historically relative rather than ingrained, as it were, in the natural scheme of things, it would make them not only more respectful of other models, but also more receptive, as and when their own limitations became apparent, to learning from them. Intellectual consistency, of course, demands the same historically open outlook from Muslim societies. There are those who might pronounce such outlook to be itself a product of 'Western' culture, hence incompatible with 'Islam'. This is where, however, one has to be exceedingly careful with terms like 'West' and 'Islam'. I put these terms in quotation marks advisedly, lest they be taken for granted, as they often are, as referring to simple, known, uniform, and contrasting essences. They are no such thing. The notion of the 'West' is more than geographical. It is also cultural. And it is also political. Which of these senses dominates a given usage is surely not irrelevant to international understanding in our times. Similarly, in talking about 'Islam', I would like to draw at least one important distinction here: namely between the historical and the ideological uses of the term. History refers us to the vision of human life as it unfolded in the Quran, revealed to Muhammad. This fundamental vision blossomed into numerous forms during a long and diverse span of history. The ideological use, on the other hand, serves the purpose of defence and retrenchment. One of its characteristics is to treat as fixed, permanent, and essential what is clearly historically relative. Thus, the stresses typical of an immigrant community's struggle for identity in a new environment take on a different aspect altogether when its ways and habits, instead of being seen as relative to the background from which the community has emerged, are declared to be features of 'Islam'. What is confined to time and place is invested with an atmosphere of permanence and absolute validity, when it is re-described as part of 'Islam'. In this way, relations between parents and children or attitudes towards women, which may be shared by communities which cut across religious differences, and reflect a pre-industrial pattern of life, rather than a theology, come to be perceived instead, both by insiders and outsiders, as part of a universal faith.

I shall return to these points. First, however, I must provide an introductory sketch, outlining some basic facts for a reader unacquainted with the necessary background.

III

The term 'Islam', commonly interpreted to mean submission to the will of God, is the faith founded by the Prophet Muhammad, who preached his message in Mecca and Medina between the years 610 and 632 AD. This message was conveyed by Muhammad as a revelation from God. Thus it was seen as the word

not of Muhammad but of God, of which Muhammad himself was only a trans-
mitter or an emissary (*rasul*), the last in the series of great prophets and messengers sent by God for the education of mankind, a series of figures like Abraham,
Moses, and others mentioned in the Old Testament as well as the New, including
Jesus Christ. The utterances of Muhammad, regarded as a direct revelation from
God, were compiled, well after his death, into the book known as the Quran, which
is the sacred scripture of all Muslims, the foundation of the beliefs and practices
of their faith.

The decades following Muhammad's death saw the Arab conquest of vast
portions of the world, beginning with the Near-Eastern lands of Palestine, Syria,
Anatolia, Iraq, and Egypt, to which Iran in the East and North Africa in the West
were soon added. Further conquests or settlements included Spain, West Africa,
what is now Afghanistan, the Indian subcontinent, and off-shore southern Asian
islands. The first seat of the empire was Damascus. This was replaced in 750
AD by a dynasty based in Baghdad. Within about two hundred years, the central authority of this dynasty was increasingly eroded by competing groups and
replaced, eventually, by rival dynasties in Spain (up to the Christian conquest of
1492), the Ottomans, who ruled a vast and powerful empire from Istanbul up to
1924, the Seljuks in Iran, and the Mughals in India, who ruled till the coming of
the British.

All these lands were governed in the name of Islam. Islam also provided a
framework for the social life and culture of the racially and linguistically diverse
people in these lands. Such a framework had to have at least three characteristics.
First, it had to be amplified considerably beyond the Quran, thus marking a transition, culturally, in the terms coined by a contemporary scholar of Islam, from the
'Quranic fact' to the 'Islamic fact'.[5]

There thus came into being schools of law, of theology, and of mysticism. The
second noteworthy feature of these developments was their attempt, at a juridical
and dogmatic level, to maintain a simplicity and a unity in the face of a mammoth
diversity. The third feature is this very diversity or plurality, which was contained
but not eliminated by the attempt at juridical and ideological unity.

This diversity, however, was not random, but united under the aegis of a coherent vision of the world. I shall mention here those elements of this vision which
have implications for the condition of society, and for the individual's relation to
society. The first of these is what one might call God-consciousness. The Muslim's life is lived with a vivid sense of the presence of God, and the inescapable
working of divine destiny. It is, in other words, anchored in a sense of an Absolute. This has important implications for values. Just as, on the level of doctrine,
atheism or agnosticism are ruled out by a rigorous monotheism, so in the sphere of
values, moral relativism is excluded by a sense of objective good and evil. Someone from a secular, liberal, modern context, engaging with Muslim communities,
is bound to be struck by the confident assurance of a difference between right and
wrong which inspires these communities. This difference has become blurred,
doubtful and equivocal in modern, secular societies.

The second noteworthy feature of the Quranic paradigm is the absence of any radical dichotomy between the world of matter and the world of spirit. It runs an entire gamut of experience, from the most sublime and metaphysical meditation on the meaning and destiny of the cosmos, to the most down-to-earth regulation of domestic and familial relationships. Similarly, its historical sweep extends from narratives of primordial times to ongoing events in Mecca and Medina. All these elements are woven into a common fabric. The spectrum is seamless, free of any fundamental cleavage. And although 'this' world is continually contrasted to 'that' world (the 'not-yet', the symbolic hereafter), the ethic of rendering to God only what is His (and not Caesar's) would sound a discordant note to a Muslim ear.

This no doubt reflects in part (and is reflected in) the contrasting milieus of Jesus and Muhammad. Rightly has Muhammad been described, in a well-known study of his life (in English) as 'Prophet and Statesman'. Possessed at once of an acute consciousness of a divine hand in human affairs, as well as of political, diplomatic, and military skills and wisdom, he united, in his life and personality, what we have nowadays come to regard as separate spheres or specialisations. In him these are not united, but rather, undivided. In brief, inherent in the Quranic model is a wholly different classification of life from its counterpart in Western modernity. The very concepts of 'religion', 'state', 'society', 'self', 'individual', etc. need to be revised when tested against an Islamic model.

The last-mentioned categories are of interest, of course, to psychology. The Quranic paradigm recognises individuality, but embeds it firmly within society. The idea that ultimately the human being stands alone under the judgement of God; the provision, in its stipulations on inheritance, for the bequest of property not only to male but (contrary to earlier custom) female heirs – these sundry references amount to a firm recognition of individuality. But individuality is one thing; individualism, another. It is not man the atom, but man the participating agent – not man, but man-in-society – who is the unit of the human community.[6]

Thus, the observer of a traditional Muslim community is apt to encounter an incomprehension – even rejection – of the notion of a self-contained individual turning his back on family or community to fulfil himself. To interpret this as a failure of individuation is – to put it charitably – to misjudge. What the mutual incomprehension highlights is not different attainments, but different evaluations, of individuality.

Finally, stemming, in part, from the acceptance of ordinary life as relatively apiece with the life of the spirit is an attitude of acceptance, as part of the human condition, of ordinary desires, appetites, and ambitions. The Islamic paradigm is more reminiscent, in this respect, of the Aristotelian warning against excess, in favour of the golden mean, than the Christian concept of inherent guilt, and the corruption of the flesh. It is right and wrong deeds, and right and wrong intentions, that mark the divide between heaven and hell. Essentially, everyone is endowed with a common humanity, potentially fallible, potentially redeemable. In the working-out of this humanity, sex, friendships, possessions and the sundry transactions of which life in society is made up, all play their part. None is in itself a cause for lament. Each is a good servant, but a bad master. In an ideal personality, they serve, not over-rule, the life of the spirit.

IV

I have so far outlined, in broad sketch, and as an 'ideal type' as it were, some of the features of the Quranic paradigm. In a specific, historical situation, however, the life of a community exhibits many features, some of which have to do with historical traditions, while others stem from an immediate environment. Of those which are historically received, moreover, many will have been transformed and re-worked in their passage through time and space. Some features, again, will reflect a culture transcending the local context, while others will reflect only the latter. Societies also tend to invoke universal principles to shelter and preserve what are, after all, local customs; just as they also seek, frequently in vain, to render permanent what is impermanent, by defining it in terms which invest the transient with the robes of the eternal.

For this reason, the description of specific situations in terms of 'Islam' must not be taken for granted. What is 'Islam' made to stand for in a particular statement? To what extent can 'Islam' be identified with a specific culture (say, of rural Egypt, a Saudi Arabian city, or an Indian village), and to what extent is it culturally unconfined? Is it ultimately logical, especially for Muslims living in the West, to define Islam, by implication, as an 'Eastern' religion, and hence incompatible with 'Western' social thought or culture? Might, perhaps, an intellectual and cultural engagement – albeit a critical engagement – between Quranically derived ideals and modern conditions not be, after all, in the same tradition as earlier Muslim encounters with Persian, Greek, Byzantine or Indian cultures?

These questions are meant to highlight the real option we have for shifting the very categories of thought, the very terms of debate which prevail today. The mental health worker in a country like the UK (or elsewhere in Europe or North America) is likely to stumble on differences in values or outlook between the immediate cultural orbit of the Muslim client, and the larger environment of the host culture. The points of this conflict will almost certainly involve relationship between the generations, troubled by parental anxiety about the seductive potential of an 'alien' culture, and the youth's attraction to this culture. Aspects of the two cultures which will stand out as mutually antipathetic will almost certainly include differing attitudes to parental authority; differing interpretations of the role of women in society; differences in moral attitudes towards sexual relations: while modern urban society regards sexual behaviour as a matter of individual choice, and tolerates – indeed, encourages – experimentation and display, traditional societies (whether Muslim or not) see sexual behaviour as subject to family and social control and regulation.

More likely than not, these issues have nothing to do specifically with Islam, but are generic to all comparable immigrant communities. They are obscured rather than illuminated by a labelling of one set of these values as 'Western', and the other as 'Islamic'. The labelling of a political or cultural stance as 'Islamic' is itself symptomatic of the political or cultural situation in which such labelling occurs. It is designed to achieve specific psychological, social, and political ends in given historical circumstances. It is, more often than not, the index of a struggle for supremacy between various constituencies – between the home and host cultures; between the old generation and the young; between men whose outlook on women will have been moulded by a patriarchal society, and women discovering the advantages of a contrary milieu. The struggle in question, then, is very often between a status quo and the tides of change.

To label one side of this equation as 'Islamic' (and 'indigenous'), and the other as 'Western' (and 'foreign'), and to identify these poles with those of tradition and modernity, or the religious and the secular, is to pre-determine how the issue is to be understood and how it might be managed. It is to preclude, in advance, alternative ways of understanding or analysing it, alternative means of dealing with it, and hence, alternative possibilities of future evolution.

Nor are these labels a matter simply of intellectual analysis. Language does not just express the mind. It conditions the mind. The terms in which a problem is stated amount to a constitution of the very problem which is being described. Moreover, when these terms have to do with the sacred – and hence with the intimate core of a person's identity – they carry immense potential for triggering and shaping powerful emotions. For this reason, a critical attention to language is of the utmost importance in the understanding of a society.

In keeping with the trend of my remarks so far, I will divide the rest of what I have to say into two parts. I shall first describe the results of a research carried out among Muslim immigrants to the USA, results which illustrate issues which are by no means peculiar to Muslims *qua* Muslims, but are typical, rather, of all immigrants in a similar situation. Subsequently, in the last part, I shall tackle some larger philosophical questions, where what I have called the Islamic paradigm, and which I have sketched in my foregoing remarks, does have a significance, though one that is not altogether dissimilar to other traditions confronting the ethos of secular modernity.

V

The study in question was based on conversations or interviews, by researchers, of subjects selected on a random basis. They were first-generation Muslim immigrants to the USA, largely from the Indian subcontinent, but also including some from the Middle East. Occupationally, they ranged from unskilled workers, owners of small businesses, property owners, professionals, officials of NGO's and political lobbyists, in several cities of the United States.[7] Many of the issues of concern to these immigrants related directly or indirectly to issues of acculturation and identity.

No sooner than the basic conditions of survival and settlement – livelihood, housing, the sense of being physically established – have been met, an immigrant community turns to the task of fostering its identity. Identity may be said to comprise three elements: first a boundary, a line of demarcation with the outside world. This is what enables the pronouns 'we' and 'they', self and other, to be used meaningfully. Second, a sense of continuity with the way of life previously followed in the country of origin. Finally, the presence of the wider community in the consciousness of its individual members. Here, identity is identification, i.e. of the individual, with the values and outlook of the community.

The challenge of an external culture stimulates changes in self-definition. How this challenge is met depends on how the culture of the host country is perceived. And this in turn is determined to a large extent by the route, the channel of transmission, through which the host culture is, so to speak, brought to the doorstep.

As far as adults are concerned, their exposure to the host culture may range from the minimal to the maximal. For the young, by contrast, the intensity is likely to be uniformly greater. An adult can count on a previously acquired talent, such as skill at business, and apply it, albeit with some anxiety and uncertainty, to the new setting which, while its rules may be unfamiliar, values the skill, and makes no demands beyond it. This is particularly true when the skill involved is technical or scientific, in that scientific technique in itself is universal and therefore culturally neutral. Although the workplace bears a reflection of the culture of the land – in the rules governing employer – employee relations, for instance – it does not demand that the immigrant be fully acculturated, only that he know the game enough to function productively at it.

The school, on the other hand, is an institution whose express purpose is to mould the child into a civic being. This means acculturation in the values of the land. One value, relevant to this inquiry, is that of egalitarianism. When, in the course of the study in the USA, the researchers asked a 13-year-old boy (who had earlier complained – at his relatively young age – of not being understood by his parents), what he had noticed about school here (which he had been attending for two years) that differed from the school back in Pakistan, he said he 'liked' the new school much better because 'here we don't have to stand up when the teacher comes into class'. He was obviously enjoying his new-found freedom, or what he in effect thought was a kind of freedom. As this child continued in school, he would be acculturated into a number of other traits and values distinctive to North American culture, possibly dissonant with, or even antagonistic to, customary values.

It is, moreover, through the youth that the external world threatens to intrude into the home culture. Indeed, youth in an immigrant community is the conduit of the external culture. Since the external culture is alien, the youth, its bearers, take on, in the eyes of their parents, the aspect of alienness. Hence arises the risk of alienation between parent and child, the risk of each becoming a stranger to the other, unable fully to comprehend, and therefore to communicate effectively with the other.

The fact that youth in an immigrant community serves as a vehicle or bearer of the host culture has the effect of creating an asymmetry, an imbalance, in the relation between parent and offspring. The parent's capacity, readiness, and opportunity to understand the new culture is relatively limited. The less his work 'penetrates' the wider society, the less Western-educated he himself is, and the less experience he has had, in a previous home, of having had to grapple with surrounding society, the hazier will be his comprehension of North American culture, for instance. Uncertain grasp of what one is reckoning with arouses anxiety. It also places the parent at a disadvantage in relation to his offspring. The child is better educated, more proficient with the English language. Where a parent has to depend on the child for such assistance as translation, something approaching a role-reversal (relative to roles in the home culture) comes to be experienced.

When a father comes from a patriarchal culture, his relative disadvantage in relation to his child, and his dependence on the latter, create an ambivalence. The ambivalence reflects the uncertain dialectic of authority and subordination. When the child has an upper edge over the father in aspects crucial to the family's progress and prosperity, when the child embodies a culture both alien as a whole, and important to be reckoned with in parts, a culture over which the father has a lesser hold, on what foundation is the father's traditional authority to be upheld?

In the USA, a middle-aged Pakistani male approached me for advice as to what career his son ought to follow. In the conversation that followed, his complex relationship to his son was revealed: a mixture of pride, dependence, anxiety, and resentment. He said his son was 'very clever'. He was clever at English. The man bought lotteries, and relied on his son to listen to TV news for winning numbers. He relied on his son to explain changes in immigration laws. His son was clever enough to understand the 'difficult English' spoken by politicians. Yet he had grown 'cheeky'. He had been refusing to come to the mosque. He was in the habit of berating his mother's cooking, asking instead for American food. And he had lately developed an appetite for designer's clothes. Who was the ruler of the household – his parents or him?

His son joined us. He reproached his father, rather strongly, for asking me about his career. It was none of his father's concern, he implied. He would figure it out himself. His father responded by accusing him of not being 'serious' – of wanting to waste away his life going to parties. His son left. His father declared he would 'send' his son to me at my hotel – could I impress upon him his religious obligation to defer to his parents? I did not, of course, expect a visit.

Parental authority is not motivated solely by a concern to uphold religious and cultural traditions. It is not self-disinterested. It is spurred as much by a concern for maintaining authority over a fast-growing child, and through that authority, maintaining a relationship with him. An interpretation of a problem of this kind, cannot, therefore, afford to take the parents' own perception of it (howsoever sincerely held) too literally. There is a natural tendency on the part of the parent, when faced by the alienness or unacceptability of a child's demands, to formulate the problem in terms of the danger that the child may drift away from the traditions of the community. Indeed, one father described to me the problem affecting his child, without elaboration, in just these terms: namely that he (now a youth of nineteen), while formerly a good, faithful, Muslim child, had now undergone a change. But the issue, on closer inquiry, turned out to be more complex. He had wanted to date a girl from outside his particular community, but had been urged by his parents not to do so. Finally, now, for several days, he had run away from home, threatening suicide.

If parent – child relations are one facet of the arduous struggle of an immigrant community for psycho-cultural comfort in a new land, the world in which youths move, as was evident to me, presents its own inherent clash of forces. Adolescent youths, in particular, have a longing for an identity which is sometimes in marked contrast to the complacency of adults. The results of the study did not bear out the assumption, sometimes voiced by adults, that youths will not seek a genuine identification with the community's religious traditions unless they are pressured to do so. The need for parents' love and approval, and the need for a sense of belonging, in addition to genuine interest in spiritual matters, ensure at least some degree of interest in these traditions.

It is useful to distinguish here between conflict-situations and conflicts. The former need not necessarily lead to the latter unless there are specific intermediate flaws. Of conflict-situations experienced by adolescent youth in the community in the American context, two may be mentioned as examples. One was occasioned by peer group attachments, the other by dating and courtship interests.

For the adolescent, peer group attachment is not simply the inevitable result of being at school. Rather, it provides an arena in which the growing youth can effect a partial and tentative separation from his parents. Hence peer group behaviour is typified by a characteristic flamboyance of style, by play-acting, and by the defiant quality, in various degrees of intensity, of gesture and action.

Behaviour of this kind has a tendency to resort to concrete items of behaviour, such as, for instance, elements of diet, dress, or social behaviour. At first sight, these may acquire disproportionate importance by appearing to be causes (rather than symbols) of conflict or confusion over identity. This process may be described as 'symbolic abbreviation'. By symbolic abbreviation is meant the psychologically understandable tendency to focus on concrete practices which are correctly seen as a problem, but which unconsciously stand, through association, for less tangible horizons. For the Muslim communities in North America and the West generally, items of behaviour such as the consumption of alcohol, codes of dress, or intimacy between the sexes have a propensity to become highly loaded symbols of a larger disequilibrium caused by the encounter of cultures.

These examples of cultural discrepancy can be extended to include other sets of relationships, like those of gender. To do this, however, would be beyond the scope of this discussion, and the few examples cited above should suffice as a basis for several conclusions. They show, first of all, that the kind of social anomalies or conflicts that may compound or aggravate personal distress, have a basis in highly specific situations. The issues affecting some Muslim immigrants in North America show the specificity of the context. This example also suggests, however, that in the idiom of traditional communities, the specificity is liable to be generalised. A historically and geographically topical conflict, between specific traditions and a new environment, may well come to be seen as a conflict between 'Islamic' and 'Western' values.

VI

However, it would be wrong simply to dismiss these terms as baseless. I have already indicated, above, a difference in general paradigms. We need, therefore, to ask whether what is at stake here, after all, is not a fundamental incompatibility between a religious, monotheistic, scripturally-based religion and a secular, demythologised – in Max Weber's words, 'disenchanted' – view of the world. Might psychiatry not be, after all, the microcosm of a larger historical drama?

A reflection on history indicates that this is indeed the case. The world view of Judaic, Christian, and Islamic societies has a two-fold basis: a spiritual, mythically charged vision on one hand, and Greek (and Hellenistic) rationalism on the other. Both saw the world as a unity. The spiritual principles of the three great Semitic religions addressed, in part, the existential conditions of life – 'limit situations'[8] like birth, death, the relation of the individual to nature and to society, power and helplessness, good and evil, and the quest for meaning – through a symbolism of the sacred. The subsequent discovery of Greek reason was a source of tension, but also of creative attempts at reconciliation between the rational and mytho-poetic strands in civilisation. In all the societies inspired by the three faiths, the spiritual and mytho-poetic legacy blossomed, in largely unbroken continuity until the modern age, in literature, painting, architecture, ritual, and religious belief and ceremonial.

The advent of the modern age saw the supremacy of a narrow model of reason, inspired by a positivist philosophy of science. The ascendancy of a narrow rationalism has served to deprive the sciences of man, including psychiatry, of intellectual tools subtle enough to take account of the role of the sacred imagination in society. This is a great handicap, for the simple reason that concern with the sacred is by all evidence a strongly rooted, ineradicable part of the human condition. A long age of resolute secularism has not succeeded in stamping out the spiritual urge. On the contrary, it might well have given it a redoubled urgency, if only by way of a reaction. When considered in this light, secular fundamentalism proves to be out of touch with, and hence a diminished rendering of the human condition.

All religious communities which draw their identity and inspiration from a book – what Arkoun, the Islamist scholar, terms 'Societies of the Book' (a variant of the Quranic expression, 'people of the Book') – face the perennial question, heightened at times of environmental instability, of how they are to 'read' the Book. This question amounts, in fact, to one of how they are to 'read' the past; of how they are to 'read' the present; and of how they are to 'read' the present in terms of the past. A vital religious tradition is alive to the presentness of the past, as opposed to a sense – ultimately an illusory sense – of a past secured only at the price of a disregard of the present. This is a powerful challenge, pointing ahead to both rewards and pitfalls along the way. But liberal secularism cannot afford to play the complacent bystander, and see the problem as something that exists on the other side of the neighbour's fence. Like charity, intellectual enlightenment begins at home.

In the storm that followed the publication of Salman Rushdie's book, secular fundamentalists routinely invoked the term 'freedom of speech' without, for the most part, enough sensitivity to the view that if freedom is to be meaningful to human beings, it must be grounded in a view of life as a whole. Without a culture of values, freedom is an empty concept. Without the vision of a cohesive and fulfilling society, freedom is a mere ideological slogan. Without a philosophy of the good, rights can be a pretext for self-indulgence.

These issues have a direct bearing on psychiatry. In so far as its intellectual affiliation is to a narrow, positivist model of science, modern psychiatry is bound to have a limited capacity for genuine grasp of the spiritual core at the heart of Judaic, Christian and Islamic history. This limitation may be irrelevant to strictly clinical situations. But in all those contexts which involve cultural values, such as the social delivery of health care, community care, individual, family, or group psychotherapy, this lack may well prove a great weakness.

If psychiatry is to be self-critical in this respect, and if it is to re-examine its cultural and philosophical foundations, it will find very definite issues of which it has so far been inadequately cognisant, and on which the Islamic, Christian or Jewish world views, among others, have important things to say. One such issue is what I might call the 'belonging' of man.

The history of modern culture shows a progressive severance of the person, conceptually, from nature as well as society. In part, this was an offshoot of the scientific conquest of nature (leading to its demythologisation), and of a rational, capitalist economy (which called for an ethic of individualism). In psychiatry, this ethic is reflected in the value it takes for granted of individual autonomy. A mere glance at manuals of popular psychology on bookshelves is sufficient to show how being original, self-driven (and indeed, self-seeking) is assumed, without further ado (as if it were the most self-evident of truths) as the sign of a fulfilled personality. The more assertive one is, the more easy one is with the expression of anger and aggression, and the more independent one is of all influences of tradition, community, or culture, the more 'healthy' one is. Even relationships are measured on the yardsticks of one's needs, likes, and preferences, and of these alone. In this scheme, notions like altruism, self-sacrifice, loyalty, constancy of devotion and purpose, so deeply rooted in the great cultural traditions of mankind over so long a period, appear at best quaint and obsolete, and at worst weaknesses: failures of 'individuation'.

At the bottom of this scheme of values there lies a Hobbesian view of man. What Hobbes called the 'state of nature' is a war of all against all. Human beings compete with one another for aggrandisement and the satisfaction of instinctual needs. In the drive for self-fulfilment, men will readily trample on one another. Society exists to restrain the individual, in search of his goods, from destroying, in the process, the individual next to him, in search, likewise, of his goods. This is its sole function. It is in order to guarantee this reciprocal liberty, that, in the words of John Locke, 'man put himself in society'. The form of Locke's statement deserves precise notice. To say that man 'put' himself in society (at a hypothetical moment), is to imply that man exists, as a finished being, before and independently of his membership of society. He does not belong to society. He is, rather, its member. No matter how supremely important society may be, it is external to the individual. Community is a human contrivance. It does not belong to the human essence.

The view of man embodied in many of the great religions, and certainly in the Islamic paradigm, is diametrically opposite to the Hobbesian picture. Man, in this view, is a relational being. This does not mean only that relationships are important to a human being; it means that relationality is the substance of the human person. Before one becomes an individual, one is defined in relation to God, nature, culture, and community. No doubt, in the course of life, one may (as individuals do) transcend and free oneself from specific communal ties; from specific cultural affiliations; and so, from particular identities. But one cannot transcend, in this view, the basic fact of one's embeddedness in nature, culture, and community. And even where one transcends, symbolically, ties to society (as at death, or at the death before death of which the mystics speak (like the Sufis in Islam)) – the death, namely, of the social ego – this renunciation is but accompanied by a heightening of the supreme bond, between self and God. At no point in the religious view may the self be conceived as a self-enclosed atom.

Might psychiatry, in the future, move towards a more relational rather than an individualistic ontology? If it does, its very conception of the ideal personality will undergo a corresponding shift. Indeed, features of the contemporary world which call for some such adjustment are by no means lacking. The hazards of environmental insensitivity, of urban alienation and gratuitous rather than acquisitive crime, seem to compel a revision of our image and estimation of human nature. In this, religious as well as secular communities will have to be partners in dialogue, debate, and the exploration of new frontiers of thought and imagination.

What is called for, in this connection, is not mutual rivalry but mutual engagement. It is not the point, for instance, that there is an Islamic (or Christian, or Buddhist, or Marxist) alternative psychotherapy. I myself regard the search for spiritual alternatives to modern psychiatry as beside the point, and even regressive. It is not by rejecting the insights of modern medicine and science that the science of the mind will move forward. It is not by a return to pre-scientific or pre-modern systems that our knowledge of human nature will advance. It is from a joint engagement between various cultural communities, in re-assessing the philosophical ground beneath modern medicine (and, by extension, other professions) that the next advance will come. It is not through a battle for cultural supremacy between religion and science, nor between 'Islam' and the 'West', nor, therefore, between 'Islamic' and 'Western' psychology, that new horizons will come to light. If there is to be progress, it will come neither out of cultural combat nor out of cultural alternatives, but out of inter-cultural creativity.

What implications does this have, finally, for the philosophy of psychiatry? The first point to acknowledge is the very legitimacy and importance of philosophical reflection. Psychiatry as a field cannot (though individual practitioners, of course, can) focus on practice to the exclusion of a reflection on its foundations and frontiers. Second, this philosophical reflection is unlikely to come – or to come entirely – from the profession of academic philosophy. For a start, it must take account of culture at large. Beyond this, it must also reckon with the concrete life of communities. Nor can modern psychology afford to stop at a recognition of cultural differences – to glory, that is, in cultural pluralism or relativism. Cultures are not static or insulated wholes. It is not in the best intellectual interests of medical anthropology to be inspired by what has been called the politics of recognition – a recognition of the rights of 'other' cultures to be themselves. It is not 'otherness' which is significant. It is with an eye to the politics of recognition that I spoke, at the outset, of the blindness that can result from the very concept of culture. This concept encourages us to see cultures as self-contained, self-sustaining wholes. But this is an artificial, relativist view of the world. It is, rather, to a joint engagement of various views of the world which have proved their durability in history – in which self-criticism based on equality and respect, will go hand in hand – that we must look today. In psychiatry the questions must surely be: what is the model of personality, for the purposes of this science, which does justice to the full range of concerns that affect the mind – spiritual as well as material, rational as well as affective, and individual as well as relational? And what corrective insights and wisdom are to be gained, for this purpose, from the various philosophies by which men have lived in history, secular as well as religious, so that there may emerge, out of these, new and more comprehensive insights and wisdom for the future?

NOTES

1 This is the revised version of a lecture entitled 'Islam in Mental Health', delivered at the Institute of Psychiatry, University of London in May 1991.
2 For the purpose of this discussion, I use the terms 'psychiatry', 'psychotherapy' and 'clinical psychology' interchangeably. While I am aware of the differences in professional training and – equally important – professional culture, implied by each of these terms, these differences are irrelevant to my purpose here.
3 See Freud, S. (1927) 'Project for a scientific psychology', in *The Standard Edition of the Complete Psychological Works of Sigmund Freud*, vol. 1, trans. and ed. by James Strachey, London: The Hogarth Press and The Institute of Psychoanalysis, pp. 295–387.
4 See Kleinman, A. (1980) *Patients and Healers in the Context of Culture*, Berkeley, CA: University of California Press.
5 Arkoun, M. (1979) *La Pensée Arabe*, Paris: Presses Universitaires de France, p. 18.
6 I use 'man' as a generic term here, in accordance with established English usage, to include – on equal terms, I might add – womanhood. One does not have to twist

language into awkward expressions in order to subscribe to the equal value and dignity of the sexes.

7 The results of the survey were analysed in an unpublished paper by the author.

8 The phrase is Karl Jaspers'. See his *Philosophy*, (1969–71) vol. 2, trans. E. B. Ashton, University of Chicago Press, pp. 203–9.

Part III

Psychopathology, psychiatry and religion

Chapter 11

Psychiatry and religion

A general psychiatrist's perspective

John L. Cox

> Any psychiatry must lead man to the door of spiritual being.
>
> Karan Singh, former Indian Ambassador to the United Nations

INTRODUCTION

To understand fully the nature of the relationship between psychiatry and religion is a complex task because of difficulty concisely defining these subjects and the need to recognise the limitations of an author's particular perspective. Furthermore, for some psychiatrists any attempt to explore the nature of this relationship is regarded as an irrelevant luxury and religious belief may be ignored or even pathologised. These considerations may therefore partially explain why most psychiatrists do not readily discuss their own religious belief even when they are profound expressions of their personality or cultural background and when they may influence their approach to medical ethics and determine their 'Weltanschauung'.

A Western psychiatrist when attending a conference in India or Pakistan may therefore be surprised when religious practice (including prayer, song and exhortation) is included in a scientific programme. Such an experience being an acute reminder of the extent of secularisation within Western society in which religious practices are now less commonly encountered in hospitals or professional meetings, and the announcement of Sunday worship schedules, arrangements for an emergency baptism and the Hospital Carol Service may remain as the only reminder of the Christian philanthropy which previously directly influenced hospital care. Nevertheless, in North America (Lukoff *et al.*, 1992) a survey found that over 80 per cent of the population believed in a God or spiritual force although they did not necessarily practise any specific religion. Mental health professionals, on the other hand, were less likely than their patients to practise religion or to hold a religious belief. This distance between the religious belief of a health professional and patient is referred to as the 'religiosity gap'. It is also evidence of an 'unmet need' for patients as the relevance of their own spirituality to the understanding of their 'illness' may not be recognised by an unsympathetic health worker. Mental health services for a multicultural society, however, are now required by Government to take into account the values and beliefs of ethnic minorities as well as the religious beliefs of the majority community: a requirement which places the teaching of Transcultural Psychiatry and aspects of Comparative Religion as a core content for the training of psychiatrists, and other mental health professionals.

However, this need to consider spiritual values and ethical mores as well as religious practice to provide a comprehensive mental health service is somewhat novel, yet is increasingly emphasised by the lay public. The Prince of Wales, Patron of the Royal College of Psychiatrists, in his address to the Annual Meeting in 1991, carefully and appropriately articulated this necessity:

> I do believe that we are in danger of cutting ourselves off into a world that recognises only mind and body. But in the treatment of mental illness we must surely recognise the importance of understanding and respecting the culture and beliefs of the individuals concerned and of those close to them. When – as is too often the case in our generation – there seems to be no beliefs but simply a spiritual vacuum, there are no foundations on which to build an acceptance of our own weakness, respect for the unique worth of others, and a reconciliation between those classed as mentally ill and society in which we must all live.
>
> Training people for your profession and maintaining your professional skills are not simply about understanding and administering the latest drugs but about therapy in the original sense of healing – physical, mental and spiritual. If you lose that foundation as a profession, I believe there is a danger you will ultimately lose your way.

These themes were prominent also in the valedictory address delivered by the outgoing College President (Sims, 1994) who likewise recognised that understanding spiritual aspects of human nature, as well as physical and social ones, was necessary for a 'holistic' client-centred clinical practice. This lecture was regarded as courageous by psychiatrists already sympathetic to these ideas but as controversial by those with humanist beliefs which underpinned their clinical work without an expressed need for a 'spiritual' understanding.

It can be argued, however, that if mental health services in a multicultural society are to become more responsive to 'user' needs then eliciting this 'religious history' with any linked spiritual meanings should be a routine component of a psychiatric assessment, and of preparing a more culturally sensitive 'Care Plan'.

TRANSCULTURAL FACETS

Issues of classification

The limitations of International Classifications of Mental Disorder which are designed in Western countries for use in cross-cultural settings are now more widely acknowledged (Littlewood, 1992). In the criteria of the *Diagnostic and*

Statistics Manual-IV for Mental Disorders (1994), for example it is recognised that a clinician who is unfamiliar with the 'nuances of an individual's cultural frame of reference' may incorrectly regard as psychopathology those normal variations of behaviour, belief or experience which are particular to the individual's culture. The examples quoted are relevant to this chapter although for an experienced clinician they would seem obvious and simplistic, e.g. 'a religious practice or belief, such as the hearing or seeing a deceased relative during bereavement (which) could be misdiagnosed as a manifestation of a psychotic disorder'.

Nevertheless a useful new category is proposed: 'Other conditions that may be a focus of clinical attention'. This category included a sub-category 'Religious or Spiritual problems' which merged two distinct reasons for a medical consultation – the psycho-religious and psycho-spiritual. Psycho-religious problems are those restricted to the beliefs and practices of organised churches or religious institutions (e.g. Christian, Muslim, Hindu), such as loss of faith, intensification of religious practice and conversion to a new faith. Whereas psycho-spiritual problems include a person's reported relationship with a Transcendent Being or Force which is not necessarily related to participation in an organised church, or other religious organisation.

There is a definite need for more subtle multidimensional measures of religiosity in epidemiological studies to include, for example, a more detailed description of the ideological, emotional and sacramental aspects of Christianity. It is certainly questionable whether the social descriptor 'Religion' used in community surveys is useful at all, as frequently this category is misused to denote a Christian denomination, such as 'Methodist', rather than to indicate a specific religion. Furthermore, without a detailed enquiry about the extent to which the religion is practised such survey data is limited and could be very misleading.

Transcultural psychiatry

Although Transcultural Psychiatry is recognised as a specialist area of academic and clinical interest within General Psychiatry, it is, however, difficult to define succinctly and was therefore restricted by Wittkower and Rin (1965) to a research comparative perspective only when the vista of an observer extended from 'one cultural unit to another'. Linton (1956), on the other hand, emphasised the continuity between generations of values and beliefs as central to Culture and defined Transcultural Psychiatry as 'Social Heredity'.

Transcultural Psychiatry thus gains its theoretical 'momentum' and clinical relevance from an interest in similarities and differences between cultures which may determine referral pathways to health care, symptom choice and management plans. Understanding the culture of the majority as well as of the minority is central to a comprehensive and accessible psychiatric service. A simplistic grasp of Cultural Psychiatry, however, which ignores the political dimension of an inequality of power between majority and minority can lead to a too superficial understanding and to a paternalistic attitude towards the religious beliefs of ethnic minorities.

Nevertheless an understanding of Transcultural Psychiatry is relevant to this chapter because religion is indeed a 'container of culture' and therefore has to be more fully understood. The rituals, beliefs and taboos of religion are profoundly important to the nature and structure of society and are vehicles whereby values, attitudes and beliefs are transmitted between generations.

Lewis (1976) in a definition of culture included religion as well as language as a specific vehicle of cultural transmission.

> For our purposes, culture is simply a convenient term to describe the sum of learned knowledge and skills – *including religion and language* – that distinguishes one community from another and which, subject to the vagaries of innovation and change, passes on in a recognizable form from generation to generation. Culture thus transcends the lives of its living exponents in any one generation: if it did not it could not survive. Its component elements are absorbed in the first few years of life largely unconsciously, and later more deliberately by informal and formal processes. Socialization inevitably takes place within and through the medium of a particular cultural tradition. When people do not know how to bring up, or what to teach, their children their cultural heritage is indeed in jeopardy [emphasis added].

This definition emphasises the responsibility of the family for transmitting cultural variables between generations, and the importance of the parent – infant relationship. Any decrease in the content and frequency of Christian education carried out by a church or school, and less general knowledge about the tenets of Christian faith will diminish the transmission of religious values and beliefs between generations.

For this writer a transcultural perspective to an understanding of mental disorder provides a historic and pragmatic way to consider the relationship of religious beliefs to psychiatric practice. However, central to this approach is a non-judgemental attitude; to be a 'participant observer' when describing the values and beliefs of others especially when different to those of the observer is essential. 'Cultural relativity' is an important additional socio-anthropological principle in this context.

Desmond Pond (1974), R. A. Lambourne (1963), Dennis Martin (1958), Frank Lake (1966), John Young (1993) were psychiatrists who understood from the inside the Christian religion and yet were able to retain objectivity in their writings, and were also aware of the 'seamy side of religious belief' (Pruyser, 1991) when exploring the relationship of psychiatry to religion. Likewise Paul Tournier (1957, 1962), a Swiss doctor with psychotherapy training, was particularly influential in recognising a specifically biblical holistic understanding of medical practice which emphasised the patient as a 'person' and the doctor's need to be sensitive to the spiritual aspects of medical work.

A greater understanding of the transcultural perspective to the practice of psychiatry will arise therefore from a greater sensitivity to the cultural and religious assumptions of health practitioners and patients. This approach also provides a bridge to understanding the relevance of religious beliefs to mental health service delivery. Transcultural Psychiatry which was once a marginalised subject is now central to clinical practice and is recognised as necessary for training Mental Health Act Commissioners, Approved Social Workers as well as other mental health professionals. Indeed, the NHS reforms which had introduced 'alien' elements of financial competition, nevertheless made more central the understanding of 'unmet need', of referral pathways and the choice of professional or folk healer.

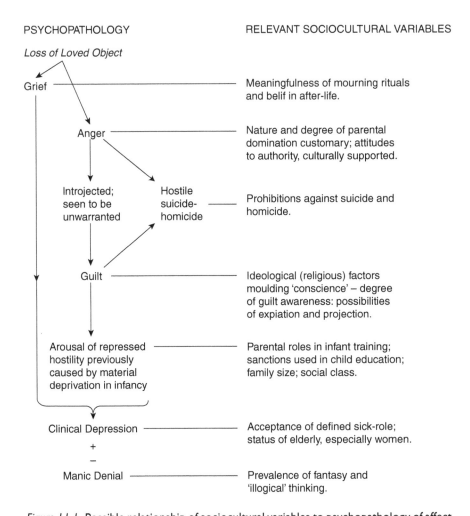

PSYCHOPATHOLOGY

RELEVANT SOCIOCULTURAL VARIABLES

Loss of Loved Object

Grief ——————————————— Meaningfulness of mourning rituals and belif in after-life.

Anger ——————————— Nature and degree of parental domination customary; attitudes to authority, culturally supported.

Introjected; seen to be unwarranted / Hostile suicide-homicide ——— Prohibitions against suicide and homicide.

Guilt ——————————— Ideological (religious) factors moulding 'conscience' – degree of guilt awareness: possibilities of expiation and projection.

Arousal of repressed hostility previously caused by material deprivation in infancy ——————— Parental roles in infant training; sanctions used in child education; family size; social class.

Clinical Depression ——————— Acceptance of defined sick-role; status of elderly, especially women.
+
–

Manic Denial ——————— Prevalence of fantasy and 'illogical' thinking.

Figure 11.1 Possible relationship of sociocultural variables to psychopathology of affect

Social psychiatry and epidemiology are more 'centre stage' in health service delivery, and their link with established Transcultural Psychiatry research literature is more widely recognised. Kleinman (1980) lucidly described reasons for understanding the 'meaning' of illness as it is constructed by patients (their Explanatory Model), as well as the reason for their choice of 'healer' whether popular, folk or professional. The overlap between 'healers', and the possibility of a simultaneous consultation is shown in Figure 11.1.

When this author was teaching a small group of first year Edinburgh medical students they were taken to non-medical healing centres and a survey carried out to determine the proportion of psychiatric patients in In-patient or Out-patient settings who had consulted 'alternative healers' during the previous months. A quarter of patients currently attending mental health facilities were found to have consulted such healers.

During this survey a Church of Scotland minister who regularly conducted healing services in the church opposite to the Royal Edinburgh Psychiatric Hospital was asked whether he would allow three students to attend a healing service as part of their training in the sociology of health care. He readily expressed a willingness to collaborate but in return asked me a favour – would I advise about how to manage those few patients with schizophrenia from the hospital who disrupted the healing services?

Other examples of collaboration are provided by Yap (1965) who described how an understanding of religious beliefs was necessary for a full grasp of the psychopathology of depression in China. In a CIBA symposium he explained how such understanding about the nature of depressive symptoms and the cause of manic-depressive illness was only possible if there was sensitivity to religious variables. In particular Yap drew attention to the meaningfulness of rituals and belief in the afterlife which determined the extent of grief and of internalised anger (see also Nayani and Bhugra, this volume). Religious prohibitions against suicide and homicide as well as the religious moulding of conscience were other central aspects of clinical depression which required an understanding of local values and beliefs. The nature of guilt was linked to a failure to appease parental figures or ancestors. In the West such guilt is more closely associated with the Christian emphasis on atonement for sins (see Figure 11.2). To quote Yap, 'The individualistic, competitive and aggressively striving Protestant cultures may specifically produce unusual psychological distress, and the belief in original sin probably intensified depressive self-reproach in a superficial pathoplastic manner' (for further discussion see Nayani and Bhugra, this volume).

PRIESTS, MINISTERS AND PSYCHIATRISTS

As noted above, the nature and extent of collaboration between ministers, priests and psychiatrists is discussed within the context of their use of differing Explanatory Models (EMs) for mental disorder and the explanations for mental disorder used by parishioners as well as patients. Confrontation between psychiatrists and

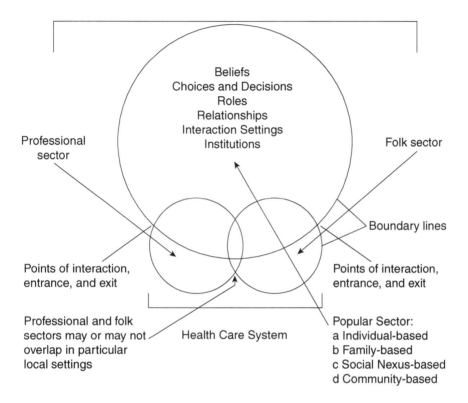

Figure 11.2 Local health care system: internal structure

ministers of religion can occur when the minister's EM for mental disorder is restricted to a spiritual framework only with no awareness of biological or social causes. Similarly, when a psychiatrist has no understanding of the relevance of religious belief or spirituality to a mental health problem then confrontation is also more likely.

Collaboration occurs when the EM of the priest includes an awareness of the complex nature of mental disorder, including biological factors, and when there is a familiarity with the range of treatments including medication and psychotherapy. Psychiatrists with a respect for the theological insights of a priest and a sympathy with the 'healing ministry' of a church and aware of the ubiquity of spiritual beliefs are more likely to work closely with a minister of religion. Indeed, a psychiatrist who values a theological and sacramental reflection, and a priest who seeks professional help for himself, a colleague or relative will also have much in common to discuss and evaluate.

Most psychiatrists readily recall depressed patients whose management was complicated because of an over-involved and uninformed minister or church member, or when a lack of faith due to the anhedonia of a depressive illness was regarded as a punishment for a misdemeanour reversed only by prayer and confession. In this instance religious belief had generated neurotic guilt. Several writers such as Pierre Solignac (1982) in his book *The Christian Neurosis* and Hans Kung (1987) *Why I am still a Christian* point their finger at anxiety-generating authoritarian prohibitions within the Catholic Church. Gerrard Hughes (1985), on the other hand, was aware of how excessive Protestant religiosity could provoke a mental health disorder. He quoted Frank Lake who described a 'Christian' disorder 'hardening of the oughteries'. Some charismatic worship is based excessively on the inculcation of true guilt for real sin and yet can also exacerbate neurotic (false) guilt. The former requires exoneration and forgiveness but such emphases may exacerbate rather than relieve the guilt which is a characteristic symptom of a depressive illness.

Joint explorations between priests and psychiatrist could nevertheless include an evaluation of a 'true' Christian experience and how it can be distinguished from an entirely neurotic form. Attempts to clarify the distinction between True and False guilt and the nature and causes of religious delusions are other areas of common enquiry. The 'religious' guilt and the 'clinical' guilt have some common features and some differences. The latter is associated with a clinical illness and the former may present itself as a complicating factor linked with 'religiosity' and specific religious values.

Having a religious counsellor as a member of a multidisciplinary team is usually beneficial although some psychiatrists find their presence difficult because of their unusual 'line management'. Ministers and hospital chaplains can also be encouraged to maintain a sacramental pastoral ministry for mental health workers; although this role is more difficult if the chaplain has become a counsellor or psychotherapist, or has diminished the pastoral oversight of health professionals (see Sutherland, this volume). Nevertheless, such a ministry within the health service, whether hospital-or community-based, can help to reduce 'burn-out'. A rigid compartmentalisation between psychiatric practice and religious belief especially when a separation occurs between public and private, is often disadvantageous and discourages recognising the contribution of religious thought to psychiatric theory.

CONCLUSION

For this author a transcultural perspective with an implicit cultural relativism together with a sympathy for interfaith dialogue provide a pragmatic platform for the further exploration of these ideas. Lambourne (1963) anticipated a coming together of psychiatry and religion in an influential book *Community Church and Healing*. He wrote:

For the local church a careful assessment of the needs of the neighbourhood, and a plan for their amelioration which includes an imaginative correlation of secular administration, practical measures, prayer and witness and sacrament is no optional extra but is the very ground of the churches' being.

A sectorised mental health service linked to the activity of Christian churches as well as other religious centres could indeed increase 'care in the community' and help restore an idealism and morality to a health service which has in turn borrowed a pseudo-religious language to underpin its secular reforms.

To the extent that the reforms encourage mental health services to be responsive to patient's needs and have not driven a wedge between doctor and patient, they may have enabled an increased dialogue between ministers of religion and health professionals – as well as between parishioners and patients. Purchasers and providers of health care who neglect this facet of service delivery are disadvantaged in the internal market and have encouraged a too secular service delivery.

Philanthropy and altruism cannot be sustained by the incentive of financial gain or 'Trust' enhancement alone. Some psychiatrists may therefore expect theologians to assist in maintaining such idealism and to provide a spiritual reflection on what otherwise is an entirely secular task.

REFERENCES

American Psychiatric Association (1994) *DSM-IV*, Washington: American Psychiatric Association.

Hughes, G. W. (1985) *God of Surprises*, London: Darton, Longman & Todd.

Kleinman, A. (1980) *Patients and Healers in the Context of Culture*, Berkeley, CA: University of California Press.

Kung, H. (1987) *Why I am still a Christian*, Edinburgh: T. & T. Clark Ltd.

Lake, F. (1966) *Clinical Theology*, London: Darton, Longman & Todd.

Lambourne, R. A. (1963) *Community, Church and Healing*, London: Darton, Longman & Todd.

Lewis, I. M. (1976) *Social Anthropology in Perspective*, London: Pelican Books.

Linton, R. (1956) *Culture and Mental Disorder*, Springfield, IL: Charles C. Thomas.

Littlewood, R. (1992) 'DSM-IV and culture: is the classification internationally valid?', *Psychiatric Bulletin* 16: 257–61.

Lukoff, D., Francis, L., Turner, R. (1992) 'Towards a more culturally sensitive DSM-IV. Psychoreligious and psychospiritual problems', *Journal of Nervous and Mental Disease* 180: 673–82.

Martin, D. V. (1958) *The Church as a Healing Community*, Guild Health, 26 Queen Anne Street, London.

Pond, D. A. (1974) *The Gifford Lectures*, University of Newcastle on Tyne, Oxford: Oxford University Press.

Prince of Wales (1991) '150th Anniversary Lecture', *British Journal of Psychiatry* 159: 763–7.

Pruyser, P. W. (1991) 'The seamy side of religious belief', in H. M. Malony and B. Spilka (eds) *Religion in Psychodynamic Perspective*, Oxford: Oxford University Press.

Sims, A. (1994) 'Psyche – spirit as well as mind?', *British Journal of Psychiatry* 165: 441–6.

Solignac, P. (1982) *The Christian Neurosis*, London: SCM Press.

Tournier, P. (1957) *The Meaning of Persons: Reflections on a Psychiatrist's Casebook*, London: SCM Press.

Tournier, P. (1962) *A Doctor's Casebook in the Light of the Bible*, London: SCM Press.

Wittkower, E. D. and Rin, H. (1965) 'Transcultural Psychiatry', *Archives of General Psychiatry* 13: 387–94.

Yap, P. M. (1965) 'Phenomenology of affective disorders in Chinese and other cultures', in *CIBA Symposium: Transcultural Psychiatry*, London: Little Brown & Co.

Young, J. (1993) 'Health, healing and communications', in H. Montefiore (ed.) *The Gospel and Contemporary Culture*, London: Cassells.

Chapter 12

The neurophysiology of religious experience

Peter Fenwick

INTRODUCTION

'When we come out of our house on a beautiful April morning and see the tulips in bloom, the blossom and blue sky overhead, our hearts expand with this vision of nature.' Clearly this is a relative statement, for were it a recently bereaved widow who stood on her doorstep, in her depressed mood the world would still seem grey and drab. Emotional value and feelings are relative to the state of mind of the perceiver. So it is with religious experience: one man's god is another's idol. Our view of the world is conditioned by our personal philosophy and system of beliefs. As yet from the point of view of science there is little to support the view that mind is more than neural nets and neurological processes. Science demands a neurocognitive explanation for all subjective experience. The difficulty is that as yet we have no comprehensive explanation of subjectivity. There is no explanation of how the beautiful morning comes into subjective experience.

THE MODERN DILEMMA

The problem for neuropsychiatry is that there appears to be no place in the brain for consciousness or mind. This has led many scientists to claim that mind cannot exist as a separate entity. For many centuries there has seemed to be no place in the physical universe for consciousness. Newton mechanics, in the eighteenth century, assumed a totally materialistic universe, without consciousness, and evolving according to a set of immutable physical laws. Descartes had a vision in which he saw the extended thing of the world and the universe fulfilling mathematical principles. The mathematician Laplace said that if he knew the position and momentum of every particle in the universe, he could predict how the world would evolve.

The idea of a mechanical universe which excludes consciousness is unsatisfactory from an experiential point of view. Both psychology and psychiatry suffer from the lack of a satisfactory theoretical framework for the explanation and investigation of consciousness. If you cut a brain you cannot find the soul, for soul-stuff and brain-stuff are different. The unitary 'I' of the Middle Ages and of our own experience has become fractionated into a multifaceted psychological structure with numerous functions, such as memory, language, spatial ability, facial recognition, etc.

The electrical probe of the neurophysiologist defines only the objective electrical mechanisms of cellular action, while the psychologist defines the objective aspects of subjective experience. There is yet no clear understanding of how these two are linked. In order to understand why, it is important to understand how consciousness came to be excluded from our science.

THE EXTENDED THING AND THE THINKING THING

Descartes, in the seventeenth century, maintained that there are two radically different kinds of substance, the *res extensa* – the extended substance, that which has length, breadth and depth, and can therefore be measured and divided; and a thinking substance, the *res cogitans*, which is unextended and indivisible. The external world of which the human body is a part belongs to the first category, while the internal world of the mind belongs to the second.

Our science is based on the rationalism of Descartes, Galileo, Locke and Newton. Galileo defined a two-stuff universe: matter and energy. These stuffs, he said, had primary and secondary qualities. The primary qualities were those aspects of nature that could be measured, such as velocity, acceleration, weight, mass, etc. There were also secondary qualities, the qualities of subjective experience, such as smell, vision, truth, beauty, love, etc. Galileo maintained that the domain of science was the domain of primary qualities. Secondary qualities were non-scientific.

Galileo in *The Assayer* said:

> To excite in us tastes, odours and sounds, I believe that nothing is required in external bodies except shapes, numbers, and slow or rapid movements. I think that if ears, tongues, and noses were removed, shapes and numbers and motions would remain, but not odours or tastes or sounds. The latter, I believe, are nothing more than names when separated from living beings, just as tickling and titillation are nothing but names in the absence of such things as noses and armpits.

(Galileo, 1623)

This view has conditioned science ever since and has led to the rejection by science of secondary qualities or subjective experience.

Einstein's recognition that mass and energy could be precisely equated changed Galileo's two-stuff universe into a one-stuff universe, the universe that we have today. The advent of quantum mechanics has done something to redress this balance, as matter, rather than being seen as discrete particles, can also exist in wave pockets, each one of which is distributed throughout the universe, but has a statistical probability of appearing in space time where the particle is. There is thus a possibility that effects in this matter are not necessarily limited to one specific area but may be non-local. Quantum mechanics also asserts that the presence of an observer in a quantum mechanical experiment interacts with the experiment and its outcome. Although this is a matter of debate among physicists at the present time, it would suggest that subjective experience may be a necessary part of the objective world.

PHILOSOPHIES OF MIND

There is as yet no explanation of religious experience that satisfies both those who have had the experiences and those who seek a scientific basis for them. Two major philosophical schools currently attempt to explain brain function. Dennett's neuro-philosophy characterises one extreme. He argues that consciousness and subjective experience are just the functions of neural nets. Nothing is required to explain personal and religious consciousness except a detailed knowledge of neural nets. This is clearly a reductionist approach, equating subjective experience with neural mechanisms (Dennett, 1991).

The other extreme is characterised by the philosophy of Nagel (1974), who argues that it is never possible to learn from an objective third-person point of view what it is like to have a first-person experience. Subjective experience is not available to the scientific method, as it is not in the third person and cannot be validated in the public domain. Nagel argues that however much we understand about the neurophysiology of the functioning of a bat's brain, we will never know what it is like to be a bat. This view suggests that the explanation of subjective experience requires a new principle which is beyond neural nets.

Searle (1992) argues from an intermediate position. He regards subjective experience as being a property of neural nets, but he does not agree with Dennett that a full understanding of neural net functioning is sufficient to explain subjective experience. Searle's view is that we need a Newton of neurophysiology to produce an entirely new principle – a synthesis between first-and third-person experience.

Until there is a satisfactory philosophical explanation of the nature of mind, it will not be possible to answer questions relating to the nature of subjective experience, religious experience and the possibility of extrasensory perception. This field is by definition still beyond the confines of science. At present, any scientific theory must explain everything in terms of brain function. However, I expect there are many people who, like Schrodinger (1967), feel claustrophobic when asked to accept that the broad sweep of the soul is contained only within the grey porridge of the brain. Will soul-stuff ever be probed by the microelectrode?

BELIEF IN HEAVEN AND HELL

In 1982 Gallup conducted a poll on a sample population of 1500 American adults over 18, to look at people's beliefs about life after death. Of their sample, 67 per cent said they did believe in an afterlife, 27 per cent did not. This correlated quite strongly with the level of religious belief in the sample as a whole – 70 per cent had some religious belief, 20 per cent did not. Gallup also found that levels of belief varied widely among different sections of the population, for example only 32 per cent of doctors and 16 per cent of scientists thought there was an afterlife.

Gallup found that 71 per cent believed in a Heaven and 64 per cent thought their chances of getting there were good (only 4 per cent rated them as 'poor'). Not every section of the population questioned was quite so sanguine about its chances as 24 per cent of doctors and only 8 per cent of scientists believed in the existence of Heaven. However, belief in Hell is considerably less common. Just over half of the whole sample (53 per cent) believed in Hell, 15 per cent of the doctors and only 4 per cent of the scientists. It seems that a belief in Heaven is considerably easier (or more comfortable) to sustain than a belief in Hell.

FREQUENCY OF RELIGIOUS EXPERIENCE

Religious experience is very common in the population and there are many studies of mystical or religious experience. Gloch and Stark (1965) showed that over 45 per cent of Protestants, and 43 per cent of Roman Catholics had had 'a feeling that you are somehow in the presence of God'. Gallup surveys in the United States by Back and Bourque in 1963, 1966 and 1967 showed that 20.5 per cent, 32 per cent and 44 per cent respectively had had 'religious or mystical experiences, and the percentage increased as the decade advanced' (Back and Bourque, 1970). However, by 1978 the Princeton Religion Research Center found, in answer to a similar question, that the positive response was down to 35 per cent, possibly a reflection of a waning of popular interest in the mystical. In Britain, David Hay organised a NOP survey in 1976, asking a similar question, and found a similar rate of reply: about 36 per cent gave positive responses. Of interest is the finding that although about a third of all people have had the experience, only 18 per cent have had it more than twice and only 8 per cent 'often' and more. There was no correlation with age, but positive replies were commonest in those whose education went beyond 20, e.g. the more articulate university graduates. There was also, interestingly, a sex difference: 41 per cent of women gave positive replies, against 31 per cent of men. Also, 51 per cent said their experience lasted between seconds and minutes, 74 per cent that it lasted less than a day.

Ecstatic mystical states, in which the subject describes a feeling of universal love, occur much less often. These states can occur spontaneously, but they, or fragments of them, may also occur in other circumstances, as in the near death experience, for example. They can occasionally occur in temporal lobe epilepsy, and frequently in psychosis, when they are usually associated with an elevation of mood. Some drugs can induce similar experiences. It therefore seems probable that the ability to experience these wide mystical states is a normal part of brain function, and, indeed, there are techniques in many Eastern religions directed at inducing these wide feelings of universal love at will (see de Silva, this volume).

Bucke, nineteenth-century Canadian psychiatrist, was one of the first Western scientists to attempt to define mystical experience. In his book *Cosmic Consciousness* he examined mainly very deep experiences:

> Now came a period of rapture so intense that the Universe stood still as if amazed at the unutterable majesty of the spectacle: only one in all the infinite universe. The all-caring, perfect one, perfect wisdom, truth, love and purity: and with rapture came insight. In that same wonderful moment of what might be called supernal bliss came illumination . . . what joy when I saw that there was no break in the chain – not a link left out – everything in its place and time. Worlds, systems, all blended in one harmonious world, universal, synonymous with universal love.

Bucke and other authors have listed nine features which categorise the main elements of the mystical experience. These are:

1 Feelings of unity.
2 Feelings of objectivity and reality.
3 Transcendence of space and time.
4 A sense of sacredness.
5 Deeply felt positive mood – joy, blessedness, peace, and bliss.
6 Paradoxicality. Mystical consciousness which is often felt to be true in spite of violating Aristotelian logic.
7 Ineffability. Language is inadequate to express the experiences.
8 Transiency.
9 Positive change in attitude or behaviour.

Although all these features are quoted widely in mystical literature, they are not in any way limited to rare, spontaneous mystical states, but are part of everyday experience. They are also a feature of pathological experiences such as psychoses. If mystical experience is so common, then it is logical to assume that there must be a brain mechanism which allows the expression of the experience. The question then is, what mechanism? Much of the evidence we have about the brain mechanisms which mediate such states has been acquired through the study of pathologically-induced mystical experiences. Epileptic states are one such example.

A MAINLY RIGHT HEMISPHERE EXPERIENCE?

Because emotional synthesis appears to be predominantly a function of the right hemisphere it has been argued that changes in right hemisphere function may be the basis of mystical experience. The evidence for this is as follows. The ineffability of the experience would suggest that there insufficient words to categorise it. Left hemisphere function is known to be associated with categorisation and thus the absence of categories and words for the experience could suggest that the right hemisphere plays a leading role.

A major feature of the experience is the loss of boundaries, both spatial and personal. When looking at the world there is a deep feeling of unity. Spatial integration is known to be a function of the right hemisphere, and thus loss of spatial boundaries is probably due to an alteration in right hemisphere function. Time alters during the experience and is usually stretched out to form an eternity. Disorientation in time and misordering of events in time is a right hemisphere, either right temporal or right parietal, function (Davidson, 1941; Wagner, 1943). Speeding up and slowing down of subjective time are found in right-sided temporal lobe seizures and with right temporal damage (Penfield and Perot, 1963; Pichler, 1943).

In many mystical experiences and also in some near death experiences where the experiencer enters a heavenly scene, heavenly music is heard. When asked what heavenly music is like, people often describe it as traditional church music as sung by angelic choirs. Traditional church music is essentially concordant and rhythmic music, as it is not until the twentieth century that discordant arrhythmic music has come to be widely played. I have yet to hear of an experience in which heavenly music was described as being discordant. In a limited study by Weiser (1986) in a patient undergoing epilepsy surgery who had implanted foramen ovale electrodes which came to lie alongside right and left medial temporal structures, it was found that concordant tones stimulated the right hippocampus and discordant tones the left hippocampus.

Although the extent to which this finding is applicable to the general population is not known, the finding does suggest that in musically naive subjects the right hemisphere may be involved with the appreciation and synthesis of concordant music. Additional evidence for the involvement of right hemisphere structures in music is that amusia follows right temporal damage (Milner, 1962) and there are occasional case reports in the literature of amusia following right temporal seizures. Rhythmic is also thought to be a right temporal function and thus rhythmic concordant music, the music of the heavenly experience, is most likely to be due to right hemisphere function. Intra-carotid sodium amytal which puts one hemisphere of the brain to sleep, shows that injections into the left carotid artery in a subject who is singing affects the words, while an injection into the right carotid artery affects the melody.

There is evidence that the hemisphere is the dominant one for emotion. The left ear which goes to the right hemisphere has an advantage for the appreciation of emotional sounds (Beaton, 1979; Carmon and Nachson, 1973). The right hemisphere has an advantage with visual emotion (Habid, 1986). Right intracarotid sodium amytal injections can lead to an elevation of mood (Terzian, 1964) and there is some evidence for elevation of mood after right temporal damage and right-sided fits (Hurwitz *et al.*, 1985).

The attribution of certainty and familiarity to ongoing perception is thought to be a function of the right temporal lobe. Patients who suffer from *déjà vu*, that is real *déjà vu* in which there is an emotional involvement of the experiencer in the *déjà vu* perception, show right-sided temporal lobe seizures. Weaker *déjà vu* experiences can arise from either temporal lobe but the strong emotional experiences are exclusively right-sided (Gupta *et al.*, 1983; Mullan and Penfield, 1959).

All this evidence points towards a major right hemisphere contribution to mystical experiences. It is thus likely that fragments of the mystical experience would be found in patients who have either damage to or right temporal lobe pathology.

TEMPORAL LOBE EPILEPSY (TLE) AND MYSTICAL EXPERIENCE

The prime example of a mystical experience associated with an epileptic seizure is that of Prince Mishkin in Dostoevsky's *The Idiot*:

> He was thinking . . . there was a moment or two in his epileptic condition . . . when suddenly amid the sadness, spiritual darkness, and depression, his brain seemed to catch fire at brief moments . . . all his agitation, all his doubts and worries seemed composed in a twinkling, culminating in a great calm, full of serene and harmonious joy and hope, full of understanding and knowledge of the final cause.

Dostoevsky was known to have epilepsy and so it seems reasonable to assume that he was describing his own experience. However, others have suggested that the experience occurred independently of a seizure, but in fictionalising it he ascribed it to the epilepsy.

In any event, positive experiences as part of the temporal lobe aura are extremely rare. In Gowers' (1881) study of 505 epileptic auras only 3 per cent were said to be emotional, and none positive. Lennox (1960), in a study of 1017 auras, found only 9 were said to be pleasant (0.9 per cent) and of these, 'only a few showed positive pleasure'. Penfield and Kristiansen (1951) cite only one case of an aura with a pleasant sensation, followed by an epigastric feeling of discomfort. However, in 1982 Cirignotta *et al.* (1980) published an account of a patient who had an aura similar to that described by Dostoevsky before a temporal lobe seizure arising in his right temporal lobe. There is thus evidence that such auras do exist prior to a seizure and that they are likely to be associated with the right side of the brain. A patient of mine had an almost similar aura to that described above and had been having it for a number of years before he sought medical care after having experienced his first grand mal seizure. MRI and EEG investigation showed his seizures to be arising from the right temporal lobe and he was started on Carbamazepine. Since that time he has been seizure-free and in the clinic he looks longingly back to the time when he could experience his auras. However, he is so frightened of having another grand mal seizure that despite the sense of loss he still takes his Carbamazepine.

It is not uncommon to find fragments of this experience in the epileptic aura. They often occur in patients who have had a psychotic episode and are associated with seizures arising usually but not exclusively in the left temporal lobe. A standard question to ask a patient is whether, during their auras, they have spoken to God. It is surprising how often the answer is yes. These findings demonstrate again a link between psychosis and temporal lobe function and between temporal lobe function and mystical experience.

Dewhurst and Beard (1970) looked at cases of temporal lobe epilepsy collected from the Maudsley and Queen Square Hospitals which showed religious conversion. The conversion usually occurred suddenly and was not always related to a mystical aura. Of greater interest, the majority of their cases had previously had a psychotic illness. It was thus difficult to know whether their experience was related to their epilepsy or their psychosis.

Work by Waxman and Geschwind (1975), Geschwind (1979), Bear (1979), Bear and Fedio (1977) gave a strong impetus to the link between temporal pathology and religious experience. Subsequent studies controlling for brain damage, psychiatric morbidity and type of epilepsy have not found the same relationship (Bear *et al.*, 1982; Mungus, 1982).

It seems that the temporal lobe is to some extent involved in the synthesis of mystical feelings and states, but that these states are associated equally with normal brain function and in illness with psychosis. A parsimonious view would be that mystical experiences are normal and that temporal lobe structures are involved with their synthesis but that their expression in fragmented form is frequently associated with pathology.

THE MAUDSLEY HOSPITAL STUDY

Sensky and Fenwick (1982) were interested in whether the American experience relating to temporal lobe epilepsy and religious experience could cross the Atlantic. Confusion with regard to terminology rages unchecked through the literature. Religiosity, religious interest, mystical states and ecstatic states, have been frequently used as synonyms or left undefined. In this study, this was taken into account, using standard questions. Subjects were taken from the Maudsley Hospital Epilepsy Clinic and the subjects were compared with national samples of the general population obtained from other studies.

Mystical states were assessed by questionnaire; the questions included 'Did your faith come gradually or was there a point at which you suddenly "saw the light" and "Have you ever felt at one with the Universe and in touch with the Universal?" If the responses were thought to occur as part of a psychotic illness they were discounted. There was a 76 per cent response rate to the questionnaire. Of the 55 responders, 28 were male and 27 female and 14 patients had generalised epilepsy (26 per cent) and 30 (56 per cent) had a diagnosis of TLE. Of the TLE, 16 had dominant foci, 7 non-dominant, and 7 bilateral. The results are shown in Table 12.1.

These results show that our subjects with TLE are no more inclined towards religion than those with generalised epilepsy. Nor did they report more frequently a belief in, or an experience of, mystical or psychic states. Of more importance, the epileptics under-report mystical and psychic states compared to the general population. This finding would seem to be at variance with the American workers who find 'religiosity' over-represented in their temporal lobe epileptics. It does suggest that the term religiosity may not be travelling across the Atlantic very well and that part of the confusion is a confusion of terminology.

Table 12.1 Reported belief in, and experience of, mystical and other psychic phenomena according to diagnosis

	% of respondents		
	TLE	*Generalised epilepsy*	*General population controls**
	(N=30)	*(N=16)*	*(N=1865)*
Religious	56	72	57
Mystical experience			
Sudden gaining of faith	40	62	42
In touch with universe	12	33	19
Other psychic states			
Belief in	54	100	65
Experience of	4	36	20

*Data from Hay and Morisy (1978) based on a specified sample of the UK population, cited in Sensky and Fenwick (1982).

CONCLUSION

What is clear from this evidence is that there are structures within the brain which seem to mediate all aspects of the mystical experience. Many of these structures lie in the right hemisphere, predominantly in the right temporal lobe. Does this force us into the position that the soul is also within the right temporal lobe?

The view you take will depend entirely on the philosophical underpinnings of the universe that are being used to explain physiological and psychological phenomena, brain and mind (see Fulford, this volume). The scientific view must lead to the rejection of a soul and soul-stuff in the universe, and to a total explanation by cerebral mechanism. Non-scientific views such as dualism or even a monistic view with the unitary stuff of the world being consciousness and manifesting itself in its various forms as mind and matter, lead to theories with little predictive power. But yet these theories do retain the possibility of the soul and universal soul-stuff.

If the scientific view is adhered to, several consequences have to be faced. This view implies that the brain is essentially a deterministic system. The full range of experience, the joy and delight of living, and the pain of loss and suffering, are no more than complex fields produced within neural nets. This deterministic philosophy must lead to the recognition that actions taken by an individual are in no sense free. The concept of free will becomes untenable. This absence of free will has implications for the relationship of the individual to the universe. Science argues for a universe in which there are universal laws and constants and which although it is always expanding is not evolving. Its laws are immutable and in it there can be no free will. The individual will have a biological responsibility and a cultural responsibility, but there can be no personal responsibility. Because the system is essentially deterministic, what an individual does matters not, providing the social and biological responsibilities are satisfied. The universe of science is thus amoral.

However, should the universe not be determinate, and the laws of nature not immutable, then a truly creative universe becomes possible. Subjective experience can then be part of the universal stuff of the universe in a way that is denied by science. When consciousness is built into the fabric of the universe, free will becomes possible. As the universe is now freely directed by individual consciousness, its history is memory. There is now individual conscious responsibility which transcends both culture and biology. Within this philosophical framework, religious experience has another explanation. It is the consciousness of the individual, seeing through into the very nature of the universe and thus experiencing the truly universal. Brain structure is clearly involved in this process, but consciousness and subjective experience are contained within this model, and the soul removed from the right temporal lobe, as Schrodinger wished.

REFERENCES

Back, K. and Bourque, L. B. (1970) 'Can feelings be enumerated?' *Behavioural Science* 15: 487–96.

Bear, D. (1979) 'Temporal lobe epilepsy: a syndrome of sensory–limbic hypoconnection', *Cortex* 15: 357–84.

Bear, D. and Fedio, P. (1977) 'Quantitative analysis of inter-ictal behaviour in temporal lobe epilepsy', *Archives of Neurology* 34: 454–67.

Bear, D., Levin, K., Blumer, D., Chetham, D. and Ryder, J. (1982) 'Interictal behaviour in hospitalised temporal lobe epileptics: relationship to idiopathic psychiatric syndromes', *Journal of Neurology, Neurosurgery and Psychiatry* 45: 481–8.

Beaton, A. (1979) 'Hemispheric emotional asymmetry in a dichotic listening task', *Acta Psychologica* 43: 103–9.

Bucke, R. (1961) *Cosmic Consciousness: A study in the Evolution of the Human Mind*, Concord, MA: Ye Old Depot Press.

Carmon, A. and Nachson, I. (1973) 'Ear symmetry in perception of emotional non-verbal stimuli', *Acta Psychologica* 37: 351–7.

Cirignotta, F., Todesco, C. and Lugaresi, E. (1980) 'Dostoievskian epilepsy', *Epilepsia* 21: 705–10.

Davidson, G. M. (1941) 'A syndrome of time-agnosia', *Journal of Nervous and Mental Disease* 94: 336–43.

Dennett, D. C. (1991) *Consciousness Explained*, London: Penguin.

Dewhurst, K. and Beard, A. W. (1970) 'Sudden religious conversions in temporal lobe epilepsy', *British Journal Psychiatry* 117: 497–507.

Dostoevsky, F. M. (1914) *The Idiot*, London: Penguin.

Galileo, Saggiatore (1623) 'Letters on the sunspots . . . (abridged)', in D. Stillman (1955) *Discoveries and Opinions of Galileo*, New York: Anchor Press.

Geschwind, N. (1979) 'Behavioural changes in temporal lobe epilepsy', *Psychological Medicine* 9: 217–19.

Gloch, C. Y. and Stark, R. (1965) *Religion and Society in Tension*, Chicago: Rand McNally.

Gowers, W. R. (1881) *Epilepsy and Other Chronic Convulsive Disorders*, London: Churchill.

Gupta, A. K., Jeavons, P. M., Hughes, R. C. and Covanis, A. (1983) 'Aura in temporal lobe epilepsy: clinical and electroencephalographic correlation', *Journal of Neurology, Neurosurgery and Psychiatry* 46: 1079–83.

Habid, M. (1986) 'Visual hypoemotionality and prosopagnosia associated with right temporal lobe isolation', *Neuropsychologica* 24: 577–82.

Hurwitz, T. A., Wada, J. A., Kosaka, B. A. and Strauss, E. H. (1985) 'Cerebral organisation of affect suggested by temporal lobe seizures', *Neurology* 35: 1335–7.

Lennox, W. (1960) *Epilepsy and Related Disorders*, 2 vols., London: Churchill.

Milner, B. (1962) 'Laterality effects in audition', in V. B. Mountcastle (ed.) *Interhemispheric Relations and Cerebral Dominance*, Baltimore: Johns Hopkins University Press.

Mullan, S. and Penfield, W. (1959) 'Illusions of comparative interpretation and emotion', *Archives of Neurology and Psychiatry* 81: 269–84.

Mungus, D. (1982) 'Interictal behaviour abnormality in temporal lobe epilepsy', *Archives of General Psychiatry* 39: 108–11.

Nagel, T. (1974) 'What is it like to be a bat?', *Philosophical Review* 83: 435–50.

Penfield, W. and Kristiansen, K. (1951) *Epileptic Seizure Patterns*, Springfield, IL: Charles C. Thomas.

Penfield, W. and Perot, P. (1963) 'The brain's record of auditory and visual experience', *Brain* 86: 595–696.

Pichler, E. (1943), 'Über Störungen des Raum-und Zeiterlebens bei Verletzungen des Hinterhauptlappens', *Zeitschrift für die gesamte Neurologie und Psychiatrie* 176: 434–64.

Schrodinger, E. (1967) *What is Life?/Mind and Matter*, Cambridge: Cambridge University Press.

Searle, J. (1992) 'The problem of consciousness', in P. Nagel (ed.) *CIBA Foundation Symposium no. 174* Experimental and Theoretical Studies of Consciousness, Chicester: John Wiley, pp. 61–80.

Sensky, T. and Fenwick, P. (1982) 'Religiosity, mystical experience and epilepsy', in C. Rose (ed.) *Progress in Epilepsy*, London: Pitman.

Terzian, H. (1964) 'Behavioral and EEG effects of intracarotid sodium amytal injection', *Acta Neurochirurgica* 12: 230–9.

Wagner, W. (1943) 'Anisognosie (sic: sc. Anosognosie), Zeitrafferphänomen und Uhrzeitagnosie als Symptome der Störungen im rechten Parieto-Occipitallappen', *Nervenarzt* 16: 49–57.

Waxman, S. G. and Geschwind, N. (1975) 'The interictal behaviour syndrome of temporal lobe epilepsy', *Archives of General Psychiatry* 32, 1580–6.

Weiser, H. G. (1986) 'Selective amygdalo-hippocampectomy: indications, investigative technique and results', *Advances and Technical Standards in Neurosurgery* 13: 39–133.

Chapter 13

Psychopathology, embodiment and religious innovation

An historical instance

Roland Littlewood

> When myths so wish, they are perfectly capable of depicting mental disorders.
>
> (Claude Lévi-Strauss, 1985, p. 179)

MENTAL ILLNESS AND MORAL AGENCY

The academic study of religion and the investigation of mental illness employ rather different approaches. The former generally aligns itself with the humanities, on occasion with social psychology, while the latter has usually preferred to seek an affinity with the biomedical sciences. We may characterise the procedures of religious studies as personalistic: as concerned with the intentions and experiences of individuals in particular cultural contexts, to be understood through the same empathetic and critical procedures as those we employ when interpreting literature or history. By contrast, academic psychiatry endeavours to follow the procedures of contemporary science in ascertaining cause-and-effect relationships in a naturalistic world which is usually opaque to human awareness, but which is rule-governed and predictable, and potentially accessible to direct and unmediated observation.

Personalistic and naturalistic paradigms are not altogether contradictory. At certain points they slide into each other, certainly providing many of the ironies and ambiguities of everyday clinical medicine.[1] Is the depressed person who takes an overdose acting as a moral agent, perhaps intending certain consequences, and thus conventionally to be held responsible for their actions? Or do we take the act as the symptoms of an underlying disease for which they cannot, in any everyday sense, be held accountable? Even with mental illnesses where psychiatry presumes some biological disease process as causal, the patient is hardly regarded as passive matter, for practical clinical and legal assumptions are made as to their particular degree of volition and moral accountability. Similar ambiguities occur with such illnesses as the chronic pain syndromes: do we take the patient as 'malingering'. Do they have a 'real' illness? When dealing with religious experiences and ideas in the course of mental illness, psychiatrists place priority on an underlying pathology which simply employs any cultural values as the material through which abnormal beliefs are elaborated or which are the 'normal' responses anyone might have to such an extraordinary experience (Schneider, 1928).[2]

This conventional distinction between the naturalistic and the personalistic has been eroded in twentieth-century physics and cognitive science (Johnson, 1993), whilst the epistemological claims of natural science to directly reflect reality have been challenged as themselves culturally constructed (Rorty, 1980). From their side, social theorists have argued that a full account of human life requires not only an understanding of how we act to create social institutions, but an explanation of how these institutions may be said to determine us through providing the necessary, indeed possible, limits through which our lives are lived (Bourdieu, 1977; Lévi-Strauss, 1968). Understanding and explaining: neither is completely true, nor false.[3] Yet as practised academic knowledge they generally remain distinct.

A number of twentieth-century disciplines have attempted to reconcile the naturalistic and the personalistic, notably psychoanalysis, phenomenology, cybernetics and sociobiology. Psychoanalysis has some claim to our interest here for Freud (1972) argued that novel social institutions, particularly religious innovations, are simply individual psychopathology writ large, and that this psychopathology would ultimately be understood in naturalistic terms. Psychoanalysts, as well as those historians and literary critics influenced by psychoanalysis, have produced a number of accounts of religious change by examining the personal lives of their innovators, a procedure more popular in North American scholarship than elsewhere, and which has come to be called psychohistory or psychobiography. Its classic instance is Erikson's study of Martin Luther (1958); as in other psychodynamic studies of personal adjustment and religion (Schumaker, 1992; Witztum *et al.*, 1990), the novel beliefs are taken as expressly therapeutic.

My concern here is rather different. We may fault psychoanalysis for failing to keep both naturalistic and personalistic knowledge in play; it has abandoned its claims to naturalistic explanation, and now employs the idioms of descriptive psychiatry – paranoid, manic, and so forth – simply as moral metaphors for everyday life. Whatever its earlier claims (Grunbaum, 1984), psychoanalysis has become hermeneutics – an interpretive procedure which seeks to uncover meaning rather than to provide a causal explanation of disease (Ewing, 1992). Any attempt to keep in play both a descriptive clinical psychiatry which ultimately situates its claims to knowledge in biology, simultaneously with an understanding of religious experience and institutions, needs to proceed on both our two levels; inevitably, it will be dialogic in attempting to do justice to both types of knowledge rather than seeking an elision which in practice reduces the one to the other. Mental illness is not just a literary trope, nor can human experience be predicated on neurophysiology alone.

THE IMITATION OF MADNESS

Can the individual experiences of mental illness be recognised in the genesis of shared, here religious, institutions? To demonstrate the very possibility we need ideally to restrict our argument to instances where we have both empirical evidence of some biological difference (and can thus avoid the recursive use of 'madness' as a literary image), and also where psychopathology can be considered according to the conventional procedures of descriptive clinical psychiatry. If we do not, at least, try to hold these two goals in mind we are likely to slide into the banal pathologisation of whole historical eras and their representative figures which have justly led to the dubious reputation of psychobiography among historians and social theorists (for an extreme instance, see La Barre, 1970).[4]

Elsewhere I have described how the experiences of a young woman during a brief psychotic episode associated with thyrotoxicosis and congestive cardiac failure were reinterpreted by her to become the charter of a new religious group; resonance with aspects of her experience became normative experiences for its members (Littlewood, 1993). Formal clinical interviews with messianic leaders are unlikely in the general run of things, and here I shall take a less reliable instance – one of an historical figure, but for whom we do have documented day-to-day accounts of his experiences and actions. Whether we consider this simply as another instance of the banal pathologisation of religious institutions depends on how closely it can be said to follow the above constraints. I am not concerned with demonstrating any necessary psychopathological impetus for religious change, but with considering the very possibility.

We can identify five general situations in which the communication of personal psychopathology (in its descriptive, biomedical sense) might be the occasion for innovation:

1   The individual. The one who develops a mental illness is already socially influential. Something like this lies behind the popular idea of Hitler or Jim Jones as charismatic madmen; it is recognised in the clinical instance of *folie à deux* where, in a close but socially isolated family, a dominant individual develops psychotic beliefs which other family members accept and seek to validate. This situation is probably short-lived, for severe psychopathology is held by psychiatrists to lead to a loss of social competence, and what for others is initially an arbitrary but not altogether unacceptable idea or action may later come to be disowned as simply insanity. At the same time, some already valued status for the innovator seems necessary for them not to be dismissed initially as insane or malicious.

2   The disease. If it is short-lived or periodic, in between the episodes or after recovery the individual returns to the shared social reality through which they interpret their arbitrary experience, and thus work them up in a conventionalised form which is accessible to others. The Amerindian or circum-Polar shaman – to take a well-studied instance – may on occasion structure a psychotic or delirious episode through the idiom of other-worldly experience, and any innovations are presented to others within this idiom. This is not so very different from the more routinised achievement of altered states of

consciousness through psychoactive substances. Psychiatric instances would include early psychosis, toxic psychoses or other deliria, manic-depressive psychosis, epilepsy and perhaps migraine. Rothenberg (1990) and Hershman and Lieb (1988) argue that manic – depression and cyclothymia have a close link to innovation precisely through their phasic pattern, and a number of Western writers have been critically examined as manic-depressives.[5]

3 The illness. 'He's mad but . . .' Innovation is not just an imitation[6] of idiosyncratic communication but a communication which has some consequences for those who take up the idea. Psychotic communications are as likely to be simply expressive (unintended communication) as instrumental yet they may nonetheless be significant for others. In certain situations the insane source of the communication may be allowed while some valid meaning is still recognised: as in our readings of Nietzsche, Strindberg and Artaud (described psychiatrically as experiencing, respectively, cerebral syphilis, paranoia and schizophrenia). We may argue that it is in the areas of art and religion that psychosis may provide valid new departures; unlike practical and discrete technical innovations, the response to the 'totalising' experiences of psychotic illness has immediate affinities with contemporary Western aesthetics and with religious cosmologies which provide radical revisions of our everyday world (Littlewood, 1993).

4 The time. Desperate times need desperate remedies. At times of experienced social crisis or dislocating change, there may be an openness to communications from unusual sources. During the Civil War and Commonwealth, seventeenth-century England was swept with a number of millennial prophecies and expectations, many of them coming from individuals who were recognised by their contemporaries as frankly insane (Hill, 1975). Yet the meaning which emerged through others' resonance with these ideas was – in these 'periods of singularity' as Edwin Ardener calls them – legitimate. 'If they were too often a moving cloud of smoke by day', Coleridge wrote of the Puritan radicals, 'yet they were always a pillar of fire by night.' Doubts as to the value of technological changes in the late twentieth century have led us again to seek wisdom from Third World shamans and (for the anti-psychiatrists of the 1960s) the insane. The themes of any psychotic experience are of course likely to include current shared concerns, whose transformation may then appear as unique solutions to others.

5 The people. Certain societies, or groups within them, may be particularly open to what for others are idiosyncratic communications. It has been argued that for subdominant groups in Western societies – Irish, Jews, Blacks, or even women in general – the mad person stands emblematically for their own identity as fey, stiff-necked, peculiar or emotional people. The Quakers, Rastas and the 1960s counter-culture may also have a wider empathy with individuals otherwise dismissed as mad. And such empathy may become generalised, as has happened with the modern movement in literature and art: the work of such psychotic artists and poets as Adolf Wölffi or Christopher

Smart are now more generally accepted as valid; and their images, tropes, style and argument become emblematic for a wider set of cultural values (for example, Sass, 1992).

My five possibilities all postulate a dual process: communication of psychotic experience and acts, followed by others' response. They are not mutually exclusive possibilities but ideal types. Communication of a set of cognitive or experiential possibilities is likely to be overdetermined: through opposition as well as identification; as iconic, indexical and symbolic; and, as in the instance below, through bodily mimesis as well as through discrete ideas. If we take biologically understood changes in the brain as arbitrary, 'natural' events, then such events have novel social consequences only if they are recognised as affecting the situations and decisions of others. As for any understanding of communication, we need to consider the prior preoccupations and motivations of the innovator, the personal experiences through which innovation draws its imagery from the shared culture, the actual genesis of the new themes, the formal techniques they employ putting the experience into circulation, and the ways in which these themes are received and modified by others. We cannot assume that any psychotic innovation must be a discrete set of worked-out ideas neatly presented to others and then adopted as a whole; such ideas (or actions or fragmentary images or even physical experiences) may provide just a minor variant from the store of dominant cultural representations, or an image or experience appropriate to quite another group but whose importance is signalled by personal conviction, extraordinary actions and local expectations. They may evoke similar experiential and mimetic resonances in others, or alternatively the very novelty of the situation and the impossibility of personal resonance with it may generate a further arrangement of the shared conceptualisations or even a universalising perspective which lies 'beyond' them.

   Our innovator may thus be a relatively minor figure. Extraordinary experiences, acts and images may be taken up and employed in a multitude of ways, from a fully-formed proposition, to the situation where the psychotic person simply serves as an emblem for others' preoccupations. It is in the gap between our desire to resonate with another's experiences and the actual limits of our empathy that the experience may become objectified as a principal in itself rather than as a personal mimesis. Or else the refiguring has long since floated free of its nominal originator. And it is in the details and context that we must seek to show how such an innovation may be plausible.

COGNITION AND EMBODIMENT: AN HISTORICAL INSTANCE

The origins of the contemporary Hasidic groups have been said to lie in a response to certain claimants to messiahship whose advent shook the foundations of European Jewry in the seventeenth and eighteenth centuries.[7] The exile of the Jews at the beginning of the Christian era had scattered an autonomous nation with its religious identification with its own land into a series of complementary relationships with Christian and, later, Islamic communities. Rabbinical tradition elaborated the original Law into a set of teachings which defined the relations between Jew and non-Jew, and interpreted the exile from the promised land as a necessary interlude before the messianic redemption. One image of the Messiah was of the conquering king who would re-establish the kingdom of David and Solomon in an apocalyptic destruction of the old order. Alternatively he was to be the suffering and rejected divine servant who held a message even for the Gentiles. For others, the exile was only one of a personal separation from God, with the promised redemption as purely 'spiritual'.

These ideas were all to be found in the Kabbalah, the collection of mystical teachings spread throughout the medieval Jewish world by Iberian Jews who had been forcibly, if often temporarily, converted to Christianity (Scholem, 1978). Like Christian and Islamic mysticism, the Kabbalah emphasised a near-pantheism. God existed in all His creation including humanity, but the failure to recognise this hidden divinity by reliance on the letter of the Law alone had resulted in our disharmonious world. One argument asserted that the Messiah would come when the existence of the Jewish community was threatened by internal sin and external violence; in another, only when Man had deliberately entered into the sinful world to release the divine sparks trapped there. The Kabbalah deployed figures of human morphology, sickness and sexual relations to describe the universe and its various conjunctions and oppositions: thus that part of God now exiled in the physical world was conceptualised as female (Littlewood and Dein, 1995).

With the emergence of local ethnic nationalism in the early modern period, the Jewish accommodation in Eastern Europe became precarious (Levine, 1993). Deprived of even the uncertain protection of feudal lords, the Jews were open to repeated pogroms by the Polish peasantry and the neighbouring Cossacks; their physical identity was threatened by assimilation and attrition. Forced conversion and massacre accounted for perhaps half a million Polish Jews in the 1640s.

Sabbatai Svi (1626–76) was a devout young rabbi in Smyrna, then part of the Ottoman empire. He practised frequent fasts, lengthy ritual purifications and night-long prayer but, after two successive marriages were annulled for non-consummation, he turned to increasingly improper actions. One kabbalistic tradition had asserted that as the Messiah was to redeem evil he was in some measure evil himself, and Sabbatai offered a new public prayer: 'Praised be Thou O Lord who permits the forbidden'. In 1665 he was proclaimed Messiah by a respected scholar, Nathan of Gaza, and millennial expectations spread rapidly through Jewish communities from Western Asia to the Caribbean. In London, as elsewhere, Jewish merchants abandoned their businesses in imminent expectation of the messianic age.[8] Sabbatianism, as we now call it, was characterised by miracles, prophecies, shared visions, states of possession and ecstatic confession, public penance, fasts to death and even self-burials. Its leader invented new ceremonies and elaborate titles: the days of ritual mourning became days of rejoicing and the Law was deliberately subverted, Sabbatai himself marrying a reputed prostitute to unite with the female (worldly) aspect of divinity. He encouraged women to publicly read the Torah; free love, public nudity and incest were encouraged for the messianic redemption could only be born through the pains of sin.

Within a year Sabbatai was arrested for sedition by the Sultan, had converted to Islam under pain of death, and was then pensioned off under house arrest in a provincial town. Most followers now abandoned him for his rejection of Judaism and they returned to traditional rabbinical teachings, but for others his apostasy embodied the ultimate messianic descent for 'The Lord was but veiled and waiting'. A few followed him to Islam, others apparently converted to Christianity. Many continued as ostensibly orthodox Jews, conducting Sabbatian rites in private and making obscure reference to their convictions in apparently orthodox writings, In the eighteenth century a Sabbatian, Jacob Frank, proclaimed himself Messiah and claimed to end the Law so the Kingdom of God could emerge in innocence. Sabbatian sects may have persisted with secret initiations until the twentieth century (Scholem, 1973); many leading rabbis continued to be accused (sometimes with good reason) of Sabbatian leanings.

Taking the biomedical perspective, it is plausible to argue that Sabbatai Svi experienced something like manic-depression. He was 'constantly depressed without being able to say what is the nature of this pain' (ibid.: 129). This extreme apathy and withdrawal, known as The Hiding of The Face, alternated with periods of illumination – infectious elation and enthusiasm, restlessness and a refusal to eat or sleep, accompanied by practical jokes and flights of apparent nonsense. Both appear to have predated any messianic claims. Examining his biography, it appears that Sabbatai had periodic mood swings, every half year or so.[9] He was born in 1626. At the age of sixteen he was tormented by sexual longings, and at eighteen turned to a life of asceticism and kabbalistic study. When he was twenty he started to alternate between long periods locked alone in his room and outrageous 'childish acts' including public claims that he could levitate. In 1648, after news of the Polish massacres, he heard a voice telling him he was the awaited Messiah. Between 1651 and 1654 he was forced to leave Smyrna for Salonika, from whence he was expelled after marrying himself to the Torah (Bible) under a bridal canopy. In Constantinople he was whipped for placing a fish in a cradle, saying, after an existing tradition, that the Messiah would come under the sign of Pisces. In 1658 he celebrated three different religious festivals in the same week and declared the Law finally abrogated. In between these episodes he was still respected as a quiet and pious scholar, albeit one who was periodically unbalanced. Expelled from Constantinople back to Smyrna for his 'strange acts' (as he himself called them when not illuminated), and thence to Egypt and Jerusalem between 1659 and 1663, he continued to fast six days out of seven. During a period of illumination in 1663–4 he returned to Cairo to suddenly marry Sarah, a young woman of doubtful reputation. He remained euthymic between 1664 and early 1665 which he credited to a self-exorcism; and laughed off Nathan's first suggestion that he was the Messiah. Sadness in early 1665 was succeeded again by illumination and acceptance of Nathan's idea in May. Miracles followed in July when he sent out letters signed 'God'; this ascription of divinity to the Messiah was an unacceptable innovation and he was finally excommunicated by the rabbinate in Jerusalem. By September of that year he was again withdrawn but another 'high' in December lasted until February 1666 when he was arrested in Constantinople and imprisoned in Gallipoli, now possibly depressed, possibly 'normal'. By September, when he apostatised, he had experienced two more 'highs' in custody. We know nothing about his mental state when recanting but subsequent 'highs' corresponded with further prosyletisation, now for Islam, and they continued to alternate with depression until his death from intestinal obstruction in 1676.

We may argue that the jokes, tricks and inversions of customary behaviour make an individual with periodic manic-depressive psychosis a particularly well-placed person to invert and transform traditional beliefs and rituals through paradoxical acts. As Scholem observes, Sabbatai 'took over items of Jewish tradition but stood them on their heads'. But the idiom of any religious message is also an embodied one: it would be a mistake to see religion in purely abstracted intellectual terms (Eilberg-Schwartz, 1992). Religious ideas resonate with the personal experiences of those who adopt them, with their selves as embodied beings, physically experiencing their lives as well as comprehending them. They employ what Mark Johnson terms an embodied schema – 'a recurring dynamic pattern of our perceptual interactions and motor programmes that gives coherence and structure to our experience' (Johnson, 1987; Lakoff and Johnson, 1980). Physical experience of our bodies in space already provides us with schemata such as verticality or containment which can serve as metaphorical projections to structure other domains of experience. 'Up' is 'more'; 'up' is also 'better' and an attribute of power, sanctity, divinity and heaven (Bevan, 1935:28 et sequ.), as well as of 'superior' secular authority – those of higher status supervise the lower classes, etc. (Cohen 1980:58–62). Ascent is arduous, descent precipitous. A virtually universal religious schema is that the other world of ultimate authority stands above us.[10] Shamans too describe other-worldly experiences as a high or as a flight, whilst female prophets may prefer, like Mother Ann of the Shakers, Mother Earth of the Earth People, or St Theresa, an idiom of entry of divinity into them (Littlewood, 1993). To be high is arguably a more accessible experiential metaphor for male prophets; being a container of unfolding creation for women (ibid.).

What we now code as experiences analogous to 'elation' and 'depression' in changes of mood are not necessarily articulated as verticality. 'Depression' (Latin de-premere) as a mood state seems only to have become a common term in English in the eighteenth century, and Shweder (1985) argues that a more common experience in melancholy employs an idiom of containment and emptying, in which something is removed or lost out of ourselves. Whilst the sense of oppression, pressure, constraint and limitation we experience in 'lowered' mood states might now seem intrinsically coded by such a spatial idiom, others may employ quite different embodied schemata.[11] If a existing religious cosmology already employs high/low as the dimensions of divine presence, then in a context where we seek a religious meaning for our experiences, a verticality schema may provide the most appropriate idiom.[12]

Judaism already used the schema of high/low to refer to nearness to/absence from God (Eilberg-Schwartz, 1992:30, 32), and Sabbatai employed this verticality to objectivise[13] his experiences as religious communion: 'high' was associated with spiritual mission, 'low' with self-doubt. For orthodox Jews, melancholy is still represented as a falling from God (Weisel, 1978). In the experience of contemporary manic-depressive patients it is usual for any religious preoccupations to occur simply with the manic phase.[14] But not always so. An orthodox Jewish patient from East London under the care of Maurice Lipsedge and myself became a fervent evangelical Christian (of the 'Jews for Jesus' persuasion) when manic; when depressed he fell into gloomy textual ruminations about his apostasy.

Sabbatai's followers not only accepted his own interpretation of his mood swings intellectually but they seem to have resonated with them, themselves experiencing episodes of religious exultation and despair which became normative experiences for many. Not so for Nathan, whose actions at all times appeared to have remained those of a quiet and restrained rabbi, anchoring Sabbatai's explanations within the habitual system of understanding. Sabbatai's experiences provided a bodily representation of the kabbalistic teaching, together with a firm conviction, when 'high', of his messiahship, although this was generally established by the acclamation of Nathan. Scholem (1973) suggests many earlier kabbalistic scholars may have privately wondered if they themselves were the messiah but waited for such an external validation.[15] For others, Sabbatai's experiences offered an interpretation of the fluctuating relations between God and Man, and thus the waxing and waning of the movement.

SABBATAI SVI AND THE HASIDIM

The influence and persistence of Sabbatian ideas after his apostasy suggest that the movement 'reached down to the layer of common heritage' of Eastern European Jewry (Scholem, 1973:3). For orthodox Jews, residence, family life, daily activities and education remain strictly determined by religious law and its commentaries (Zborowski and Herzog, 1962). Conversation, cooking, eating, bathing, bodily movements, excretion and sexual relations were ordered in conformity with established ritual – which always opposed itself to non-Jewish society – and within the constraints of a rigid spatio-temporal system: the order of daily activities in the household, the celebration of the Sabbath and the annual festivals, and a history reworked in telling the innumerable tales of the lives, wit and teaching of scholars. Nothing outside the community could be considered entirely wholesome; when a Jew converted to Christianity, funeral prayers were offered.

As in all forms of Judaism, men were dominant in religious life. They conducted the services in the prayer house; women, if they attended at all, concealed themselves behind a partition. From an early age boys and girls learnt to avoid each other, for male and female domains were always distinct. Whilst a girl's interest was directed towards her household, her brother spent long hours in religious study. Initially he learned by rote but later gained considerable freedom for disputation with others; human conduct should always conform to the Law but this was open to the varied interpretations of older men whose authority was in their knowledge. A man gained more respect by such debate than he did by lineage, age or wealth, and after marriage he continued to study for a few years supported by his father-in-law before he turned to earning a living. A woman's role was as guardian of health, home and family, and through her care in this she safeguarded the bodily purity of the men. The geography of prayer house, home, room, clothes and body complemented and commented on each other, and the Law gave specific instructions for every activity. Through a complex numerology employing the numerical value of alphabetical letters, cardinal numbers (the number of good or bad deeds, gifts, objects, alms) and ordinal numbers (of a text or birth order), it enclosed the social and physical worlds in a tight cognitive network. *Kosher* was a term which was applied simultaneously to food, clothes, non-menstruating women, books and ideas.

It will be apparent that I have represented Jewish culture as a dual classification, anchored politically in the community's distinction between Jew and Gentile, and internally between men and women. Jewish life has indeed been regarded by many (Freud, Bakan, Mintz, Zborowski and Herzog) as experientially dual, as perhaps life is among any subdominant groups which constitute a permanent minority (Littlewood, 1993). Arranging some of the key elements as a polythetic model gives us Jew: Gentile :: Observance of the Law (*mitsva*): Violation of the Law (*aveyreh*) :: Sacred: Mundane :: High: Low :: Male: Female :: Learned (*sheyn*): Simple (*prost*) – a schema which opposes the centrality of the inside male to the values of the wider society.[16] From the outside, it may be taken as a subdominant schema vis-à-vis the Gentiles, but in its self-aware historical continuity it places the Jew as central.

Sabbatai can be seen as inverting certain of these pairs through his own actions and subsequent justifications: certain pairs alone, for there was no way he could cease being Jewish – until his apostasy. This type of cognitive inversion was available to interpretation by his community in various ways. Even from the start of his 'strange acts', before he accepted the title of Messiah, Sabbatai's actions were regarded as concealing some hidden, higher, meaning; and one which was taken by some as perhaps the dawn of the messianic age. The overturning of an external Law may have been particularly attractive to the dispersed Iberian *marranos* who had been forcibly baptised as Christians whilst retaining a private Jewish identity: Sabbatianism legitimated their own external apostasy. Following Sabbatai's own adoption of the turban, the majority of Jews returned to rabbinical orthodoxy – but often of an attenuated, less rigorous, type. Scholem (1971) has suggested that the antinomian attack on the Law by the Sabbatians both reflected and hastened the development of modern secular Judaism: freed from its existing social structurings, the method of criticism and argument perfected in the ghetto passed out into a more universal and secular rationalism.[17]

If some Sabbatians used the contravention of the Law as a passage to a now increasingly secularised Gentile society, others reappropriated the messianic moment back into rabbinical orthodoxy. The relationship of the Sabbatians to the Hasidic movement of the eighteenth century remains controversial. Hasidism has been described as 'neutralisation of messianic elements into mainstream Judaism' (Scholem, 1971), and even as a 'a dialectical synthesis' of the two (Bakan, 1958).[18] It appears to have crystallised out of the mystical – pietist groups influenced by Sabbatai Svi: many early leaders were ex-Sabbatians and continued some of his ritual reinterpretations whilst opponents condemned it as a continuation of the heresy. Although now adhering strictly to the accepted body of Jewish Law and tradition, Hasidim differ from other orthodox Jews in two characteristic features: their cultivation of ecstatic states and the role of the dynastic leader, the *Rebbe* or *Zadik*. The movement was developed among the small Jewish communities of Poland, by wandering preachers *Zadikim*, who emphasised the presence of God in all creation and in all human activity: every person however uneducated could communicate with Him through prayer or contemplation. Hasidim originally used intoxicants and tobacco, and turned somersaults in their prayers, and there is still encouragement of a body mysticism through shouting, singing, clapping and joyful dancing in the prayer houses, punctuated by trembling and rapturous prayer.

The movement spread rapidly during a period of economic crisis and endemic anti-semitism despite fierce opposition from other orthodox Jews. In the 1930s perhaps half of the eight million Jews in Eastern Europe were associated with Hasidism. The vast majority died in Nazi concentration camps. The many different groups which survived and settled in England, Belgium, North America, and more recently Israel, have varied traditions but each is characterised by the reverence paid to its *Rebbe*. The life of the community is rooted in him as the mediator with the external world. Surrounded by a constant crowd of attendants and petitioners, he holds court for his awed followers who closely follow his advice and teaching. He foretells misfortune, heals infertility and disease, and performs daily miracles through the talismans he distributes. During communal meals the food he leaves on his plate is distributed to the followers, after which he may offer homilies in a joyful trance-like state. Many *Rebbes* claim to alter the course of world events and despite disclaimers to the contrary, the *Rebbe's* powers are taken as personal rather than derived from God. Hasidim consult him on how and when to travel, which job to take, whether to divorce, or to invest in a particular project, whom their children should marry, the ultimate cause of their sickness, which doctor to consult (for examples see Littlewood and Dein, 1995). Some orthodox Jews (for whom the rabbi is only a teacher, however gifted) have viewed Hasidic *Rebbes* with distaste – 'the wretched ringleaders of a widely spread delusion' says Schechter. For many Jews, however, the Hasidim remain a guarantee of the permanence of Yiddish culture, and were regarded by liberals with affectionate amusement until the rise of political ultra-orthodoxy in Israel in the 1980s; one group, Lubavitch, now proselytise actively among non-observant Jews (ibid.).

To what extent did Sabbatai's ascetic and antinomian actions become routinised models in Hasidism? Hasidic texts to the present day include ambivalent injunctions against excessive asceticism, for these practices continued. To avoid military service which would have prevented them carrying out ritual observances, Eastern European Hasidim fasted to near starvation or mutilated themselves contrary to conventional orthodoxy. Hasidic men still study the Kabbalah with its cryptic references to the unreality of evil. Judaism has always emphasised the neutralisation rather than the rejection of evil: sorrow is necessary for joy, evil for good, and Hasidim take this paradox further: 'The subversion of the Torah is its true fulfilment', 'Great is sin committed for its own sake'. Evil is less a force to be avoided than a divinity in exile which must be restituted so that its scattered aspects can finally be united. In the last, argue some, even Jesus may be redeemed. The descent into evil to raise the imprisoned sparks of divinity is dangerous: it is easy to go down and not return. The descent is reserved for the *Rebbe* alone and many groups privately argue that their own leader is indeed the Messiah (see Note 15). As mediator between Hasid and Gentile he is in constant contact with evil. Hasidic tales are full of inversions of the Law by the *Rebbes* – always motivated, often ironic yet always with a deeper moral purpose beyond the Law and beyond its inversion. It is as if the *Rebbe* were so pure he could sin without sinning; he could eat pork without impurity. In practice he does not and indeed usually conforms to all traditional observances, but his saintliness gains by close association with evil.

The interpretation I have offered argues a progression from an individual inversion mediated by Sabbatai's psychopathology through which a whole community is turned upside-down temporarily, to one located in the permanent social order – the *Rebbe*. Hasidim, in spite of fluctuating messianic expectations, live in a continuous biblical present. The *Rebbe* sees across space and time, and he may be the incarnation of a prophet; life is organised around cyclical festivals; children are named after the dead and take on their identity; the dead remain with us in other ways, as revenants, in dreams and in visions. Hasidic teaching contains the opposing principles of the rabbinical Law and their inversion in Sabbatian antinomianism: the Law can be contravened for greater ends by select individuals at certain carefully controlled times and the licence to invert it is only gained by its conspicuous observance at all other times. Whether we see Hasidism primarily as a continuation of Sabbatian messianism or as a reaction against it, it appears to be an appropriation of certain active messianic elements by orthodoxy: the emphasis on the Law coexists with the 'deep' possibility of overturning it. The two persist together in a dynamic tension which provides a remarkably consistent pattern of culture: one which articulates the relationship of *Rebbe* to follower, male to female, and Hasid to the outside world.

In summary, then, the Jewish exile was understood as a preparation for the messianic arrival, When the political accommodation with the Gentiles was threatened in the early modern period, the messianic moment abrogated the Law and introduced the fabled redemption into the mundane world. The frustration of the active messianic impulse resulted in a return to an orthodoxy which was constantly threatened by anti-semitism and assimilation. Hasidism internalises and accommodates active messianism within the traditional framework, whilst Zionism essays a millennium without the Messiah. More recently, some Hasidim in Israel have again emphasised a political messianism in association with the 'religious' turn in Zionism. Each development – rabbinical orthodoxy, Hasidism or Zionism, even Sabbatianism – is bound by (and for) the persistence of the group as a distinct ethnic entity. Each offers a solution to the dangerous relationship with the non-Jewish majority.

To what extent does Sabbatianism meet the five conditions I suggested for 'the imitation of madness' (p. 180)? Sabbatai was certainly respected as a promising scholar before his controversial actions and it is not easy to see how he could have been taken seriously otherwise; he was not, however, so influential that his community would fully accept all outrageous ideas immediately (paragraph 1, p. 180). His respectability established his acts as antinomian – as meaningful and motivated contraventions of a now otiose Law – rather than as a simple refusal to follow it. His experiences were periodic, enabling him to explain their meaning later within the common shared assumptions (paragraph 2): 'behaviour' became 'action'. The audience did not have a restricted concept of psychopathology (Gradek, 1976), nor did they recognise Sabbatai's actions as 'mad but . . .' (paragraphs 5,3). Opponents certainly characterised him as insane but his followers usually refuted this, although at times they cited Isaiah's vision of the Messiah as 'a man of pains and acquainted with disease' (Isa. 53, cf. A.V. 'a man of sorrows and acquainted with grief') (Scholem, 1973:629, 130, 54). Eastern European Jews arguably took themselves as living in 'desperate times' (paragraph 4) given the Chmielnicki massacres. The movement was most significant, however, not among the surviving Polish Jews but among those in Palestine under Turkish rule where Jews were more secure than in Christian countries, although Sabbatai himself dated the onset of his mission to 1648, the year of the massacres. Sabbatian adherents were as likely to come from the affluent and assimilated sections of the Jewish community as from among the pauperised and marginal.[19]

Our conclusions must remain tentative. My example is limited by the usual problems of conjectural psychohistory: the ascription of psychopathology across culture and across time. Any assumption of Sabbatai Svi's manic-depression is based on sources compiled by his followers. That his 'highs' and 'lows' could be so neatly interpreted in kabbalistic terms may lead us to wonder whether the interpretation was not prior to what were not altogether arbitrary physiological experiences; perhaps

Sabbatai was just amplifying periods of everyday cheerfulness and sadness? His mood swings, however, seem generally unrelated to external events, and at times of crisis or communal fervour he was often nowhere to be found. The movement largely developed away from the messianic presence: Sabbatai was not a charismatic leader who firmly placed the stamp of his own personality on all its aspects. Instead, his audience appear to have found in his unseemly actions the physical locus through which to rework their own preoccupations.

NOTES

1 What one might loosely term an academic Cartesian dualism conforms to our own everyday experience. We do not experience our bodies simply as the agents of our will but as also subject to arbitrary processes outside our volition, whether pain and sickness, emotion, physiological processes mediated by the autonomic nervous system, or the consequences of external events. Beyond our agency, they appear as some 'other' opposed to our self. Leder (1990) argues that the experience of everyday physical actions is usually characterised by a rupture between goal and process; and that dualism is derived from this. The extent to which Judaeo-Christian theologies themselves reinforced such a folk dualism, and their subsequent transformation into contemporary psychiatric epistemology is considered in Littlewood and Dein (1995).
2 As form or content in the conventional psychiatric idiom, derived from, but somewhat curiously reversing Kant's antinomy of cognitive versus material.
3 Samuel (1990), Leder (1990), and Lawson and McCauley (1990) have argued that the distinction between 'understanding' in the humanities, and 'explaining' in the natural sciences (suggested by Kant and commonly used in psychiatric texts following the terminology of Karl Jaspers (1963)) is not absolute. In a more inclusive model of human knowledge which owes much to Bateson's early cybernetics, Samuel claims that a non-causal interpretive approach may still have explanatory and predictive power, whilst Leder advocates an embodied phenomenology. The epistemological justifications of the current anti-dualist debate are beyond the scope of this chapter which is concerned rather with the interpenetration of practical knowledge from the two approaches; each may be taken as a valid map of reality, constructed for a particular purpose, and each remains grounded in its customary procedures whilst entailing the other – what I have termed elsewhere an ironic simultaneity (Littlewood, 1993). This may recall the 'dual aspect' theories of Spinoza or Nagel (or even Feyerabend's 'eliminative materialism'), but it is procedural not epistemological. Caramagno (1992) provides an example in the area of literary criticism. By contrast, the common procedure in the human sciences since Foucault is to interpret both religion and psychiatric illness alike as culturally constructed domains of inquiry which have become reified, with consequent problems of establishing associations or causalities between them (e.g. Csordas, 1992).
4 La Barre argues that all religious ideas have originated in psychosis. More sophisticated approaches to the psychobiology of religious experience are provided by Comfort (1981), and on the biological adaptiveness of religious institutions by Reynolds and Tanner (1983), whilst Mazlish (1990) offers a more interpretive psycho-analytical view in arguing that the melancholy of Puritan New England should be read as 'a form of discourse' rather than as a pathology. On the general absurdities of retrospective diagnosis, and for an exemplary and modest instance, see Porter (1985).
5 Virginia Woolf (Caramagno, 1992); Robert Lowell (Hamilton, 1983); for other examples see Hershman and Lieb (1988), Littlewood (1993). There is a certain amount of evidence that manic – depression is more common in 'creative' individuals

but something like a two-stage process may be found in any illness, including physical illness which calls to attention feelings and cognitions which are otherwise tacit or latent: experience plus reflection.

6 To employ Devos' (1976) term *pathomimesis*, which he takes from Theodore Schwartz's work on the 'imitation' of epilepsy in the institution of Melanesian cargo cults (cf. Girard, 1978).

7 My argument is developed from some remarks in an earlier paper (Littlewood, 1983) which may be consulted for sources and ethnographic references. As a number of colleagues have pointed out, Gershom Scholem's thesis (1971, 1973), that Hasidism may be said to appropriate or reframe a substantially Sabbatian sensibility, is by no means generally accepted. I am especially grateful to Maurice Lipsedge for having called my attention to Scholem's work; and to him, to Chimen Abramsky, Simon Dein, David Greenberg and Bernard Wasserstein for useful criticisms. Romanised transcriptions of Sabbatai's family name include Svi, Sevi, Zevi.

8 Sabbatai's father had been the agent in Smyrna for a group of English merchants and it is possible that Sabbatianism was influenced by Puritan millenialism. Sabbatianism in turn sparked off rumours among radicals in England that redemption for all was at hand (Scholem, 1973: ch. 4), for the Fifth Monarchy Men and others had predicted 1666 as the beginning of the messianic age. Many radical sectarians, such as Henry Finch (*The World's Great Restauration, or the Calling of the Jews*, 1621), already regarded the Jews as the chosen people and looked for divine events concerning them (Hill, 1975). Some Christians adhered to the Sabbatians, whilst ten years previously British Jews had declared Cromwell to be the Messiah (Stokes, 1913:219–20). At other times Jews have cast messianic glances on Huss, on Luther (later of course to be a virulent anti-semite), and even Napoleon (in common with some Christian sects).

9 Scholem (1973), whilst no enthusiast for the pathologisation of religion (La Barre, 1970:316), referred the detailed primary sources written by Sabbatai's associates to clinical colleagues: the diagnoses they offered were paranoid psychosis and manic – depression.

10 On the use of spatial representations of 'mental states' see Shweder (1985:194 esp.); Johnson (1987, 1993). Whilst among some ecstatic groups such as the Sufis, contact with divinity may be determined by one's heat (*hal*), groups may, like the American Shakers, use *high* and *hot* interchangeably to mark ecstasy. 'Deep' is often mundane, elemental and primordial (Crapanzano, 1992). The spatial metaphors favoured by the Kabbalists 'became concretely applicable only at the lowest stage of the process of divine emanation, that is, our material cosmos' (Scholem, 1973:29). Thus we have 'an ascent to God', a 'higher world', counterposed to 'lower orders of being' and 'the fall of Adam' (ibid.: 15, 28, 39). The mundane world of evil (the *qelippah*) is a fallen one but it can be raised by acts of merit (*tiqqun*). In prayer Hasidim still tie a band around the body to separate the upper spiritual half from the lower profane half. On the possible spatial representations of the kabbalistic world and their reflection in the human body see Littlewood and Dein (1995). Contemporary secular Zionists use the term *alijah* (ascent) to refer, not to a movement to God, but migration to Israel: the converse being the term for leaving Israel.

11 Rarely, a verticality schema may be used the other way: in Fiji something akin to the psychiatrists' mania is termed *matikuru*, 'low tide' (Price and Karim, 1978) (but the 'low' is perhaps an inappropriate English equivalent, and 'out to sea' may be a more apt translation).

12 The medical choice of a verticality schema in the eighteenth century seems different, perhaps related to the privileging by Enlightenment science of optical paradigms which followed the development of fixed-position perspective to become the idea of a correspondence theory of knowledge which was ascertained by the 'context-independent' scientific observer (Heelan, 1983; Howes, 1991: Introduction; Rorty,

1980): what Foucault (1973) has termed the 'clinical gaze'. Perhaps the first graphic example of verticality as the index of madness is Hogarth's engraving of *Enthusi-asms Delineated* (1761) which satirises the religious ecstasy of the Methodists. In the bottom right-hand corner of a scene of a lustful and lunatic congregation, a type of thermometer may be seen emerging from a brain, calibrated upwards from Despair, through Low Spirits, Luke Warm, Lust Hot and Ecstasy, to Revelation. In the revised plate (1762), the bottom of the scale is now labelled Suicide. From the perspective of phenomenology, the visual modality is arguably the least 'embodied' of all senses (Leder, 1990), and a common critique of contemporary academic psychiatry is that it is purely visual/verbal, missing the embodied experiences of altered patterns of sensation, kinaesthesiae, comportment and gesture, or at least translating these into a verbal checklist. Certainly many experiences of severe 'mental' illness are embodied experiences – of penetration, physical passivity, synaesthesia and altered sensory perception in different modalities including proprioception. The popular European paradigm of insanity remains cognitive – 'hearing voices' – whilst elsewhere it may be characterised primarily by physical comportment (e.g. Littlewood, 1993). Sabbatai's choice of a verticality schema may fit with a predominantly written (and thus visual) Jewish mysticism, but in biblical Hebrew words are not simply representations of external reality; they are themselves physical presences, symbols which stand for themselves (Littlewood and Dein, 1995). Howes (1991: Introduction) argues Jewish epistemology was predominantly articulated in aural rather than visual terms: truth is 'heard' not 'seen'; revealed not ascertained.

13 To use Obeyesekere's term (1981): in psychodynamic understanding, projection plus reification, by which we take our personal experiences for some entity outside ourselves which is superordinate; and through which the idea appears to transcend personal experience. Whilst the basis of 'context independent' science (see Note 12), this is argued by psychiatrists and psychoanalysts to be characteristic of messianic psychoses where individuals then identify with this external power (Jaspers, 1963; La Barre, 1970). Whether the delusional interpretation may be said to have historically facilitated the normative scientific perspective – as exemplar or biosocial change – is beyond the scope of this chapter but see Murphy (1967), Littlewood (1993), and Note 17 below.

14 'Religious delusions' are common enough in psychosis to be categorised separately, and in the Catego program of the Present State Examination are associated particularly with mania (Wing *et al.*, 1974). The sense of unbounded possibility, foreshortened time and the interconnectedness of all things which characterise mania certainly make it an apt vehicle for a millennial vision.

15 A contemporary instance is the Lubavitcher *Rebbe*, Menachem Mendel Schneersohn, who has encouraged his followers to speculate on his messiahship. His recent stroke and incapacitation led them to immediate messianic expectations: 'We want Moshiach now' (Freedland, 1993). The *Rebbe's* bodily illness is argued by them to signal the imminent messianic descent into the physical world of impurity and sickness to redeem the exiled sparks of divinity (Littlewood and Dein, 1995). By November 1993 he had been proclaimed King Messiah. He died in 1994.

16 Each pair in the chain takes a relational meaning from the elements adjacent to it. The system of social classification was so 'tight' that the bipolarities are even more context dependent than I have indicated. The Sabbath, which from my model we might presume to be male in opposition to the profane week, was female in opposition to the community which 'embraced' it (Zborowski and Herzog, 1962).

17 In terms of my model, the inversion of the chain in certain elements is interpreted as a twisting – a chiasmus (which may be pictured as akin to a double helix). Seeking to read the new schema into a now limited set of social circumstances provides a psychological and moral universalisation, beyond the conceptual chain and beyond its

inversion. And thus accessible to others outside the group in which it is elaborated. To take a Christian instance, Jesus' picking corn on the Sabbath argued a more universalised yet individualised moral dispensation, beyond a local religion of ritual attachment to the collective land. Psychoanalysis has been regarded by Bakan (1958) as a later stage of the same movement. Freud himself stated that analysis could only have evolved out of Judaism (cf. Gay, 1987; McGrath, 1986; Robert, 1974) and was at times atypically reluctant to apply his ideas to it: on the death of a Zionist colleague he wrote that 'Jewishness . . . was inaccessible to any analysis so far' (cited in Robert). Henri Ellenberger (1970) suggests that the origins of the (psychological) Oedipus complex lie in the (social) experience of anti-semitism, whilst for Kafka the revolt against the father in psychoanalysis was not against the father *per se* but the revolt of the assimilated Jew against the Jewishness of his father (ibid.): for castration read circumcision. Whether we accept that Freud consciously identified himself with Sabbatai as Bakan suggests, it is true that his family was partly Hasidic in origin and we can find certain kabbalistic themes in psychoanalysis: a monist epistemology; the physical and its numerical and linguistic representations as metaphors for each other; the transcendence of the immediate world by sexual relations with the symbolic mother; the return of the exiled past; renunciation and sublimation; the significance behind the apparently random association of ideas in dreams, jokes and parapraxes; the master – pupil relationship, and mastery through experience. For Freud, then, the concept of the libido was perhaps an image for certain social relations, a point he came close to accepting before he died. If his concerns were indeed social, if not political, he was using the available medical symbolism offered by his training and by the physical symptoms of his hysterical patients. McGrath (1986) argues that by accusing hysterics of projecting personal preoccupations on to their bodies, Freud was projecting his own cultural concerns on to a hypothetical psychology. If, as many psychiatrists argue, hysteria is best regarded as a social phenomenon, patients and doctor were not dissimilar to the native Australians described by Lévi-Strauss: 'The total system of social relations, itself bound up with a system of the universe, can be projected onto the anatomical plane' (Lévi-Strauss, 1968). If Sabbatianism was primarily concerned with articulating the relations between Jew and Gentile, then one of its successors, Hasidism, used its themes to recreate the ghetto wall, whilst the other, psychoanalysis, attempted to transcend the ghetto by universalising the principles of Jewish mysticism, principles evolved during a period of forced assimilation; for the Jew as analyst was less vulnerable to anti-semitism than the Jew as Lawgiver (Bakan, 1958).

18 Sharot (1982) summarises the current debate. The founder of Hasidism, the Baal Shem Tov, suggested that Sabbatai had a spark of holiness but had gone astray (Scholem, 1973:695).

19 Poles were not particularly conspicuous among Sabbatian adherents, but both Sabbatai and Nathan were of Askenazi rather than Sephardic origin. The Lurianic kabbalism of the Spanish exiles which was so influential in legitimating and shaping Sabbatai's actions developed in Safed in Galilee, a 'miniature distillation of the whole Jewish Diaspora' (Scholem, 1973:7); many expected the Messiah to appear there first. Yet the messianic age, sharply distinguished from the present, was to be ushered in by disaster for 'redemption arises on the ruins of history' (ibid.: 9). Any massacre or persecution might be the 'birth pangs' of the apocalypse. In quieter times the whole apocalyptic tradition had been ridiculed by scholars such as Maimonides: 'Do not think the messiah will have to . . . perform any spectacular deeds' (cited in Scholem, 1973:12–13). The common psychological explanation of messianic movements – relative deprivation – appears (as so often: Heelas and Haglund-Heelas, 1988) inadequate, despite Sabbatian grumblings after the apostasy that Sabbatai had been betrayed by the 'rich misers' (Scholem, 1973: ch. 7). Scholem himself discounts any single explanation of the movement, psychological or otherwise (ibid.: 1–8).

'Desperate times' may, however, be more than physical or personal hardship and we may consider under this gloss the internal and external pressures to assimilate recognised by Jews in the early modern period; as I have suggested above, Sabbatianism articulated the more general question of Jew/Gentile relations.

REFERENCES

Bakan, D. (1958) *Sigmund Freud and the Jewish Mystical Tradition*, Princeton: Princeton University Press.

Bevan, E. (1935) *Symbolism and Belief*, London: Allen & Unwin.

Bourdieu, P. (1977) *Outline of a Theory of Practice*, Cambridge: Cambridge University Press.

Caramagno, T. C. (1992) *The Flight of the Mind: Virginia Woolf's Art and Manic-Depressive Illness*, Berkeley, CA: University of California Press.

Cohen, P. S. (1980) 'Psychoanalysis and cultural symbolisation', in M. L. Foster and S. H. Brandes (eds) *Symbol as Sense: New Approaches to the Study of Meaning*, London: Academic Press.

Comfort, A. (1981) *I and That: Notes on the Biology of Religion*, New York: Crown.

Crapanzano, V. (1992) 'Hermeneutics and psychoanalysis', in T. Schwartz, G. M. White and C. Lutz (eds) *New Directions in Psychological Anthropology*, Cambridge: Cambridge University Press.

Csordas, T. J. (1992) 'The affliction of Martin: religious, clinical and phenomenological meaning in a case of demonic oppression', in A. D. Gaines (ed.) *Ethnopsychiatry: The Cultural Construction of Professional and Folk Psychiatries*, New York: State University of New York Press.

Devos, G. (1976) 'The interrrelationship between social and psychological structures in transcultural psychiatry', in W. P. Lebra (ed.) *Culture-Bound Syndromes, Ethnopsychiatry and Alternative Therapies*, Honolulu: University of Hawaii Press.

Eilberg-Schwartz, H. (ed.) (1992) *People of the Body: Jews and Judaism from an Embodied Perspective*, New York: State University of New York Press.

Ellenberger, H. (1970) *The Discovery of the Unconscious: The History and Evolution of Dynamic Psychiatry*, London: Allen Lane.

Erikson, E. (1958) *Young Man Luther*, New York: Norton.

Ewing, K. P. (1992) 'Is psychoanalysis relevant for anthropology?' in T. Schwartz, G. M. White and C. Lutz (eds) *New Directions in Psychological Anthropology*, Cambridge: Cambridge University Press.

Foucault, M. (1973) *The Birth of the Clinic: An Archaeology of Medical Perception*, trans., London: Tavistock.

Freedland, M. (1993) 'Brooklyn's Messiah', *The Times* (London) 15 January.

Freud, S. (1972) *The Future of An Illusion*, London: The Hogarth Press.

Gay, P. (1987) *A Godless Jew: Freud, Atheism and the Making of Psychoanalysis*, New Haven, CT: Yale University Press.

Girard, R. (1978) *To Double Business Bound: Essays on Literature, Mimesis, Anthropology*, Baltimore: Johns Hopkins University Press.

Gradek, M. (1976) 'Le concept de fou et ses implications dans la littérature talmudique et ses exégèses', *Annales Medico-Psychologiques* 134: 17–36.

Grunbaum, A. (1984) *The Foundations of Psychoanalysis: A Philosophical Critique*, Berkeley, CA: University of California Press.

Hamilton, I. (1983) *Robert Lowell: A Biography*, New York: Random House.

Heelan, P. (1983) *Space-perception and the Philosophy of Science*, Berkeley, CA: University of California Press.

Heelas, P. and Haglund-Heelas, A. M. (1988) 'The inadequacy of "deprivation" as a theory of conversion', in W. James and D. H. Johnson (eds) *Vernacular Christianity: Essays in the Social Anthropology of Religion Presented to Godfrey Lienhardt*, Oxford: JASO.

Hershman, D. J. and Lieb, J. (1988) *The Key to Genius: Manic-Depression and the Creative Life*, New York: Prometheus.

Hill, C. (1975) *The World Turned Upside Down: Radical Ideas During the English Revolution*, Harmondsworth: Penguin.

Howes, D. (ed.) (1991) *The Varieties of Sensory Experience*, Toronto: University of Toronto Press.

Jaspers, K. (1963) *General Psychopathology*, trans. of 7th edition of *Allgemeine Psychopathologie*, Berlin: Springer.

Johnson, M. (1987) *The Body in the Mind: The Bodily Basis of Meaning, Imagination and Reason*, Chicago: University of Chicago Press.

—— (1993) *Moral Imagination: Implications of Cognitive Science for Ethics*, Chicago: University of Chicago Press.

La Barre, W. (1970) *The Ghost Dance: Origins of Religion*, London: Allen & Unwin.

Lakoff, G. and Johnson, M. (1980) *Metaphors We Live By*, Chicago: Chicago University Press.

Lawson, E. T. and McCauley, R. M. (1990) *Rethinking Religion: Connecting Cognition and Culture*, Cambridge: Cambridge University Press.

Leder, D. (1990) *The Absent Body*, Chicago: Chicago University Press.

Levine, H. (1993) *Economic Origins of Antisemitism: Poland and Its Jews in the Early Modern Period*, New Haven, CT: Yale University Press.

Lévi-Strauss, C. (1968) *Structural Anthropology*, vol. 1, London: Allen Lane.

—— (1985) 'Cosmopolitanism and schizophrenia', in C. Lévi-Strauss, trans., *The View From Afar*, Oxford: Blackwell.

Littlewood, R. (1983) 'The antinomian Hasid', *British Journal of Medical Psychology* 56: 67–78.

—— (1984) 'The imitation of madness: the influence of psychopathology upon culture', *Social Science and Medicine* 19: 705–15.

—— (1993) *Pathology and Identity: The Work of Mother Earth in Trinidad*, Cambridge: Cambridge University Press.

Littlewood, R. and Dein, S. (1995) 'The effectiveness of words: religion and healing among the Lubavitch of Stamford Hill', *Culture, Medicine and Psychiatry* 19: 339–83.

McGrath, W.J. (1986) *Freud's Discovery of Psychoanalysis: The Politics of Hysteria*, Ithaca: Cornell University Press.

Mazlish, B. (1990) The iron of melancholy', in B. Mazlish (ed.) *The Leader, the Led, and the Psyche*, Hanover: Wesleyan University Press.

Mintz, J. R. (1968) *Legends of the Hasidim*, Chicago: Chicago University Press.

Murphy, H. B. M. (1967) 'Cultural aspects of the delusion', *Studium Generale* 2: 284–92.

Obeyesekere, G. (1981) *Medusa's Hair: An Essay on Personal Symbols and Religious Experience*, Chicago: Chicago University Press.

Porter, R. (1985) 'The hunger of imagination: approaching Samuel Johnson's melancholy', in W. F. Bynum, R. Porter and M. Shepherd (eds) *The Anatomy of Madness*, vol. 1, London: Tavistock.

Price, J. and Karim, I. (1978) 'Matikuru: a Fijian madness', *British Journal of Psychiatry* 133: 228–30.

Reynolds, V. and Tanner, R. E. S. (1983) *The Biology of Religion*, London: Longman.

Robert, M. (1974) *D'Oedipe à Moise: Freud et la Conscience Juive*, Paris: Calman-Levy.

Rorty, R. (1980) *Philosophy and the Mirror of Nature*, Oxford: Blackwell.

Rothenberg, A. (1990) *Creativity and Madness: New Findings and Old Stereotypes*, Baltimore: Johns Hopkins University Press.

Samuel, G. (1990) *Mind, Body and Culture: Anthropology and the Biological Interface*, Cambridge: Cambridge University Press.

Sass, L. A. (1992) *Madness and Modernity: Insanity in the Light of Modern Art, Literature, and Thought*, New York: Basic Books.

Schechter, S. (1970) 'The Chassidim', in S. Schechter, *Studies in Judaism*, New York: Atheneum.

Schneider, K. (1928) *Zur Einführung in die Religionspsychopathologie*, Tübingen: Mohr.

Scholem, G. C. (1971) *The Messianic Idea in Judaism*, London: Allen & Unwin.

—— (1973) *Sabbatai Sevi*, London: Routledge & Kegan Paul.

—— (1978) *Kabbalah*, New York: Meridian.

Schumaker, J. F. (ed.) (1992) *Religion and Mental Health*, New York: Oxford University Press.

Sharot, S. (1982) *Messianism, Mysticism and Magic: A Sociological Analysis of Jewish Religious Movements*, Chapel Hill, NC: University of North Carolina Press.

Shweder, R. (1985) 'Menstrual pollution, soul loss and the comparative study of emotions', in A. Kleinman and B. Good (eds) *Culture and Depression*, Berkeley, CA: University of California Press.

Stokes, H. P. (1913) *Studies in Anglo-Jewish History*, Edinburgh: Ballantyne.

Strauss, E. W. (1958) 'Aesthesiology and hallucinations', trans. in R. May, E. Angel and H. F. Ellenberger (eds) *Existence*, New York: Basic Books.

Weisel, E. (1978) *Four Hasidic Masters and their Struggle against Melancholy*, London: Notre Dame.

Wing, J.K., Cooper, J. E. and Sartorius, N. (1974) *The Measurement and Classification of Psychiatric Symptoms*, Cambridge: Cambridge University Press.

Witztum, E., Greenberg, D. and Dasberg, H. (1990) 'Mental illness and religious change', *British Journal of Medical Psychology* 63:33–41.

Zborowski, M. and Herzog, E. (1962) *Life is with People: The Culture of the Stetl*, New York: Schocken.

Chapter 14

Guilt, religion and ritual

Tony Nayani and Dinesh Bhugra

INTRODUCTION

Among various emotions experienced by humankind, experience of guilt occupies a uniquely central role at the meeting point of social and psychological theory. It combines a conception of a psychic component (remorse and self-reproach) with a social one (the transgression of a moral principle). It is this observation that leads, as we shall see in the first part of this chapter, to attempts to provide a theoretical overview of different approaches to this problem and to direct contemplation of the nature of emotional experience, its socio-cultural function, and the inter-relation of these domains. However, the practising psychiatrist who describes in a patient, with clinical disinterest, the existence of guilt as a phenomenological entity, may be surprised to experience that this function is eclipsed in a subtle and mysterious way by the need of the patient to engage his clinician as confessor, absolver, or judge. This phenomenon, again perhaps unique in the explication of guilt, raises important questions about the religious role of the psychiatrist in secular society and the function of ritual in psychiatric, particularly psychoanalytic, practice: these considerations will be addressed in the second part of the chapter when the relationship of the experience of shame and guilt is considered.

One of the major issues in discussing guilt as a phenomenon is that pathological guilt, as seen by the clinician, is defined as:

> subject blames himself too much for some peccadillo which most people will not take seriously. He realises that his guilt is exaggerated but cannot help feeling it all the same . . . . Guilt must be unpleasant, beyond voluntary control, and out of proportion to the situation.
>
> (Wing *et al.*, 1974)

Guilt in religion has a different meaning. For example, when we consider guilt in the Christian tradition it means that the guilt has a different quality and it is also a result of replacement of love and attitude of understanding towards Christ by vicarious atonement and fear encouraging 'compulsive formations of a collective neurotic character' (Pfister, 1944). There is no doubt that sometimes religious passion may pass over into pathology where it may take on the form of depressive guilt (in melancholia), or exaltation where a transitory and relative passive state may be marked by intense feelings of love (Ribot, 1884; 1896). Sometimes it is difficult to differentiate between religious and pathological guilt. Yao (1987) has argued that in the 'shattered faith syndrome', where evangelical or fundamentalist Christians have left the church, yet another type of chronic guilt may emerge which is associated with anxiety and depression, low self-esteem, loneliness, distrust, anger and bitterness, lack of basic social skills and sexual difficulties including guilt over sexual desire. Under these circumstances the difference between 'religious' and 'clinical' guilt may be difficult to discern. Clinical guilt may be secondary to an underlying psychiatric disease, whereas religious guilt may be linked with religious rituals or lack of perceived forgiveness in the subject's mind.

THEORETICAL PERSPECTIVES

Psychodynamic accounts

With breathtaking boldness, Freud proposed in 'Totem and Taboo' (1912–13) a psychoanalytical account of primitive religious organisation which, as constituted by the emergent Oedipal complex, he used to provide the keystone of his architecture of mind. The scheme of his reasoning was wide and embraced early anthropological speculations as articulated by Darwin in his theory of evolution. The suggestion that early social relations between humans may have been characterised by small aggregates of people living closely together in a hoard led Darwin to speculate that such a group may have been dominated by an elderly, powerful male who exercised his authority to control access to sexual relations with the female members of the group. Younger males, spurred by instincts of competitive rebellion and jealousy, commit an act of collective murder when they slay the father (figure). In consequence, feelings of guilt and remorse arise in them and in atonement for their terrible crime they deify the slain figure, identifying him with the totemic ancestor of the clan. The second expiatory act which issues from this grief was their renouncement of the right of sexual relations with the female members of the group. In this way, the two fundamental taboos of totemism were declared, to be echoed in all social organisation in perpetuity: the prohibitions of patricide and incest.

The singular importance to psychoanalytical theory of these speculations about the psychological life of early Man resides in Freud's articulation concerning the resolution of the nascent Oedipal anxiety with the formation of the superego (Freud, 1924). This process entails the combination of identification and projective mechanisms and leads in essence to the incorporation of the parental figure as an internal censor. In this way, the formal mechanism that leads to the experience of guilt is established in the mind of the developing infant. It is important to emphasise the dimensions of this emotion which implies something far greater than simple fear of punishment, and is akin to the absolute dread that arises when the natural cosmological order is perturbed. This awesome apprehension of the violation of the world is contained in the idea of taboo, and as such constitutes the essential basis of any ethical framework, any moral order. The vigilance of the internalised superego scrutinises not only errant action but unacceptable instinct, and in this way the tendency of the Ego to stray invites the consequence of imminent punishment.

In Freud's view, the impress of the Oedipus complex remains in all later religious forms and practices. Each succeeding generation inherits the sense of guilt resulting from having killed and devoured the father (see Wulff, 1991, for further discussion). Freud maintained that the Christian doctrine of atonement represents an undisguised acknowledgement of the 'guilty primeval deed'. This is reflected in Christianity where the ancient totemic meal in the form of Eucharist is the symbolic consumption of the body and blood of Christ to expiate the deed of sacrifice of God's son. Guilt feelings resulting from forbidden wishes and ambivalent feelings are among' the most powerful tools of religion' and may be fostered by the religious traditions (Ostow and Schaferstein, 1954).

This account given by Freud has met with much criticism and revision. Melanie Klein, for instance, located the origin of the superego and reparative instinct (1928) at a much earlier developmental stage when the new-born infant struggles with the Breast deploying primitive defence in the process: at this stage, the first intimations of guilt arise in reaction to intense oral – sadistic attacks on the breast. By stressing the mimetic or identificatory instincts of the developing child, Girard (1977) meditates on the nature of desire and reaches the conclusion that at its heart is a double-bind which contains the injunction to imitate (and thereby seize the object of desire) but not to imitate (because of the threat of rivalrous violence). Furthermore, the resolution of this contradiction, he suggests, lies in the division of the world into two spheres, anticipating the polarity of the Sacred and Profane. In the Jungian scheme (Jung, 1938), the base instincts, the darker side of Man, are incarnated in the archetype of the Shadow which in turn derives much in substance from the collective unconscious.

The coincidence of psychological and sociological theory to be found in 'Totem and taboo' has attracted the attention of cultural anthropologists since the 1920s who were able to examine Freud's assertions in the natural context of primitive societies. The most celebrated of these critiques was adduced by Malinowski (1929, 1930, 1960) in his description of familial organisation in the Coral Archipelago of New Guinea. Here, the function of the authoritarian patriarch is assumed by the maternal uncle whose role it is to instruct the children and guide them through rites of passage; the father meanwhile is contracted to play as befriender and kindly assistant to his children. The contrast with the familiar patriarchal society is clear and, while the existence of distinct incestuous taboos (focused in the main on sibling sexuality) in the matriarchal society of New Guinea seems to support Freudian notions of infantile sexuality, the existence of civilised forms of society in which the Oedipal configuration is seemingly absent betrays the argument that it is the emergence of the patriarchal superego that provides the necessary foundation of civilisation. The response of the psychoanalytic movement to this charge was articulated by Jones (1924) who argued that the affective colour (threat, power, dread, and so on) that imbues the internalised psychic father figure is retained in society. However, the maternal uncle comes to occupy the corresponding social role, thereby relieving the biological father of this function. Jung (1958) argued that Christianity was responsible for an increase in the sense of guilt in the West, although others (e.g. Pfister, 1944) have argued the opposite. However, the psychoanalytical theories cannot be applied blindly across cultures. Projection and introjection have both been described as the underlying principles in the development of guilt, but we need to understand the application of these principles in different cultures and religions prior to seeing these as universally applicable hypotheses.

In summary, classic Freudian theory identified the emergence of the Oedipal complex with the strictures of instinctual repression and control and proposes that this permits the emergence of authoritarian social structures, and the divergence of libidinal energy into cultural aspiration and creativity. Others (e.g. Fromm, 1990) demur and conceive this form of instinctual repression to be the consequence of patriarchal social organisation.

Some authorities (Suttie, 1988) discern a distinct matriarchal lineage epitomised in the cults of the Earth Mother that came to be superseded by the later development of patriarchal form. It is argued that the punishing, even cruel, manifestation of the superego was yet present in the Matriarch (the Witch) but the quibbling intense preoccupations of the neurotically repressed, stifled by layer upon layer of prohibition, may have been absent in this earlier social structure.

THEOLOGICAL ACCOUNTS

We have alluded to the dread fear that constitutes taboo, and we have suggested that it is this fear that underpins the psychodynamic understanding of guilt. The theological construct of sin illuminates two additional refinements of this concept which emphasise the central function of the emotion of guilt in psychosocial theory. Primitive conceptions of evil contain the notion of defilement and impurity. Ritual cleansing and ablution serve not only the function of ridding the individual of the sinful blemish but reinforce for the social group the sometimes ambivalent pole of the Sacred and Profane (Ricoeur, 1970). Here the schemata of divinity and that of disease assume an identity that still ramifies in modern conceptions of contagion and plague (Suttie, 1988). Again of interest is the hypothesis adduced by Douglas (1988) that 'bodily control is an expression of social control' the physical governance of the body by sanctified authority in the unfolding drama of the ritual echoes the psychoanalytical account of infantile mental development through the medium of the maturing physical form. The complex relation between the Self and Authority condensed into sinew and tissue is a theme that Canetti (1962) explores with great insight.

The transformation of the notion of sin from the implication of impurity to that of guilt marks an important development, suggesting the emergence of the individual agent as author for the misdeed (Ricoeur, 19709). The Covenant of God and Man, in the Hebrew tradition, altered the conception of sin in this way, where the emergence of a relationship between the deity and his followers implies the assumption of responsibility by them to keep the Law. The purpose of punishment in this framework was to expiate God and restore the Covenant; both sacrifice and scapegoating (Grinberg, 1992) were used to accomplish this end.

The Biblical account of Original Sin in the mythology of Eden and the serpent locates the tendency to sinfulness in Man. Yet distinct from him is the agency of the snake. Baptism is viewed as the purifying rite to neutralise this state and the restoration of the *tabula rasa* is achieved. In the Catholic faith, the relationship of God and Man is mediated by the church. whose provenance and privilege it is to observe the rituals of the sacrament and by delivering absolution through confession restores the individual to grace (see Sutherland, this volume). The précis contains an important general principle concerning guilt: we meet the notion of a process that leads either through punishment or forgiveness to the dissolution of the burden of guilt. It seems that it is implicit in the experience of this emotion that it will endure until some positive action is taken to abolish it; again, the ubiquitous and varied cultural forms of expiation signify the depth of this need.

Sociological accounts

Inspired by ethnographic data originating from field studies of Australia, Durkheim outlined his project to develop a sociological theory of religion (1915). The quest encompassed an ambition to reveal the societal constitution of those ethical strictures that Kant (1949) alluded to in the moral imperative. His analysis of totemic society shared with Freud a prejudice that the unsophisticated structure of religious life in the aboriginal community afforded the opportunity to inspect religious observation in its earliest forms. (This view is no longer tenable since it has been shown that totemic ideas can coexist with other religious institutions.) Again, like Freud, Durkheim was struck by the power of the Totem, both as the organising principle of social life and as the repository and source of the sacred attitude that combined veneration, devotion and coercion. The ceremonial aspects of religious life serve the essential function of delineating the Sacred: the investment of sanctity in objects employed in rituals shows the potency of symbolic transformation. According to Durkheim, the roots of all religious feeling stem from the Society, which is to say, to totemic principles. The awesome forces that are sensed to pervade the rites and rituals that distinguish the religious life of the community, are, in essence, no more than the representation of the social group to itself. Furthermore, it is the form of the organisation of the social group that comes to constitute the epistemology of the society and informs the cosmological and mythical components of the ritual.

In this sociological account of the phenomena of religious life, the psychological dimension is occluded; it becomes redundant to speculate about the tendency to divine feeling when the presumption of a social instinct constitutes this experience. But as Girard (1977) demonstrates with great eloquence and force, it is precisely with the logic of emotion that the structure and impulse of the social institution are to be found. For example, Girard argues that in those societies in which the institution of the judiciary is absent, the ritual of sacrifice, carried by the instinct for vengeance, comes to occupy a central role. Sacrifice enables the dangerous impulse of violence to be expelled from the group; as Girard put it: 'between vengeance, sacrifice, and legal punishment, it is important to recognise their fundamental identity'. The beauty of this argument is that the inspiration of the Sacred is traced not to the nebulous apprehension of Society, but rather finds its locus in the specific human agency of violence and the terror that it inspires. The incarnation of these fears in the mythology of the culture lends form and substance to these anxieties and, of course, in psychodynamic terms, represents their projection (see also Sartre, 1948, Frankl 1989).

Psychological accounts

A distinct alternative approach to the general problem posed by emotion, and the difficulties that are encountered when the phenomena under scrutiny seem to necessarily arch two domains (the psychosocial), is to be found in the Social Constructivist viewpoint. According to this theory, emotions are 'characterised by attitudes such as beliefs, systems of cultural belief (Coulter, 1979). The traditional and still commonplace opinion that emotions are exclusively inner processes, non-cognitive and similar to sensations, appears to be untenable when, as Wittgenstein (1980) argues, they form a part of a shared language. Again, the implication of an external relation in the expression of an emotion (I am angry with x; I love y) denotes a series of rules that come to be engaged when these words are used. The link between the emotional state and the external referent is given by the cognitive activity of believing (I believe x is better than me, and I feel envy). The assumption that these beliefs are learnt, the belief/emotion complex is culturally determined and acquired, represents a radical departure from the orthodoxy of the psychodynamic school (although the conception of agency that constitutes the experience of emotion finds its echo in Object-relations theory). This presumption about the nature of emotion leads naturally to a functional account of emotional behaviour where the meaning of the emotion is to be found in the socio-cultural system (Averill, 1980). The demonstration of the use of this approach can be found in developmental (Averill, 1980) and transcultural analyses (Crespo, 1986).

The social construct that informs the experience of guilt would be, according to this perspective, inculcated into the developing child by innumerable and densely interconnecting references that would form a mutable but coherent lexicon for this emotion.

In an important sense, it is assumed that the phenomenological features of this experience are irreducible, although presumably a (psycho-biological) disposition to this affect-state must be implied (Kraepelin 1904). In theory, a social form could be imagined in which this emotion is not known as its function in this society is superfluous. Again, the deliberate enhancement of the experience of guilt may serve social functions in particular instances and one would expect to find situations when this may be apparent. Armon-Jones (1986) argues that the religious confessional may serve this purpose. A practical application of this methodology is to be found in the use of cognitive therapy (Beck, 1976) for the treatment of depression: the hypothesis that the depressed individual suffers from disordered thinking, which includes, for example, the exaggeration of the sense of responsibility for deeds, real or imagined, in the experience of guilt, carries the implication that by training the individual to recognise and change these distortions the emotional experience can be altered.

By drawing on these different perspectives concerning the nature of guilt, the central role of this emotion in different conceptual schemes becomes apparent. The psychodynamic, theological and anthropological accounts have a respect for the absolute nature of this experience, the imminent awareness of which provides an ontological basis for the organisation of the psychosocial world. It is the experience of guilt that alerts us to the fine moral structure of the world; we may move bodily in dimensions of space and time, but psychologically we move in a medium of ethical consideration and, barely distant from this, a world of dread and awe which inspires the Taboo. The notion of ritual is inherently bound to that of guilt and by observing the performance of these rites, we can gain direct insight into the structure of cosmologies both in their social-cultural manifestation and in terms of the internalised psychological fantasy: the symmetry of these accounts may signify the origin of an epistemology or a transcendent psychology (Jung, 1937). The constructivist account of guilt, in contrast, denies itself such grand ambition: the stress on the social functions of emotion seems to lead inexorably to a cultural relativism. The immediate advantage of this project, as it eschews the intricate theoretical constructs of, say, the psychodynamic account, is that it lends itself to empirical methods; its weakness, on the other hand, reflects its gaunt humility, when the absence of an absolute prejudice about the existential status of emotion seems to obscure something essential about this experience.

PSYCHIATRY, RELIGION AND GUILT

Experimental interest in the study of guilt has in the main rested upon techniques which attempt to quantify the experience. Projective techniques (Miller and Swanson, 1966), self-report inventories (Buss and Durkee, 1957) and the assessment of moral standards (Mosher, 1966) have all been employed (see Kugler and Jones, 1992, for a useful review of this area). The psychiatrist is most likely to encounter guilt in the context of a depressive disorder (Berrios *et al.*, 1992) where the judgement concerning the pathological nature of this experience will encompass evaluations about its appropriateness, its duration and its intensity. Illusions of guilt can dominate the clinical presentation and may represent morbid exaggerations of pre-existing personality traits or culturally informed notions of culpability or sinfulness; some authors have suggested that these manifestations of delusional guilt may now be less prevalent than before (Hamilton, 1982). Pathological guilt may also occur as part of a grief response and may indicate a poor prognosis (Parkes, 1991). The association of this emotion with experience of mourning was anticipated by Freud's seminal speculations about the nature of depression (Freud, 1917). In contrast, the inappropriate absence of guilt marks the boundary of psychopathic disorder (Cleckley, 1964) when the individual may commit acts of arresting cruelty and yet profess to feeling no remorse at the harm inflicted. Evil, according to Parkin (1985), was once conceived of as the positive presence of malevolence and vile intent, perhaps then in the imagination of the popular contemporary culture the intimation for the lack of guilty feeling has come to epitomise the capacity for evil now.

In the first part of this chapter the constructivist theory of emotion was described: the implication of a social determination for emotional behaviour raises important questions about the validity of experimental and clinical judgements when the observer and the observed come from different backgrounds (Lutz, 1985). For example, one of the earliest ethno-psychological observations can be attributed to Kraepelin, who, whilst visiting Indonesia, remarked upon the nature of depression there as being 'usually mild and fleeting', and that 'feelings of guilt were never experienced'. Many transcultural studies have alluded to the relative absence of psychological symptoms in some cultures when it appears that somatic manifestation of depression may predominate (for instance, Kleinman, 1982). Some authors have argued that it is the form of social organisation, particularly the degree to which a self-individualistic culture arises, that determines the degree of the psychological component to these expressions of distress (Leff, 1981). Others, whilst accepting that the explicit declaration of guilty feelings may be less common in certain cultures, argue that this does not mean that they are not present but rather that they are masked by culturally determined patterns of, say, projecting blame on to others (El-Islam, 1969; also see Bhugra *et al.*, 1995 for further discussion).

It has been believed that some cultures and religions are likely to experience shame rather than guilt when depressed (Yap, 1965). The alleged rarity of depression in illiterate Africans had been ascribed to the absence of self-reproach and a sense of personal responsibility (especially towards the family and the community) along with a fatalistic attitude (external locus of control) (Tooth, 1950). A lack of individualistic competition was also put forward as a possible explanation (Carothers, 1948). Other possible explanations suggested a failure to introject hostility (Benedict and Jacks, 1954) and a fault in the mechanism of repression (Carothers, 1948). One of the major problems in making sense of the symptoms of 'depression' across cultures is because the concepts of depression and presentation may differ across various cultures. The other problem that needs

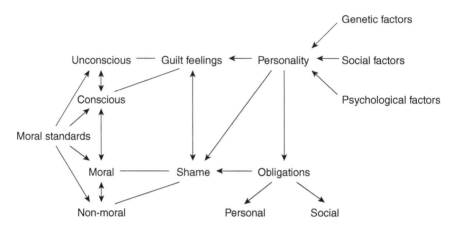

Figure 14.1 Notions of guilt and shame

to be emphasised is the distinction between shame and guilt. Although various authors (e.g. Benedict, 1947; Mead, 1937, 1950) have made an attempt to distinguish between the two, these have not always been very successful because of semantic difficulties as well as lack of agreed criteria for identifying the two experiences (e.g., Bandura and Walters, 1963; Piers and Singer, 1953).

Yap (1965) had proposed a linear ordering of unconscious guilt feelings, conscious guilt feelings and conscious moral shame (generated by an anticipation of discovery of the wrong conduct by others). A distinction between the three is important to identify the exact feelings, emotion and experience. In addition, non-moral shame may have some role to play under certain circumstances.

Guilt feelings may be related to certain religious rituals. Concepts of 'face loss' and an obligation to one's family, community, elders and religion may be relevant. Where all these feelings are enforced and encouraged by the society, a sense of moral obligation exists. This related to the work ethic and belief in the original sin may, in conjunction with social forces and moral values, contribute to the feelings of guilt (see Figure 14.1).

Some earlier work (see Chance, 1964; Murphy et al., 1964) suggested that self-reproachful depression was more common in socially cohesive groups. Murphy (1978) noting the psychological similarities between seventeenth-century England and twentieth-century Africa, observed that guilt was becoming more apparent in the latter. He argued that one possible explanation for this is the development of entrepreneurship and more individualisation. He pointed out that the lack of a traditional base is more likely to increase the guilt feelings in depression.

Where religion teaches that human nature is evil from a supernatural cause, it also provides the means for absolution and atonement and the relief of guilt in the individual (Yap, 1965). There is no doubt that religion forms an important part of one's life and culture, and some authors (e.g. Westermeyer, 1984) have gone as far as to suggest that religion is a part of the individual's ethnicity. Wulff (1991) argues that those suffering from anxiety and guilt are understandably drawn to resources that promise forgiveness, love and moral support.

The distinct emotional experience of shame, it is suggested (Kleinman and Good, 1985), may exist on a spectrum of experience which has quiet at the other pole. Tangey *et al.* (1992) argue that there are important phenomenological features which distinguish these emotions: the essence of guilt derives from a sense of having done something wrong; the emotion of shame, on the other hand, denotes a sense of being a bad person. The sense of exposure and vulnerability that distinguishes the feeling of shame stems both from the expectation of ridicule from others as much as it does from the harsh gaze of the punishing Self. Thus, Lewis (1971) employs the notion of the 'internalised other'. Freud (1905) perhaps paid less attention to the emotion of shame than might have been expected given the direction of his general argument concerning the repression of instinct by authoritarian society; he suggested that shame owed its origin primarily to the exposure of genital exhibition, and hence in pathological terms, signifies the occurrence of reaction formation to exhibitionistic fantasy.

If we accept the argument that the guilt – shame constellation may provide an axis of emotional experience, the question arises as to whether the relative expression of these emotions may be determined culturally. Certainly, some authors (Broucek, 1991) have argued that it is precisely the shamelessness of post-industrial Western society that is the source of the familiar litany of social ills to which these cultures seem to be prone. Hong and Chiu (1992) performed a study on a group of Chinese Hong Kong students that led them to conclude that the constructs of shame and guilt are similar across cultures (for example, guilt would be expected to be associated with the violation of a moral norm in any society). If then the understanding of the meaning of these terms is universally shared, differences in the use and expression of these emotional states among cultures may imply that, in some general sense, it is the specific behaviours that are associated with each emotion that occur to a differing degree. It seems clear that the psychiatrist who works with patients who originate from alien cultures may mistake the emotional signals that denote the inner experience of the patient. However, the prejudice that emotion arises in specific and universal context (the experience of yearning, say, which arises from loss) will alert the clinician to the necessity of seeking the meaning of the emotional expression in the natural form that is dictated by the conventions of the particular culture. The alternative view, which denies the possibility of contact between alien cultures inevitably leads to a barren solipsism which appears in sullen opposition to the steadily accumulating understanding (deriving from sources as diverse as genetics and structural linguistics) of the universal matrix from which diversity seems to stem.

There is no doubt that guilt does form a part of the depressive syndrome. The epidemiology of affective disorders is well analysed elsewhere (see Bebbington, 1978; 1993; Singer, 1975). The role of religion in this field has to be appreciated. There is evidence that Jews were less hostile and less guilt-ridden than Catholics and Protestants respectively (Fernando, 1966; 1967; also see Cooper, this volume). This difference has been attributed to the closer kinship ties in Jewish families. Depression is reinforced by factors like early formative influences, culture change like industrialisation, social cohesion, role deprivation and other factors (see Singer, 1975, for a detailed discussion) and counteracted by rituals and beliefs, extended family systems and status provision. For our purposes rituals and beliefs are an important factor. Fernando (1966) among others has argued that confession among Roman Catholics was a means of relieving guilt. Cultures may also provide means of 'status reversal rituals' (ritual humiliation of the powerful) and 'cathartic strategies' (like feasts, fasts, carnivals, etc.) (Wittkower, 1971). Mourning rituals and rites of passage also enable individuals to prepare for the possible depressive episode and cope with losses.

It has been argued that there is a lot in common in rituals related to religion and those related to obsessive compulsive disorders. Although Freud (1907) argues that there are parallels between neurotic ceremonials and religious actions characterised by careful attention to detail, conducted in isolation, and neglect is followed by anxiety or guilt. However, to complicate this argument further, there are distinct differences between the two. The formation of religion is based upon the suppression and the renunciation of certain instinctual impulses. Greenberg (1984) reported on religious compulsions in four patients, and demonstrated that there were phenomenological similarities and differences between the two and advised that therapists need to modify their behavioural regime accordingly. Milbert et al. (1991) pointed out that the thoughts of state of deprivation (of self-denial) provoked by religious ritual practice were an important feature in the obsessional neurosis. They argued that, unlike the latter, where the ritual becomes a pathological cycle, the severe deprivation in the former becomes an integral part of the liberation felt after the mystical ecstasy has subsided. Steketee et al. (1991) examined thirty-three patients with obsessive compulsive disorder (OCD) and twenty-four patients with other anxiety disorders. They observed that OCDs were more likely to have no religion or feel more guilt, although severity of OCD pathology was positively correlated with both religiosity and guilt. Social anxiety was linked with guilt but not with religiosity. Obviously, with such small numbers it is very difficult to make generalised observations, but this is an area that needs to be explored further.

We may then accept that there exists a core of human experience of which guilt is one strand constituted by the instinctive demands of the developing child, the expression of which comes to be shaped by cultural structures that in turn, owing to their fundamental importance as an organising principle of behaviour, inform the development of these structures. The question of the jeopardy of translating subjective experience between cultures has been alluded to, but we may state it more precisely now: if we accept that psychiatric knowledge (with its innumerable roots in other scientific disciplines) constitutes a cultural system in its own right, then what particular problems might we expect when this emerging culture comes into contact with, or indeed supersedes, older cultural forms which we may loosely designate as religious (see also Cox, this volume)?

Nelson (1973) explores the ramifications of this problem: he argues that psychiatry, which includes psychotherapy, has come to absorb many of the familiar functions of religion in modern society. He cites, for instance, the growth of existential psychotherapy as a consequence of general dissatisfaction with the traditional response of the Church (in its many guises) to anodyne pleas about ultimate meaning. Again, he proposes that the ritualistic function of religion has come to be obscured by the structural manifestations of psychiatric culture including the community health centre and the psychotherapist's suite! The author of this critique was careful not to inform the reader of his judgement about the desirability of these changes, but Bergin (1980) is less inscrutable when arguing that the importance of religious values should be recognised by the therapeutic establishment and incorporated both into clinical practice and theoretical frameworks. There is no doubt that knowledge about the nature of the patient's faith can help the therapist to understand his/her inner world and the observation of pathology can only be accurately made when this understanding is reached.

CONCLUSION

In the first part of this chapter different perspectives about the nature of guilt were offered: the central importance of this emotion is psychic architecture and social structure was intimated. We saw that guilt, sometimes as an emotional state of ferocious potency, serves to bind the individual into ethical structures upon which society is built. Furthermore, we saw that the origin of this emotion and that of primitive social organisation can be traced symmetrically to a common source in the conception of the Taboo. We also noted that there may exist a basic instance arising from a neuro-genetic substrate which leads to the unfolding of the experience of guilt in the developing infant, and that this instinctive component may be pathologically disturbed both in exaggeration and absence in some individuals. Finally, we speculated that the instinctive basis of this emotion may manifest itself in other forms that might include the experience of shame, but that cultural convention may dictate the degree to which guilt is made manifest in any one society. In this respect, the problem of understanding the emotional language of an alien culture was mentioned, and the specific problem of the imposition of the psychiatric frame upon other value systems was referred to.

In conclusion, we may now consider the functions of the psychiatrist when apprehending guilt in a patient. Perhaps, unlike the ephemeral emotions of fear or joy that normally arise in response to specific stimuli and that perish soon after the stimuli are perceived to have gone, the emotion of guilt shares with hatred and love an enduring quality that extends through time and is in a sense carried within. The feature that marks these durable emotions is their root in activity and therefore in agency: guilt implies the occurrence (in reality or fantasy) of a transgressive act and it is the lingering quality of the memory of this act (consciously or subconsciously known) that sustains the emotional tone.

As Greenberg *et al.* (1992) remark, it is important for the examining psychiatrist to be aware of cultural background and issues. It is apparent in their small sample that hallucinations, grandiose and paranoid delusions, and social withdrawal and phenomena do not (necessarily) distinguish the psychotic from the mystic, though diagnosis of psychosis is made based on duration of the state, ability to control entry into the state, and the associated deterioration of habits, particularly neglect of religious duties. The psychiatrist, when dealing with strictly religious patients, should attempt to cooperate with the patients' spiritual mentor; examine his/her own religious attitudes to modify feelings of counter-transference and acquire knowledge of the patients' religion to facilitate interviewing (Greenberg and Witztum, 1991).

However if guilt arises from activity, it also compels us to act in turn: guilt contains necessarily the instinct of reparation and repair (Klein, 1940). The very intolerability of the knowledge of harm seems to provide the impetus for this force; it is important to note, however, that socially sanctioned hatred in the form of, say, warfare may relieve the individual of this burden. The numerous cultural manifestations of the experience of guilt, particularly in their religious form, have been alluded to; it is perhaps obvious that many of the rituals and practices of expiation which are given formal structure in these faiths derive from the need to achieve reparation. Within the dimension of intersubjectivity, this impetus is known to us in acts of forgiveness (Smedslund, 1991). In forgiveness we come to know that the harm inflicted has been repaired, that the disturbance caused by the transgressive act is nullified, and that the natural order of things is reinstated: punishment, in the experience of guilt, can come to an end.

There is, then, within the experience of guilt a condensation of a story that arises from an act and seeks inevitably its release in another act. The psychiatrist who listens to the beat of the guilty heart cannot help but become embroiled in the sad quest for peace. It seems to be of little import whether this function is conceptualised as the manifestation of the transference or the supplanting of spiritual authority, the ineluctable impulse of the guilty mind is to find a figure who is whole and undamaged. The placing of careful boundaries in psychotherapeutic practice and the imposition of order on the chaos of disease by the psychiatrist both convey the pristine authority that is seen to have survived the earliest attack on the Totem.

REFERENCES

Armon-Jones, C. (1986) 'The social functions of emotion', in R. Harre (ed.) *The Social Construction of Emotions*, London: Blackwell.

Averill, J. (1980) 'A constructivist theory of emotions', in R. Plutich and H. Kellerman (eds) *Emotion, Theory, Research and Experience*, New York: Academic Press.

—— (1986) 'The acquisition of emotions during adulthood', in R. Harre (ed.) *The Social Construction of Emotions*, London: Blackwell.

Bandura, A. and Walters, R. H. (1963) *Social Learning and Personality*, New York: Holt, Rinehart & Winston.

Bebbington, P. E. (1978) 'The epidemiology of depressive disorder', *Culture, Medicine and Psychiatry* 2: 297–341.

—— (1993) 'Transcultural aspects of affective disorders', *International Review of Psychiatry* 5(2/3): 145–56.

Beck, A. (1976) *Cognitive Therapy and the Emotional Disorders*, New York: Meridian-New American Library.

Benedict, P. and Jacks, I. (1954) 'Mental illness in primitive societies', *Psychiatry* 17: 377.

Benedict, R. (1947) *The Chrysanthemum and the Sword*, London: Secker & Warburg.

Bergin, A. (1980) 'Psychotherapy and religious values', *Journal of Consulting and Clinical Psychology* 48: 95–105.

Berrios, G., Bulbera, A., Bakshim, N., Dening, T., Jenaway, H., Markar, H., Martin-Santos, R. and Mitchell, S. (1992) 'Feelings of guilt in major depression', *British Journal of Psychiatry* 160: 781–7.

Bhugra, D., Gupta, K. R. and Wright, B. (1995) *Depression in North India*, submitted for publication.

Broucek, B. (1991) *Shame and Self*, London: Guilford Press.

Buss, A. and Durkee, A. (1957) 'An inventory for assessing different kinds of hostility', *Journal of Consulting Psychology* 21: 343–9.

Canetti, E. (1962) *Crowds and Power*, London: Penguin.

Carothers, J. C. (1948) 'A study of mental derangement in Africans and an attempt to explain its peculiarities', *Psychiatry* 11: 47–80.

Chance, N. A. (1964) 'A cross cultural study of social cohesion and depression', *Transcultural Psychiatry Research Review* 1: 19–21.

Cleckley, H. (1964) *The Mask of Sanity: An Attempt to Clarify Issues About the So-Called Psychopathic Personality* 4th edition, St Louis: Mosby.

Coulter, J. (1979) *The Social Construction of Mind*, London: Macmillan.

Crespo, E. (1986) 'A regional variation: emotions in Spain', in R. Harre (ed.) *The Social Construction of Emotions*, London: Blackwell.

Douglas, M. (1988) *Purity and Danger: An Analysis of the Concepts of Pollution and Taboo*, London: Ark Paperbacks.

Durkheim, E. (1915) *The Elementary Forms of the Religious Life: A Study in Religious Sociology*, London: Allen & Unwin.

El-Islam, F. (1969) 'Depression and guilt: a study at an Arab psychiatric centre', *Social Psychiatry* 4: 56–8.

Fernando, S. (1966) 'Depressive illness in Jews and non-Jews', *British Journal of Psychiatry* 112: 991.

—— (1967) 'Cultural differences in the hostility of depressive patients', *British Journal of Psychiatry* 42: 67.

Frankl, G. (1989) *The Social History of the Unconscious*, Amersham, Bucks: Halson & Co. Ltd.

Freud, S. (1905) 'Three essays on the theory of sexuality', in *The Standard Edition*, vol.7, London: The Hogarth Press, pp. 153–243.

—— (1907) 'Obsessive actions and religious practices', in *The Standard Edition*, vol. 9, London: The Hogarth Press, pp. 115–29.

—— (1912–13) 'Totem and taboo', in *The Standard Edition*, vol. 13, London: The Hogarth Press, pp. 1–162.

—— (1917) 'Mourning and melancholia', in *The Complete Psychological Works of Sigmund Freud*, vol. 14, London: The Hogarth Press.

—— (1924) 'The dissolution of the Oedipus Complex', in *The Standard Edition*, vol. 19, London: The Hogarth Press, pp. 173–83.

Fromm, E. (1990) *The Anatomy of Human Destructiveness*, Harmondsworth: Penguin.

Girard, R. (1977) *Violence and the Sacred*, trans. P. Gregory, London: Johns Hopkins University Press.

Greenberg, D. (1984) 'Are religious compulsions religious or compulsive?: a phenomenological study', *American Journal of Psychotherapy* 38: 524–32.

Greenberg, D. and Witztum, E. (1991) 'Problems in the treatment of religious patients', *American Journal of Psychotherapy* 45: 554–65.

Greenberg, D., Witztum, E. and Buchbinder, J. T. (1992) 'Mysticism and psychosis: the fate of Ben Zoma', *British Journal of Medical Psychology* 65: 223–35.

Grinberg, L. (1992) *Guilt and Depression*, London: Karac Books.

Hamilton, M. (1982) 'Symptoms and assessment of depression', in E. Paykel (ed.) *Handbook of Affective Disorders*, London: Churchill Livingstone.

Hong, Y. and Chiu, C. (1992) 'A study of the comparative structure of guilt and shame in Chinese society', *Journal of Psychology* 126: 171–9.

Jones, E. (1924) 'Psychoanalysis and anthropology', in (1951) *Essays in Applied Psychoanalysis*, vol. II, London: The Hogarth Press.

Jung, C. (1937) *Religious Ideas in Alchemy*, London: Routledge & Kegan Paul.

Jung, C. (1938) *Psychology and Religion* (The Terry Lectures), London: Routledge & Kegan Paul.

—— (1958) 'Answer to job', in *Collected Works of C. G. Jung*, trans. F. R. C. Hull, vol.11, London: Routledge & Kegan Paul.

Kant, I. (1949) *Critique of Practical Reason*, Chicago: University of Chicago Press.

Klein, M. (1928) 'Early stages of the Oedipus complex', in *The Writings of Melanie Klein*, London: The Hogarth Press.

—— (1940) 'Mourning and its relation to manic-depressive states', in *The Writings of Melanie Klein*, London: The Hogarth Press.

Kleinman, A. (1982) 'Depression and neurasthenia in the People's Republic of China', *Culture, Medicine and Psychiatry* 6: 1–80.

Kleinman, A. and Good, B. (eds) (1985) *Culture and Depression*, Berkeley: University of California Press.

Kraepelin, E. (1904) 'Vergleichende Psychiatrie', in S. R. Hirsch and M. Shepherd (eds) *Themes and Variations in European Psychiatry*, Bristol: Wright.

Kugler, K. and Jones, W. (1992) 'On conceptualising and assessing guilt', *Journal of Personality and Social Psychology* 62: 318–27.

Leff, J. (1981) *Psychiatry Around the Globe*, New York: Marcel Dekker.

Lewis, H. (1971) *Shame and Guilt in Neurosis*, New York: International University Press.

Lutz, C. (1985) 'Depression and the translation of emotional worlds', in A. Kleinman (ed.) *Culture and Depression*, London: University of California Press.

Malinowski, B. (1929) *The Sexual Lives of Savages in North West Melanesia*, London: Routledge.

—— (1930) 'The sociology of the family', in J. Thornton and P. Skalinik (eds) *Early Writings of Broruslaw Malinowski*, Cambridge: Cambridge University Press.

—— (1960) *Sex and Repression in Savage Society*, London: Routledge.

Mead, M. (1937) *Cooperation and Competition among Primitive Peoples*, New York: McGraw-Hill.

—— (1950) in M. L. Reymert (ed.) *Feelings and Emotions*, New York: McGraw-Hill.

Milbert, F., Merinim, F., Benoit, M. (1991) 'Rituals: from obsessional neurosis to religion', *Psychological Medicine* 23: 1367–9.

Miller, D. and Swanson, G. (1966) *Inner Conflict and Defense*, New York: Schoken.

Mosher, D. L. (1966) 'The development of multi-trait, multi-method matrix analysis of three aspects of guilt', *Journal of Consulting Psychology* 30: 20–39.

Murphy, H. B. M. (1978) 'The advent of guilt feelings as a common depressive symptom: a historical comparison of two continents', *Psychiatry* 41: 229–42.

Murphy, H. B. M., Wittkower, E. D. and Chance, N. A. (1964) 'Cross-cultural enquiry into the symptomatology of depression', *International Journal of Psychiatry* 3: 6–15.

Nelson, S. (1973) 'The religious functions of psychiatry', *American Journal of Orthopsychiatry* 43: 363–7.

Ostow, M. and Schaferstein, B. (1954) *The Need to Believe: The Psychology of Religion*, New York: International University Press.

Parkes, C. (1991) *Bereavement: Studies of Grief in Adult Life*, London: Penguin.

Parkin, D. (1985) *The Anthropology of Evil*, Oxford: Blackwell.

Pfister, O. (1944) *Christianity and Fear: A Study in History and in the Psychology and Hygiene of Religion*, trans. W. H. Johnston, London: Allen & Unwin.

Piers, G. and Singer, M. (1953) *Shame and Guilt*, Springfield, IL: Free Press.

Ribot, T. (1884) *The Diseases of the Will*, trans. M. M. Snell, Chicago: Open Court.

—— (1896) *The Psychology of the Emotions*, New York: Charles Scribner & Sons.

Ricoeur, P. (1970) *Freud and Philosophy: An Essay on Interpretation*, Boston: Yale University Press.

Sartre, J.-P. (1948) *The Emotions: An Outline of a Theory*, New York: Philosophical Library.

Singer, K. (1975) 'Depressive disorders from a transcultural perspective', *Social Science and Medicine* 9: 289–301.

Smedslund, J. (1991) 'The psychology of forgiving', *Scandinavian Journal of Psychology* 32: 164–76.

Steketee, G., Quay, S. and White, K. (1991) 'Religion and guilt in OCD patients', *Journal of Anxiety Disorder* 5: 359–67.

Suttie, I. (1988) *The Origins of Love and Hate*, London: Free Association Books.

Tangey, J., Wagner, P. and Gramzow, R. (1992) 'Proneness to shame, proneness to guilt, and psychopathology', *Journal of Abnormal Psychology* 101: 469–78.

Tooth, G. (1950) 'Studies in mental illness in the Gold Coast', *Colonial Research Publications*, London: HMSO.

Westermeyer, J. (1984) 'The role of ethnicity in substance abuse', *Advances in Alcohol Substance Abuse* 4: 9–18.

Wing, J., Cooper, J. and Sartorious, N. (1974) *The Measurement and Classification of Psychiatric Symptoms*, Cambridge: Cambridge University Press.

Wittgenstein, L. (1980) *Remarks on the Philosophy of Psychology*, Oxford: Blackwell.

Wittkower, E. (1971) *Sociocultural Factors in the Prevention of Mental Illness*, paper presented at the Fifth World Psychiatry Congress, Mexico.

Wulff, D. M. (1991) *Psychology of Religion: Classic and Contemporary Views*, New York: John Wiley.

Yao, R. (1987) *An Introduction to Fundamentalists Anonymous*, New York: Fundamentalists Anonymous.

Yap, P. M. (1965) 'Phenomenology of affective disorder in Chinese and other cultures', in A. V. S. de Rueck and R. Porter (eds) *Transcultural Psychiatry*, London: J. & A. Churchill.

Chapter 15

Mental illness or life crisis?

A Christian pastoral counselling contribution

Mark Sutherland

> Kay exclaimed: 'Oh dear! I feel as if something has stabbed my heart! And now I've got something in my eye! . . .' 'I think it's gone!' he said; but it had not gone. It was one of those glass pieces from the mirror, the troll mirror, which you no doubt remember, in which everything great and good that was reflected in it became small and ugly, while everything bad and wicked became more distinct and prominent and every fault was at once noticed. Poor Kay had got one of the fragments right into his heart. It would soon become like a lump of ice. It did not cause him any pain, but it was there.
>
> (Hans Christian Andersen, *The Snow Queen 1990*)

This extract tells me something essential concerning people who experience mental health problems. 'Madness' is a term which does not necessarily mean 'illness'. It may mean 'crisis'. The 'crisis' may be one which involves the complete breakdown of a person's sense of meaning and rational functioning. It may lead in some cases to a series of such breakdowns, reoccurring at intervals throughout a lifetime. It is like the fragment of the troll mirror which being lodged in the heart becomes the frozen source of a distortion in life.

Anton Boisen (1992a), the father of the Clinical Pastoral Theology and Education Movement, described a kind of disturbance in which conflict was the likely root of the difficulty. Such conflict throws up a number of psychological phenomena, which a religious perspective understands to be evidence of an emotional reorganisation or a conversion. The psychiatrist viewing the same process identifies the characteristics of pathology, or abnormal mental functioning. Are these different ways of viewing a person's experience? Or is there a difference which would justify a distinction between the disturbances in the mental state which accompany conversion as a psychological and spiritual rite of passage, and psychiatric illness?

Jesus taught those who followed him to judge actions and experiences according to the fruits they bear (Matt. 12:33). Boisen, likewise, directs attention to the results of the experience. The same set of characteristics may result in reintegration of the personality around an enhanced capacity and purpose in life; they may equally result in defeat, demoralisation and a more permanent emotional and psychological disintegration. What is of crucial importance in this area is the capacity to judge between the two at an early enough stage before the first state results in the second.

The pastoral counsellor is a religious and psychological specialist who stands in a similar relation to the pastor as the psychiatrist does to the general practitioner. The pastoral counsellor's relationship with the psychiatrist might, therefore, be seen as one of liaison.

PASTORAL COUNSELLING AND THE RELIGIOUS TRADITION

Jacobs (1982) describes pastoral counselling as an approach which, though not always appropriate to every pastoral or counselling context, is an attempt to understand internal difficulties and conflicts inside people standing in the way of change. He contrasts this approach with those which seek external explanations finding in them external solutions. He refers to the 'fine theological tradition' behind the word 'counsel' quoting Proverbs 11:14 'Where there is no guidance a people fall; but in an abundance of counsellors there is safety.' Jacobs describes pastoral counselling as an activity which takes place within the context of religious communities where attention moves easily between human issues and spiritual and theological exploration.

A sharing of religious perspectives does not mean a protection of religion as a no-go area. Neither does it mean that religious perspectives are shared between counsellor and counselled at the same level of sophistication. People who find their way to pastoral counselling will bring internal conflicts stemming from rigid and confused understandings. However, the difference between mental health professionals and the pastoral counsellor is that the pastoral counsellor is working with rigidity and confusion, seeking to open flexibility and growth, from within the religious tradition. Macquarrie (1966) speaks to this point in drawing out the distinction between the theologian and the philosopher of religion. The philosopher of religion views religion from the outside, while the theologian is charged with reflecting upon religion as someone who shares the same faith dimension as his audience. The theologian speaks of God, religion, and religious experience as one who is at the same time a commentator on, and member of, the community of faith. The pastoral counsellor not only identifies religious belief and experience as significant factors but brings a nuanced approach utilising the tools which religious traditions have developed over time for the discernment between false and authentic spiritual experiences and theological understandings.

Pastoral counsellors have access to the same system of symbols and representations of spiritual experience as those they counsel. The difficulty for many psychiatrists in seeking to understand the religious experience of their patients is that they are often presented with a stark choice; to either reject such experience as illness, or in accepting it, to separate it out from the constellation of other presenting symptoms. The pastoral counsellor is in a better position to discern both nature and function of the patient's religious experience, neither rejecting it out of hand, nor accepting it completely at face value.

In writing from a Christian perspective, I do not want to give the impression that pastoral counselling is the exclusive preserve of Christians. As Jacobs writes:

> Philosophical, political and ethical thinking – whether Christian, Jewish, Buddhist, humanist or Marxist – contributes to the value system of the counsellor, and informs his view of man and society. If it is necessary to draw distinctions, perhaps the pastoral counsellor can be said to take a particular interest in man's search for understanding, not only of himself and his immediate context, but also of the total context in which he finds himself.
>
> (Jacobs, 1982)

This means that although the term 'pastoral' is associated with Christian practice, the activity of pastoral counselling easily takes place across a range of philosophical and religious traditions. Again, what would characterise the equivalent of pastoral counselling beyond the Judaeo-Christian context would be the application of psychologically informed practice by a counsellor occurring within and drawing on a particular religious tradition which is shared with the counsellee. However, this approach to counselling activity needs to be distinguished from more traditional care, teaching, and counselling activities which all religious leaders use in the guidance and disciplining of members of their faith communities. An example of this kind of approach would be the explicit use of religious texts to instruct a person in behaviour and attitude. The psychodynamic or humanistic psychological framework within which the pastoral counsellor usually works will separate his or her activity from forms of counselling which are attempts to give instructions and advice (also see Foskett, this volume).

PASTORAL COUNSELLORS, PSYCHOLOGY AND PSYCHIATRY

This chapter explores the nature and role of the pastoral counsellor in the lives of people whom psychiatry diagnoses as suffering from mental illness. For many psychiatrists, psychosis is a sign of deep and disturbing illness. Inherent within this notion is a belief that such disturbance is highly atypical of the human being's usual mental functioning. Characterised as an illness, psychosis is seen as something alien which attacks normal rationality and for which a cure must be sought (see Main 1957).

The pastoral counsellor will share many of the attitudes concerning mental disturbances which form the psychiatric view of madness as illness. It is, after all, the prevailing societal view in the Western world. Other cultures may view these differently (see Cox and Esmail, this volume). However, as the name suggests, the pastoral counsellor's insights will be formed by an interaction between the Judaeo-Christian theological and pastoral tradition and the developing ideas and practices of modern psychology. Within pastoral counselling the schools of theology and psychology may range widely across a spectrum from conservative to progressive, behavioural to psychodynamic. However, pastors and counsellors who use the term pastoral counselling to describe an area of their work will usually be theologically liberal and identify with psychodynamic or humanistic schools of psychology.

In viewing madness from a religious perspective, pastoral counsellors see it as part of a range of experience within which madness and sanity differ only in their creative fruitfulness and the social context in which they occur. They are also likely to have a psychological view of madness as a regression to primitive levels of psychological organisation. This regression is understood as having a purpose.

As a pastoral counsellor, I adopt a psychodynamic view of psychosis. The term 'dynamic' is significant here. It presents a picture of intrapsychic dynamism, of internal forces in a relationship to one another, characterised by fluidity of movement, sometimes ebbing, sometimes in flux, often in tension with one another and at times in outright conflict. This is a view which I feel least closes off the potential for movement and change. This view understands psychosis not as something separate from normal mental functioning but acknowledges a fluctuating movement back and forth across a borderland between a primitive 'psychotic' and more sophisticated 'rational' mental functioning. It is possible to move in and out of psychotic experience because the psychotic organisation of psychological functioning is neither a stage of development left behind, nor an abnormal state of illness. It remains a level of psychological organisation underneath rational functioning, into which a person will regress under the influences of psychological and emotional stresses. Although giving rise to behaviour we often find disturbing, this regression can be seen as an attempt to return to a more basic level of mental functioning in an attempt to deal with stress. The pastoral counsellor combines this psychological view with the traditional understanding of the Judaeo – Christian tradition which has understood lapses into madness as fulfilling a function, being associated with certain states of communication with the divine (1 Sam. 10:10; Acts 2). Anton Boisen puts it succinctly, thus:

> Psychosis, like the conversion experience, [is] a desperate attempt to resolve a sense of inner conflict . . . . [Psychosis is] characterised by marked religious concern and by the sense of mystical identification . . . . They may be looked upon as extreme manifestations of the consciousness of sin which theology has long regarded as the first step in the process of salvation. Like the fever and inflammation in the body, such disorders seem to be the manifestations of nature's power to heal.
>
> (Boisen, 1992b)

The individual's natural quest for mental health, implied above by Boisen, is equivalent in spiritual terms to the quest for 'salvation'. Salvation, in this sense, is a human issue which anticipates, and yet remains distinguishable from any subsequent theological process of dogmatic definition. In the same way the quest for mental health is a broader human issue moving far beyond any process of diagnostic definition.

The pastoral counsellor is, therefore, concerned both with salvation and diagnosis in the psychiatric context. In this chapter I will focus on manic depression to illustrate some of these points by offering two case histories. However, it will be clear from my development of the case material that my understanding of manic-depression differs from a conventional psychiatric one in ascribing an important psychological and emotional function to the manic depression experience. As a pastoral counsellor working in the area of mental health I encounter people with a variety of psychiatric diagnoses. I have chosen manic-depression because it is commonly encountered within religious communities by clergy and pastoral counsellors. One possible explanation for this is offered by Boisen (1992a) when he comments that between the psychotic and neurotic states lies an in-between area. This is the area of the 'psychoneurosis'; a state of 'unstable equilibrium' of which manic-depression is the most common example. I would go further to suggest that psychotic depression and hypomania seem from this perspective to be variations of bipolar affective and schizo-affective conditions. It is within the range of these conditions that questions concerning the ultimate realities of life will often lie concealed. Schizophrenia is the condition most associated with religious delusion and disturbance and, while far from being uncommon in the day-to-day experience of clergy and pastoral counsellors, it raises quite different issues from the ones I seek to discuss here.

The following two cases represent the work of the pastoral counsellor in both a community and institutional setting.

Simon

Simon is a 48-year-old married man with three adult children. He is a teacher by profession and lives with his wife, Philippa. Both Simon and Philippa are members of the local Christian (Anglican) community.

Seven years ago Simon had an experience which the members of his family and others around him refer to as 'his breakdown'. Although he avoided hospitalisation, he was subsequently psychiatrically diagnosed as a manicdepressive. Simon called this his 'label'. Having a label terrified him. Even after seven years, he found it hard to reconcile himself to this diagnosis. Despite his middle-class and professional background, Simon distrusted psychiatry. He complied with his prescribed lithium treatment. Yet he found it very difficult and upsetting that he was being treated as having a biological medical condition and resented being treated as a psychiatric patient. He felt somewhere inside him that his experience needed to be differently understood. Simon began to connect his mood swings to the emotional cycles of tension and pressure which were part of both his professional and domestic life. He was aware of, though not always articulate about, the connection between his mood and his family's expectations of him. These patterns of expectations stretched back into his childhood experience as well as having been reproduced in his own marriage and family life.

Simon came to me to discuss his problems about both his mood swings and his diagnosis. Although I had only recently arrived in the parish, Simon had been awaiting my arrival with a mixture of expectation and cynicism which in part was due to my colleague's hopes. Knowing of my interest and training in counselling and psychotherapy, my colleague hoped that Simon would find me of some use.

Simon and I met a number of times in the first month after my arrival. He spoke about the connections he made between his experience and the experiences described in both the biblical and spiritual writings of the Christian tradition. For Simon, his mood swings and his love of God were connected. He discovered in his reading that others before him had believed this to be so. Simon felt he had access to a way of viewing himself which avoided the 'illness' label. The Christian tradition conveyed to Simon a view of psychological disturbance as an expression of inner conflict. The direction of such conflicts indicated the possibility for psychological reintegration as well as pathological deterioration. Religious conversion had often been accompanied by the phenomenon of mental and emotional upheaval. The religious concern was less with the detail of such phenomenon and more with the nature of the fruit born out of such conflict. In the lives of Jesus, Paul and Augustine what counted was that periods of psychological conflict which modern society would view as psychiatric illness, were the experiences of break-down leading to break-through. These needed subsequently to be understood in wider terms of development of character, social helpfulness, breadth of sympathy, and the resulting strength, serenity and beauty of the personality (Boisen, 1992a).

As his parish priest my training and proximity to Simon enabled me to discern the quality and character of the direction often indicated by his mood swings. However, as a psychodynamic counsellor this very proximity ruled out a more conventional psychotherapeutic relationship. I, therefore, encouraged him to seek out psychotherapy as something separate and supportive to our relationship. This was a difficult process because of Simon's fear that this amounted to acceptance of the illness label. Had I not been his parish priest, it would have been possible for us to have worked within conventional psychodynamic boundaries. However, the need to hold these boundaries firmly for the safety of the work requires that the counsellor and client encounter one another only within the therapeutic session. As his parish priest, my relationship with Simon could not be confined in this way. Therefore, the two aspects of my identity, which while both being useful, had to be carefully and appropriately interpreted with Simon.

This was at first difficult for Simon to accept. He felt that if I couldn't be his therapist, then I was of no more use to him. This reaction reflected his two conflicting experiences of himself. When he was depressed, he felt limited and handicapped, constrained within himself. When he was elated, he felt as if there was no limit to his creativity and energy for living, constrained only by the expectations and fears of those around him. In a sense Simon and I had been thrown together in the manner of people who find themselves belonging within the same community. In first understanding the limitation this placed on us, only then could we discover the possibilities opened up by circumstances. The understanding of limitation, which did not fail to recognise possibility, was the central question concerning a successful containment of Simon's anxieties.

Others around Simon were sometimes burdened by his depressions and often frightened when he was elated. Nevertheless, his family and community were able to provide him with enough support to stay out of hospital. His psychiatrist and psychotherapist each had particular understandings of the nature of his experience as a manic-depressive person; however, Simon seemed frightened by his psychiatrist's understanding of manic-depression. The idea of a lifetime on medication left him feeling an invalid. He felt mystified by the way his psychotherapist spoke to him about the different parts of himself. I felt he was unfair to both these professionals who, while working with the most difficult and potentially dangerous aspects of his condition, could expect little thanks from him. I felt an aspect of my task was to continually facilitate and urge his continued cooperation with both psychiatric and psychotherapeutic treatment. Yet, at the same time, I could see it from his side. He wanted above everything else to feel himself as an alive human being, not a walking set of symptoms nor an enigmatic life puzzle.

PASTORAL COUNSELLING AND THE DYNAMICS OF CONTAINMENT

Simon needed someone who would understand his experience in a way which made him less afraid of himself. He wanted someone to recognise that his completeness as a human being expressed through his capacity to realise a fuller experience in life could neither be limited by, nor separated from, the manic and depressive fluctuations in his mood. Unlike his psychiatrist and psychotherapist I encountered Simon within the context of both his daily life and his religious practice. My interpretation of the role of pastoral counsellor with Simon had been to accept the structure of the pastoral context while drawing in an implicit way upon my psychodynamic understanding of his situation. In effect this meant working with him in his day-to-day struggle towards more successful living with both his depression and elation. However, this required containing the anxiety which his mood swings generated. Before looking at this process in more detail, I want to say something about the development of the pastoral counsellor's professional identity and the counsellor's investment in this.

Within my role as pastoral counsellor I have already distinguished the two separate professional identities of pastor and counsellor. Both of these identities arise from a dual process of training and formation. As clergy feel an increasing need to be able to do more than offer advice and reassurance to people with mental health issues, a trend is developing for them to acquire counselling skills. Important as these are, without the accompanying experience of receiving psychotherapy as part of training, these skills remain as superficial tools functioning more to reassure the clergy of their continued usefulness in a world which often leaves them feeling unskilled and amateur.

Being able to contain anxiety is related to the capacity to withstand both the projection of another person's fear and the evocation of a corresponding fear in one's self. The religious tradition of training for clergy until quite recently emphasised 'formation'. The priest was 'formed' by exposure to a life built around certain daily and weekly rhythms. Sustained over a period of training the young priest emerged with these rhythms internalised within. Thus he and more recently she could go out into the world able to draw upon these inner resources without needing them to be externally reproduced for him and her being. The priest is able to offer others patterns appropriate to differing life situations. These derived from his and her own deep formation in the patterns of Christian spiritual living. For the pastoral counsellor, the experience of having been 'in therapy' is the equivalent to formation. In the training of the psychiatrist, more might be made out of the long years and different stages of training as a period of formation. Theses provide an experience which has as much to do with formation of the 'person' of the psychiatrist as they do with imparting the necessary technical knowledge and skills.

Perhaps the dual implications of training and formation can be more clearly seen from the viewpoint of the way Simon approached me. By training and through public ordination I was the official representative of a tradition to which Simon looked for support. My interpretation of that tradition enabled us to give full weight to the gravity and importance of his psychiatric diagnosis, while not surrendering him to its reductive tendencies. Simon and I had access to an understanding of human experience which portrayed his situation as one of lived crises, more productive, more laden with meaning, than the notion of illness was capable of conveying. The Bible and resulting Church tradition, recording many thousands of years of lived faith experience, afforded us access to a system of symbols, ritual actions and forms of communal celebration. This drew us into an emotional and spiritual space within which the irrational and disruptive aspects of experience and feeling could be contained and healed through the transformation of perceptions (Reed, 1978). The transformation of perceptions is not the alteration of underlying dynamics, but a change in the individual's capacity for an increased tolerance of the underlying psycho-emotional tensions and conflicts. This process underlies the distinction made by religious people between healing and cure. The life outlook of a person who has matured in the spiritual life is one which does not envision life as conflict-free, but conflict managed. It is through the management of conflict that growth takes place. The relationship with God is the primary focus for the management of conflict in life. Simon did not ask for his manic-depression to be cured; he understood that this would be asking for the removal of key elements in his identity. He asked for a greater tolerance enabling a more successful negotiation of the elements which were in conflict within himself, and, by extension, between him and others. Making sense of Simon's emerging use of me as his pastoral counsellor, I came to understand that he viewed me as possessing more than the interpersonal skills normally associated with counselling and psychotherapy. As his pastoral counsellor I represented, in his mind, someone who stood in a particular relationship to him as the representative of the wider spiritual tradition which offered the means whereby perception could be continually transformed in the service of growth and more creative living.

The aspect of emotional formation of professional identity affected the way Simon and I related within a network of pastoral and personal relationships. We related to one another across a variety of contexts from causal day-to-day contacts to formal and prearranged meetings. In each of these varying situations, I responded to Simon. This response could chiefly be characterised as meeting an emotional demand from him. Both demand and response were at the level of unconscious communication between us. His psychiatrist recognised his manicdepression, but in a manner which left Simon's experience of manicdepression severed from the rest of him and the context of his life beyond the consulting room. On the other hand, the people among whom Simon lived and worked tended to deny his manic-depressive experience, leaving him with a sense that we all have when we recognise something as an issue by the atmosphere of avoidance surrounding it. Simon's demand of me was for someone to recognise his manic-depressive feelings in the context of his daily living. This decreased his anxiety and increased his sense of being in contact with the human world around him in a contained manner.

The Christian community also made a similar demand upon me. As the recognised leader, others observed both consciously and unconsciously how I related to Simon. This lowered their anxieties about him, themselves, and their own relating to him. My role as pastoral counsellor facilitated and managed the way Simon interacted with the spiritual tradition, his own self, and the community. Both Simon and his community were able to use me in this role in order to become less anxious about one another.

Both training and formation act together to enable the pastoral counsellor to sustain a particular type of availability to those he or she works with. With Simon, this meant a willingness to try to tolerate aspects of his feelings and thoughts which he knew others found much more difficult to do. Reed (1978) records in *The Dynamics of Religion* a comment by the psychiatrist and paediatrician Donald Winnicott:

> People who are ill (and we are all ill to some extent) have a drive to cure themselves. Nothing is more important than to do that. This means they experience a great need to feel real, and they only come to feel real by doing something like regression to childhood dependence, to something which can hold them. This may be localised, for example, in the Church or in music [Or in the pastoral counselling relationship.]

Psychoanalysts, psychodynamic psychotherapists, and counsellors are familiar with the containment of the patient's regression within the boundaries of the analytic or psychotherapeutic session. The regression in this context can often be quite extreme, and both therapist and patient survive this experience because of the superior ego strength of the therapist, the firmness of the boundaries to the session, and, by extension, within the analysis and psychotherapy or counselling as a whole. Winnicott is talking about this process, but what distinguishes his contribution to the discussion on regression is that he understood regression as occurring naturally. As a primary example of natural regression he drew attention to the way the mother selectively regresses in order to understand and meet the needs of her newborn infant (Winnicott, 1956). This led Reed to develop his concept of oscillation to describe the natural cycles of regression in the lives of individuals and communities. The purpose of this regression was to seek powers of renewal and transformation at the levels of psychological organisation which psychiatry recognises as the psychotic (Reed, 1978). Reed understood oscillation as a process which had both a functional and dysfunctional form of operation. When operating functionally, oscillation allowed for a process of regression which did not obliterate or overwhelm the capacity for continued conscious and rational functioning. He understood the religious leader as being invested with cultic, spiritual and pastoral authority to facilitate and to preside over a community's collective oscillation through the dynamics of ritual and worship. This function extended to the relationship between religious leader and particular individuals where a similar process of oscillation is managed and contained within prescribed sacramental, pastoral and counselling activities. Simon's manic-depression cycles were understood by me as an oscillation process in search of emotional and psychological health.

Fiona

Fiona had suffered from severe manic-depression over the last twenty years of her life. Now aged 43, she had her first breakdown while at university. The periods between breakdown over this twenty-year period fluctuated, but more recently they seemed to occur yearly. Fiona was usually hospitalised under a 'section' of the Mental Health Act. As in the past, this only happened after serious manic deterioration of her mental state had already taken place. Each new admission heralded a long period of medicated management. Fiona was well known to one of my colleagues, and when this colleague left, Fiona asked me if I would see her for what she called 'psychotherapy'. In addition to bringing her communion on Sundays, I agreed to meet her each week while she was on the ward.

Fiona and I met over the four and a half months of her hospitalisation. At first we met to talk about religious matters. Ordinarily Fiona would not have described herself as religious in any conventional sense. However, when manic, she developed along with everything else a heightened sense of the importance of God and the Bible. Quite early on in our relationship Fiona surprised me in two ways. She hated being on medication and complained bitterly both about its deleterious effects and its infringement of her liberty. Yet, she also was aware of how important and necessary it was. She like to read the Bible; yet, at the same time was aware of how the powerful images and language, while giving her the graphic means of expressing the nature of her situation, inflamed and excited her mood. I, therefore, suggested that she only read the Bible when we met together. That way she could continue to explore and use its powerful and primitive imagery while I provide some containment and interpretation of the experience.

She had the vibrancy of an uninhibited imagination. Her favourite parts of the Bible came from the Books of the Prophets. These she could bring alive through the immediacy of her own experience. My physical presence, together with my interpretation of meanings, provided a boundary for her experience.

One day, early on in our work, Fiona provided me with an image of her experience which helped me to think about the role I was taking up for her. She described herself as a person living in a house with no roof and no floor. My role in our reading of Scripture was to act as her roof and floor. As time went by, my role changed to helping her to find within herself a roof and floor.

When stable, Fiona experimented as an artist. She had her own studio, which she shared with a friend who kept things going during her periods of breakdown. She seemed unsatisfied with much of her effort, but I was impressed by her obvious creativity. Her inability to use that creativity as a source of richness in her living imposed itself forcefully upon me. Her long acquaintance with psychiatry had contributed to the internalisation of a view of herself which saw the sum total of her parts in terms only of the symptoms of manicdepression. According to this view, artistic creativity was dangerous and inflammatory. I found myself taking the opposite view to this, seeing in her creativity the best defence against manic escalation. Like most manic patients, Fiona's difficulty was that mania blocked access to her creativity. While depressed she had no creativity. Depression imposed a grey monotonous existence between narrow tram lines. She could not endure this for long before breaking out into the Technicolor fireworks of mania.

As the date of her discharge approached, she became less religious and asked me whether I would still continue to work with her. Fiona seemed to confuse religiosity with spirituality. The difference between the two is that religiosity is experienced as something separate from general life concerns, whereas spirituality is integral to ordinary everyday life preoccupations. We worked out a pattern for continuing to meet after her discharge whereby she would come to see me at prearranged times once every three weeks. We have continued in this pattern for over a year now, which is the longest interval between breakdowns for some time. At the time of writing her anti-depressant medication has been reduced with a view to her eventually coming off it completely. Fiona is also coming to terms with the limitations, frustrations, and sheer ordinariness of everyday life, something from which her manic spirals had offered her a way out.

PASTORAL COUNSELLING AND THE DYNAMICS OF INTERNAL MIRRORING

The Gospels present a picture of Jesus engaging in a wide range of activity. Of particular interest to my present purpose are the accounts of his healing those who sought him out with various dis-eases. At a popular level these accounts are often misunderstood as examples of miraculous cures. The implication here is that for those who have faith, the same is still possible today. However, this is to misunderstand the purpose these accounts play within the fabric of the Gospel writer's narrative. They are not evidence of magical curing. This alone would not have distinguished Jesus from the host of magicians and miracle workers who roamed the Palestinian countryside. They are evidence of Jesus's identity. The miracle stories are set within the wider narrative as proof of Jesus's status as Son of God. In the hands of Jesus, they are revelations of the power and majesty of God. In effect, they are a self-revelation articulating the attributes he derives from his relationship to God. Jesus's activity is not properly speaking curing, but healing. Primarily his encounters with others reveal his identity (Nineham, 1963). They are not about what he does, so much as who he is. Who he is dictates the manner in which he makes himself available. He uses the 'parable form' of story telling. 'Parables' are a specific oral genre whereby a story is created out of details drawn from the everyday run-of-the-mill lives of the story's hearers. However, the story contains a sting in its tail. This sting is an inversion of the familiar or a juxtaposition of two familiar facts to produce a conflict of images designed to draw from the hearer an acceptance, which expanded understanding (conversion) or a rejection, which confirmed spiritual blindness. Expansion of understanding meant *metanoia*, a change of heart, an internal transformation of perspective upon which the promise of fuller life is realised.

My role with Fiona was to formulate an image of what a fuller life might mean for her. This required helping her to take risks, a frightening experience. She had been taught by her life experiences somehow to fear the risks involved in living. Her mania was the ultimate in risk-taking, but because she was never in control of this process she was also unaware of the risk. In her experience of being overwhelmed by mania, she was relieved of the responsibility of taking the risks which could lead to a sustained development of her creative potential.

As the Chaplain, I was the only professional person involved with Fiona who did not carry responsibility for her treatment. I was alone in not being charged to do anything to her. I had a duty not to interfere with the treatment managed by others. Freed from the responsibility to treat her psychiatric condition, I could play a different role in her life. As her pastoral counsellor, I was to play the role of a practitioner of life skills. Life skills in this sense are not a set of learned behavioural characteristics. They are the external expression of an inner negotiation which links feelings or fragments of feeling into a meaningful whole producing more successful patterns of response and action. This negotiation of internal fragments explains the underlying dynamics present within Jesus's telling of parables. Each parable was a call to new forms of living based upon a *metanoia* of inner conversion (Boucher, 1981).

My task was to aid Fiona's creation of a bigger inhabitable space in her house. Earlier, Fiona had referred to this house as having no roof and no floor. The more usual result of psychiatric containment was to return her to a house in which she was squeezed flat in the narrow space between the floor and the foundations of the house. Even though her experience revealed that she was unable to endure it there for very long, memories of the fear she experienced during the last manic episode compelled Fiona's acceptance of such narrow but safe living space.

In one session the following exchange took place between us.

F.   Have you ever had mental illness?

M.   Why do you ask?

F.   You get things right when you describe how I feel. How else could you know?

M.   I have never been formally diagnosed as mentally ill, but listening to you I find I'm able to find faint resonances to your experience in my own. It's as if I have inside me a black and white small screen film version of your Technicolor cineramic experience of manic-depression. I find this is enough to guide me as to how to respond to what you describe from your intensified experience.

This short exchange had a great effect on both of us. For Fiona, it was the first time anybody who was not manic-depressive had linked their experience to hers. This introduced a new idea to her, namely that her experience differed not in kind, but simply in intensity from that of someone like myself. I began to speculate about what had been up to then my instinctively guided responses to her.

Winnicott (1971) wrote:

What does the baby see when he or she looks at the mother's face? I am suggesting that ordinarily, what the baby sees is himself or herself. In other words the mother is looking at the baby and *what she looks like is related to what she sees there* [emphasis added].

So often what seemed to pass between Fiona and myself was a process closely associated with Winnicott's description of the mother mirroring for the baby an experience of itself. I also closely equate this process with the activity of Jesus in the Gospels. The Gospel accounts so often tell us where Jesus looked, and at what he looked, as he worked his miracle healings (Mark 7:34; 9:20; 10:21). Looking is not simply looking at something or someone, it conveys the richer notion of mirroring contained in Winnicott's description of the mother and baby interaction.

When Fiona began to talk about her feelings, fears, and experience an identificatory response was activated inside of me. This enabled me to mirror something which she recognised as being of use to her. Menzies-Lyth (1988) describes the process which passes between carer and patient as projective identification. The plight of the patient evokes within the carer an internal representation. The process of the patient's recovery is mirrored in the carer's overcoming of their internal identified phantasy. The pastoral counsellor is able to offer himself or herself to the patient in a similar way by using their own internal state to find an internal resonance within themselves to the patient's more intense and overwhelming feeling state. The pastoral counsellor may not be particularly conscious of the process; however, he or she conducts a rehearsal of the process of negotiation between his or her own internal objects and fragments mirroring for the patient, a process which, over time, can be successfully internalised.

I use the term rehearsal to express two important aspects of this process within the pastoral counselling encounter. The first is that the pastor is operating within an area of experience which is at least known. The second aspect to note here is that this process is a triggered response to the patient's unconscious needs. The pastoral counsellor cannot have any idea about this until shown by the patient. The triggering results from the manner in which he or she makes himself or herself available to the patient. In turn, this is determined by something much closer to identity than any notion of a specific activity.

There are a number of factors which go to make up the pastoral counselling encounter. In both the processes of training and formation there comes together within the pastoral counsellor a blending of personal and professional self-identities. Added to this is his or her identification with the patient. In turn, the patient identifies with the pastoral counsellor, and both are identified with the religious tradition. My experience is that while I do not know what it is I symbolise to the patient, he or she will find a way of using what this might be for his or her own purpose.

This places the process firmly within the patient's control. Fiona was working at the frontier of her experience, while I was working within an area of experience which was at least, in greater part, familiar to me. This meant Fiona not only initiated the process, but was also protected from being used by me as someone on whom to work out my own agenda.

CONCLUSION

The two case discussions in this chapter reveal 'oscillation' and 'mirroring' to be two of the key elements in pastoral counselling. Oscillation is that process which affects nearly every aspect of human living. It can be detected in the broad movements of societies and institutions as they move between phases of activity, disintegration, and renewal. It affects the lives of individuals and my discussion of Simon rests upon my drawing out of connections between the external cyclothymic cycles in manic-depression and their internal and dynamic purpose as movements towards health.

Understood within the activity of pastoral counselling, Simon's individual experience is linked back into, and contained within, the dynamics of the religious community and its tradition. The pastoral counsellor utilises psychological understanding and practice as a recognised representative of wider spiritual tradition.

Mirroring, as Fiona's material shows, is a fundamental human experience. It retains its crucial significance from the early phase of infant life remaining present within the more complex interactions of adulthood.

Three additional factors are significant in further identifying the particular nature of pastoral counselling. These are: the psychological understanding and training of the pastoral counsellor, his or her 'therapeutic and spiritual formation' as a counsellor and as a religious person, and the pastoral counsellor's role as a participating representative of a religious tradition.

Pastoral counselling occupies an area of working which emerges out of general pastoral care on one hand, and secular psychological counselling and psychotherapy, on the other. It shares with pastoral care a world view. It uses the same symbolic and ritual elements, which it draws upon in order to open up problematic areas of experience to the potential for change and growth. From psychological counselling and psychotherapy, pastoral counselling gains boundaried structure, therapeutic space, and an understanding of intra-psychic dynamics. Substantial areas of overlap exist where the activity of the pastoral counsellor will be difficult to distinguish from that of the pastor in pastoral care or the secular counsellor or psychotherapist. However, I have tried to indicate areas in which pastoral counselling will emerge most clearly and distinctively from both pastoral care and secular psychological counselling.

For the psychiatrist, the pastoral counsellor is an ally in the work with people for whom the religious and the spiritual are powerful elements in both their life experience and their psychiatric phenomenology. As Foskett points out in an earlier chapter in this book, the ambiguity of this position has historically been the focus for open hostility and suspicion from psychiatry. This hostility shows up the mutual weakness of both the psychiatrist's and the pastor's positions. A separation between the two in the struggle to understand and combat the potentially damaging features of psychosis led Boisen (1992a) to complain that the pastor offers treatment without diagnosis, or even worse, offering neither treatment nor diagnosis, and the psychiatrist, in not understanding the significance of the religious factors in psychosis offers diagnosis and treatment without understanding.

The medical profession, approaching the problems of the individual on the basis of their experience with the seriously disturbed, have made use of the methods of science to clarify many of the principles involved and have won increasing prestige . . . . The professional servants of the Church have been performing a great and important service in the realm of mental health. But these things have been done on an intuitive and common sense basis. There has been a strange lag among [them] in the matter of applying the methods of science to the field which is distinctly their own, that of religious experience . . . and the achievement of mental, or spiritual health.

REFERENCES

Andersen, H. C. (1990), *Fairy Tales* trans. H. L. Braekstad, Oxford: Heinemann.
Boisen, A. (1992a) 'Concerning the relationship between religious experience and mental disorders', in G. Asquith (ed.) *Vision From a Little Known Country*, Atlanta, GA: Journal of Pastoral Care Publications.
—— (1992b) 'The minister as counsellor', in G. Asquith (ed.) *Vision From a Little Known Country*, Atlanta, GA: Journal of Pastoral Care Publications.
Boucher, M. I. (1981) *The Parables*, Wilmington, DE: Michael Glazier, Inc.
Jacobs, M. (1982) *Still Small Voice: An Introduction to Pastoral Counselling*, London: SPCK.
Macquarrie, J. (1966) *Principles of Christian Theology*, London: SCM.

Main, T. F. (1957) 'The ailment', reprinted in J. Johns (ed.) (1989) *The Ailment and Other Essays*, London: Free Association Books.

Mark, St. *Gospel According to*, chapter 2: 23–8, chapter 10: 17–22.

Menzies-Lyth, I. (1988) 'The functioning of social systems as a defence against anxiety', in *Containing Anxiety in Institutions*, vol. 1, London: Free Association Books.

Nineham, D. E. (1963) *Saint Mark*, Harmondsworth: Pelican Books.

Reed, B. (1978) *The Dynamics of Religion: Process and Movement in Christian Churches*, London: DLT.

Winnicott, D. W. (1956) 'Primary Maternal Preoccupation', in *Through Paediatrics to Psychoanalysis*, London: The Hogarth Press (1987).

—— (1971) *Playing and Reality*, London: Tavistock.

Conclusions

Religion, mental illness and mental health – the way forward

Dinesh Bhugra

The development of psychiatry as a branch of medicine has given it a 'scientific' context. The underlying danger has been that this approach may tend to take it further away from its humanistic and holistic concepts. One may argue that psychiatry took over from religion and created its own high church and in extraordinary developments, unlike religion, locked people away in a physical space.

There is no doubt that psychiatry and its practitioners have often been the agents of the society to curb 'deviancy'. Whereas religion has locked its practitioners in institutions of a different variety, their spiritual welfare has been its main concern. This division between spiritual and psychological well-being led to the parting of ways between religion and psychiatry. Is there a likelihood that they will come together? This was the question with which the conferences in the Institute of Psychiatry and this book started. The next step is to continue exploring commonalities and be aware of differences so that the relationship continues to grow. The competition between religion and psychiatry is probably more exacerbated now, though this competition cannot be described as healthy.

The fear among some psychiatrists has been that again religion may hijack their 'profession', thereby negating their own historical development and growth. Psychoanalytic works of Freud and Jung pay due homage to religion, and the development of guilt, sin and shame depends upon individuals, society and social expectations. Different cultures and different religions manage to support their memberships – both healthy and sick groups.

If the relationship between religion and mental illness is to flourish, the expectations of the one from the other and the limitations need to be clearly stated. Psychiatrists and religious personnel may wish to work together to develop sophisticated measures of religion, functioning and activity rather than simple religiosity and the understanding of one's faith in determining and dealing with distress. The two groups need to decide the definitions of spiritual mental or psychological health, if indeed such boundaries can be drawn. The pressure to 'pass on' the individual to another set of 'professionals', because spiritual problems end here and mental distress begins at such and such a point, is bound to be counter-productive. These two groups need to work together.

One may perceive the dialogue and dealings between psychiatry and religion as a cross-cultural dialogue and this may need taking further in a similar fashion (see Bhugra, 1993, for a basic review). Religion can be perceived as a mediating factor in culture change. Under stress, individuals become social movement leaders and with their charisma happen to shift the social chaos on to gods by redefining personal distress in religious terms. This distinction is important in understanding the emphasis that religion and psychiatry put on individuals. Spiritual beliefs, like the rest of the culture, may undergo transformations in periods of crisis, culture contact and modernisation (Bourguignon, 1992). Under these circumstances, the psychiatrist needs to question his/her beliefs in the definitions of mental illness, especially those that may be dictated socially. Thus 'deviancy' and dysfunction have to be seen in their proper context. As we have learnt, highly similar mental and behavioural states may be designated psychiatric disorders in some cultural settings and religious experiences in others. Prince (1992) suggests that within cultures that invest these unusual states with meaning and provide the individual experiencing them with institutional support, at least a proportion of these may be contained and channelled into socially valuable roles. These roles can be defined by joint workings within these two groups. Rites of mourning and anger allow management of underlying distress in a religious context. Religion considers guilt and the definitions of sin, but clinicians see this guilt as part of an underlying psychiatric illness. If the two disciplines are to work in some conceptual level, they have to define their boundaries, strengths and weaknesses in a way that is understandable to both their users and their practitioners. The two philosophies have an underlying emphasis on the understanding of the human psyche and suffering, so technically it should be possible to draw out the common ground.

The view that there are neurophysiological correlates of meditation and related states (see Kwee, 1990), although seen as genuine, means that this 'friendliness' and a nod towards religion may in the end prove to be simply reductionist. The mind – body dichotomy may actually help religion and psychiatry (Wulff, 1991). Traditional religious elements may appear sympathetic with behaviourally oriented psychologists but comparative work on human behaviour will acknowledge individual and social contexts.

Religion and psychiatry have a lot to say to each other and need to continue the dialogue to understand each other's weaknesses and strengths and work together or separately (as long as each is aware of the contribution the other can make) for the betterment of the individual who is suffering.

REFERENCES

Bhugra, D. (1993) 'Influence of culture on presentation and management of patients', in D. Bhugra and J. Leff (eds) *Principles of Social Psychiatry*, Oxford: Blackwell.
Bourguignon, E. (1992) 'Religion as a mediating factor in culture change', in J. F. Schumaker (ed.) *Religion and Mental Health*, New York: Oxford University Press.

Kwee, M. R. T. (1990) *Psychotherapy, Meditation and Health: A Cognitive – Behavioural Perspective*, London: East-West Publications.

Prince, R. H. (1992) 'Religious experience and psychopathology: cross-cultural perspectives', in J. F. Schumaker (ed.) *Religion and Mental Health*, New York: Oxford University Press.

Wulff, D. M. (1991) *Psychology of Religion: Classic and Contemporary Views*, New York: John Wiley.

Index

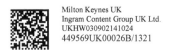

Milton Keynes UK
Ingram Content Group UK Ltd.
UKHW030902141024
449569UK00026B/1321